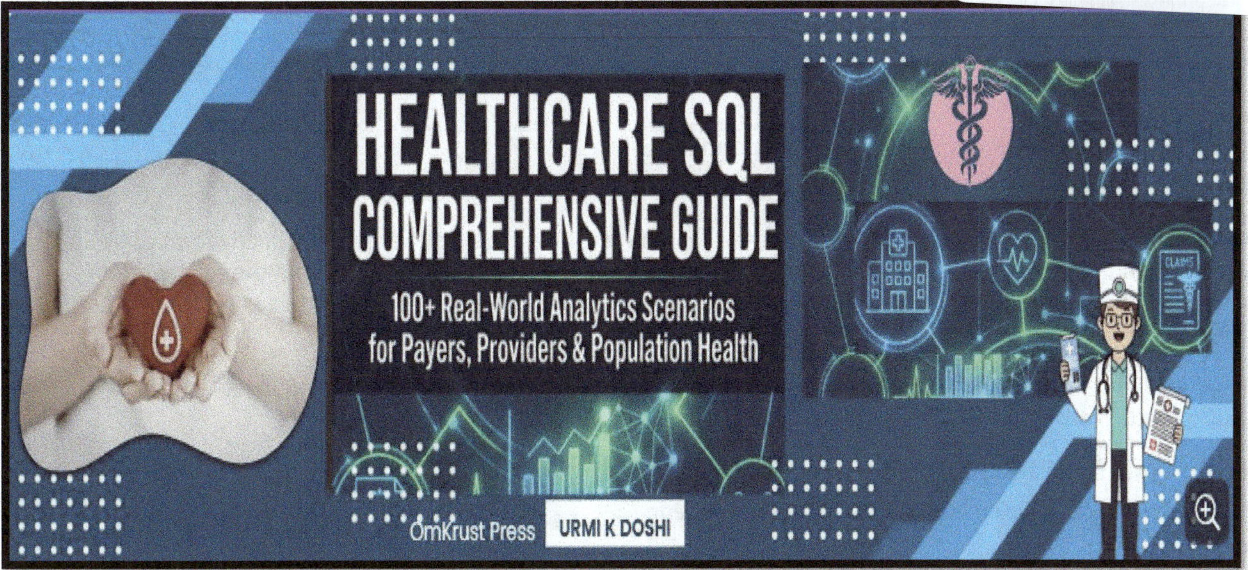

Healthcare SQL Comprehensive Guide

100+ Real-World Analytics Scenarios for Payers, Providers & Population Health

Urmi K Doshi, M.S. Health Informatics
OmKrust Press

Copyright

Published by OmKrust Press — An Imprint of Health Analytica Publishing

Permissions & Inquiries — For permission requests, speaking engagements, or bulk order inquiries: OmKrust@Gmail.com

ISBN (Paperback): 978-1-971447-19-3

First Edition: 2026 | Printed in the United States of America

OmKrust Press, FL

Disclaimer — For Educational and Informational Purposes Only

The information, SQL code, and analytical frameworks in this book are provided strictly for educational purposes. Healthcare analytics is a dynamic field. Governing bodies — including CMS, NCQA, AMA, and FDA — continuously update their specifications, value sets, and methodologies. This includes annual updates to HEDIS measures, CMS-HCC Risk Adjustment models, ICD-10-CM, CPT, MS-DRG groupings, and NDC directories.

All SQL queries and data models are illustrative examples provided on an "as-is" basis without warranty. Neither the author nor the publisher shall be held liable for any loss, damages, compliance penalties, or clinical outcomes caused by the information or code contained in this book. It is the sole responsibility of the reader to verify all logic against the official, current-year technical specifications before executing any queries in a production environment.

All patient names, provider names, member IDs, NPIs, and clinical scenarios presented in this book are entirely fictitious and computationally generated. They contain zero Protected Health Information (PHI) and operate entirely outside the scope of HIPAA. Any resemblance to actual persons or proprietary data is purely coincidental.

All product names, logos, and brands (SAS®, Microsoft SQL Server®, Epic®, Oracle®, NCQA®, HEDIS®) are the property of their respective trademark holders. Their use in this book is for identification and educational purposes only and does not imply endorsement or affiliation.

Notice of Privacy, Compliance, and Liability

HIPAA Compliance & Protected Health Information (PHI)

The datasets, patient names, provider names, identification numbers (such as Medical Record Numbers, Social Security Numbers, or NPIs), dates of birth, and specific medical histories presented in this book are entirely fictitious and simulated.

These examples have been generated synthetically solely for educational purposes to demonstrate SQL functionality and healthcare analytics methodologies. They do not represent real individuals, living or dead, nor do they reflect actual clinical records from any specific healthcare organization, payer, or provider. Because all data is 100% synthetic, it contains zero Protected Health Information (PHI) and operates entirely outside the scope of the Health Insurance Portability and Accountability Act (HIPAA). Any resemblance to actual persons or proprietary business data is purely coincidental.

Medical & Professional Disclaimer

This book is a technical manual intended for data analysts and healthcare professionals. The SQL code, clinical logic, and analytical frameworks provided herein are for informational and training purposes only. They do not constitute medical advice, clinical guidelines, or official coding recommendations (e.g., ICD-10, CPT, DRG).

While every effort has been made to ensure the accuracy of the information within this book, the author and publisher assume no responsibility for errors, omissions, or damages resulting from the use of the information contained herein. Readers must independently verify all code, logic, and value sets against their specific organizational protocols and official regulatory guidelines before implementing them in a production environment.

Trademarks

All product names, logos, and brands (e.g., SAS®, Microsoft SQL Server®, Epic®, Oracle®, NCQA®, HEDIS®) are the property of their respective trademark holders. All company, product, and service names used in this book are for identification and educational purposes only. The use of these names, logos, and brands does not imply endorsement, sponsorship, or affiliation with the author or publisher.

Educational Framework & Logic Sandbox Disclaimer

The "Logic Sandbox" Methodology

The SQL queries and data architectures provided in this manual are designed from a teaching perspective. They serve as a structural "sandbox" intended to demonstrate the sequential logic required to solve complex healthcare analytics problems.

- **Template-Based Learning:** These code snippets are templates for logic development. They are designed to illustrate specific technical concepts, regulatory inclusions, and exclusion variations. They are not "plug-and-play" production-ready scripts.
- **A "Handholding" Approach:** This manual provides the cognitive framework and the logic sequence necessary to navigate healthcare data. However, the final "real-world" execution must be adapted to your organization's unique data schema and infrastructure.
- **Production Readiness & Scrubbing:** In a live production environment, all logic must be rigorously scrubbed against the most current mandates from governing bodies (CMS, NCQA, HHS, OIG, OCR). Healthcare regulations are continually updated; the business rules of yesterday may not meet the compliance standards of today.

User Responsibility & Professional Diligence

The responsibility for the accuracy, compliance, and performance of queries in a live environment rests solely with the user.

Successful health informatics requires more than just syntax—it requires a commitment to continuous regulatory monitoring. Use these templates to build your foundational logic, but always validate your final code against the most current Source of Truth from the prevailing regulatory agencies.

Regulatory Compliance & Technical Maintenance Statement

The Requirement for Continuous Validation

While the logic provided in this text is production-grade, it is the user's responsibility to perform regular logic scrubbing against the most current technical specifications released by these governing bodies.

- **Annual Technical Updates:** Users must validate all codes (ICD-10-CM, CPT, HCPCS, LOINC) and value sets against the most recent annual releases (e.g., the NCQA Volume 2 Technical Specifications).
- **Exclusion Refinement:** Clinical and administrative exclusions are subject to change based on updated federal mandates and quality measure revisions.
- **Infrastructure Sensitivity:** These queries should be tested in a controlled QA environment before deployment to ensure they align with your organization's specific data dictionary and compliance protocols.

Liability Notice: The author and publisher provide this content for educational purposes. Success in healthcare analytics requires a commitment to continuous regulatory monitoring; the code provided is a blueprint, but the Source of Truth remains the most current documentation from the governing regulatory agencies.

Data Privacy & Synthetic Data Statement

Ethical Data Usage & HIPAA Compliance

The scenarios, datasets, and SQL queries presented in this manual are designed strictly for educational and professional development purposes. As a career-long advocate for healthcare data integrity, the author has ensured that this work adheres to the highest standards of data privacy.

100% Synthetic Data: All data utilized in this book is computationally generated. While these datasets are architected to mimic the complexity, schemas, and statistical distributions of real-world payer and provider systems, they do not represent actual patients, providers, or healthcare entities.

- **De-identification & Safe Harbor:** This manual contains no Protected Health Information (PHI) or Personally Identifiable Information (PII). All identifiers, including Member IDs, Provider NPIs, and clinical dates, are randomized and synthetic. No data in this publication can be traced back to a living individual or a specific corporate entity.
- **Regulatory Alignment:** The logic and business rules described herein (such as HEDIS, Risk Adjustment, and CMS-HCC) are based on publicly available regulatory specifications and industry-standard white papers.

Dedication

First and foremost, to God, the source of all wisdom.

To my loving family, who believed in me even when I doubted myself.

To my work family —
the analysts, nurses, managers, and leaders
I have met in the trenches of healthcare.

You are the unsung heroes of this industry.

Every conversation, every corrected error, every shared insight
was a building block.

I am the sum of your collective guidance.

FOREWORD

The Physician Has Always Been an Analyst

Before writing a single line of SQL, you must understand the world that generated the data.

The physician of antiquity had no laboratory, no imaging, and no biopsy. They observed, reasoned, and searched for patterns—practicing analytics with a sample size of one and limited ability to share knowledge. That constraint defined medicine for over 2,500 years.

That era is ending.

The physician of the future is a physician-analyst. Supported by systems trained on millions of patient records, they no longer rely solely on personal experience or manual review of literature. Instead, they can identify—at the moment of decision—whether a patient matches a cohort where a treatment has demonstrated measurable success. This is not the replacement of the physician; it is the amplification of the physician.

Medical errors remain a leading cause of preventable harm in the United States. Often-cited estimates suggest hundreds of thousands of deaths occur each year due to preventable causes. These failures are rarely due to incompetence, but rather to cognitive overload, incomplete information, and the limits of individual memory. Analytics and AI directly address these challenges.

The knowledge already exists. Decades of research and randomized controlled trials have built a vast evidence base. The challenge is no longer discovery—it is application. The role of the physician-analyst is to ensure that existing evidence is applied consistently, accurately, and at scale.

Consider the healthcare analyst who builds a HEDIS gap closure program identifying thousands of diabetic patients overdue for retinal screening. They are not discovering diabetic retinopathy. That work has already been done. They are building the bridge between what is known and what is practiced. A single well-designed query, executed against a claims database, can prevent more cases of avoidable blindness in a quarter than an individual clinician could prevent over a lifetime.

I wish I had been given this manual 20 years ago. It took me two decades to understand the full system—insurance mechanics, data architecture, regulatory frameworks, clinical domains, and financial levers—and how each piece connects. This book is the guide I needed then.

It is structured as a ladder, with each chapter building on the last. A reader who progresses from Chapter 1 through Chapter 31 will gain a comprehensive understanding of healthcare analytics within the U.S. system.

The physician of the past carried knowledge in their mind.

The physician-analyst of the future carries the knowledge of the entire system and SQL is the instrument that turns that knowledge into action.

Urmi K. Doshi, M.S. Health Informatics
OmKrust Press | 2026

TABLE OF CONTENTS

Healthcare Analytics: Comprehensive Guide

Book Overview — Nine Rungs

Table of Contents

PART I: The Healthcare Ecosystem

Rung 1 · Chapters 1–2

Part I lays the essential groundwork every healthcare analyst needs before writing a single line of SQL. Chapter 1 orients you inside the healthcare ecosystem — who the players are, how money flows, why healthcare data defies every convention you learned in other industries, and what the analyst's role actually demands. Chapter 2 goes deeper into the financial engine: how Medicare, Medicaid, and commercial plans are structured, how each program pays providers and plans, and the lifecycle of a claim from submission through remittance. Together these two chapters form the domain foundation that every subsequent SQL query in this book depends upon. You cannot write correct healthcare SQL without first understanding why the data looks the way it does.

Part I The Healthcare Ecosystem

Chapter 1: Introduction to Healthcare Analytics

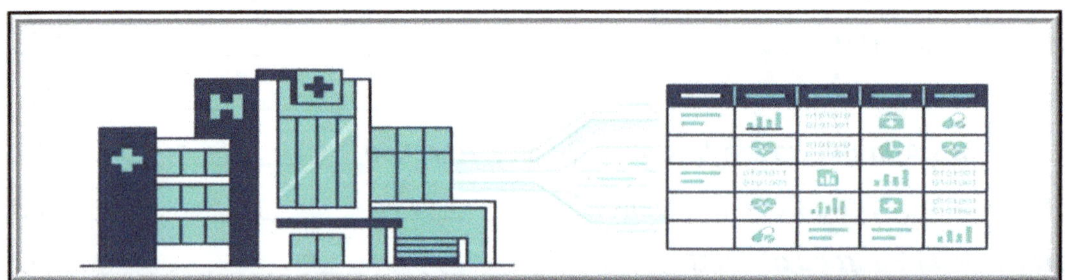

American healthcare spending reached $4.9 trillion in 2023. That's 17.3% of GDP—more than any other developed nation.

Here's a concise overview of how U.S. healthcare has evolved — from fragmented beginnings to our digital present — and where the gaps still remain.

Early foundations (pre-2000s)

For most of the 20th century, American healthcare was fee-for-service and paper-based. Employer-sponsored insurance became the norm after World War II, Medicare and Medicaid launched in 1965, and HMOs emerged in the 1970s as cost-control experiments. By 2000, the system was already the world's most expensive — yet tens of millions remained uninsured and medical records were stacked in filing cabinets.

The 2000s: quality crises and the digital push

The Institute of Medicine's landmark 2000 report *To Err Is Human* shocked the public by estimating that up to 98,000 Americans died annually from preventable medical errors — many traceable to paper records, illegible handwriting, and fragmented information. This created political will for digitization. The Bush administration began pushing for health IT adoption, but without financial incentives, hospitals moved slowly.

The ACA and HITECH (2009–2010): the twin catalysts

Two landmark laws reshaped the landscape almost simultaneously. The **Health Information Technology for Economic and Clinical Health (HITECH) Act** (embedded in the 2009 stimulus bill) committed over $30 billion in incentive payments to push hospitals and physicians to adopt **Electronic Medical Records (EMRs)**. Providers had to demonstrate "Meaningful Use" — actually using the technology to improve care — or face Medicare/Medicaid payment penalties.

Then came the **Affordable Care Act (ACA)** in 2010, which:

- Extended coverage to ~20 million previously uninsured Americans via Medicaid expansion and marketplace exchanges
- Banned denial of coverage for pre-existing conditions
- Shifted reimbursement philosophy from volume to *value* — paying for outcomes, not just procedures
- Created Accountable Care Organizations (ACOs) that required coordinated, data-driven care — impossible without EMRs

The ACA didn't mandate EMRs directly, but its value-based payment models *required* the data infrastructure that EMRs provide. The two laws were effectively symbiotic.

Let me visualize the full arc of this evolution:**EMR adoption: mission accomplished — but at a cost**

By 2015, over 95% of U.S. hospitals had adopted EMRs. Epic, Cerner, and Meditech became the dominant platforms. But adoption created its own problems: clinicians reported spending 2 hours on documentation for every 1 hour with patients. Physician burnout spiked. And the dream of seamless data sharing across systems remained elusive — hospitals on different EMR platforms often couldn't exchange records easily, defeating much of the interoperability promise.

The **21st Century Cures Act (2016)** and subsequent CMS rules tried to fix this by requiring FHIR-based APIs, giving patients legal rights to access their own data, and penalizing "information blocking."

Where we are today — and how far we still have to go

The wins are real: a physician in an ER can now pull up your medication list, allergy history, and recent labs almost instantly. Telehealth exploded during COVID-19 and permanently normalized virtual care. AI tools are beginning to automate prior authorizations, flag sepsis risk, and transcribe clinical notes in real time.

But the gaps are significant:

- **Coverage**: ~25–28 million Americans remain uninsured; 12 states still haven't expanded Medicaid under the ACA
- **Cost**: the U.S. spends ~$4.9 trillion in 2024 on healthcare — roughly double comparable wealthy nations — yet ranks poorly on life expectancy and preventable death
- **Mental health**: a national shortage of psychiatrists and therapists, with parity laws still unevenly enforced
- **Rural access**: hospital closures, provider shortages, and digital divide issues mean rural Americans have fewer options
- **Data fragmentation**: even with FHIR mandates, patient data still too often can't follow patients across state lines or into specialty networks

- **Drug pricing**: the U.S. pays 2–5x more for brand-name drugs than peer nations; the Inflation Reduction Act (2022) began Medicare negotiation but covers only a narrow set

The arc of the last 20 years is genuinely remarkable — from paper charts and 40 million uninsured to near-universal digital records and meaningful coverage gains. But the U.S. healthcare system remains uniquely expensive, fragmented, and inequitable by wealthy-nation standards. The infrastructure is finally in place; the harder work of making it work *for everyone* is still ahead.

Medicare and Medicaid are the twin pillars of U.S. public health coverage, yet they serve very different populations with different funding structures. Here's a clear breakdown.

Medicare — the age and disability program

Created in 1965 under President Lyndon Johnson as part of the Social Security Act, Medicare is a *federal* program that primarily covers Americans aged 65 and older, plus younger people with certain disabilities or end-stage renal disease. It is not income-based — you earn it through work history (payroll taxes), regardless of wealth.

Medicare is organized into four parts. Part A covers inpatient hospital care, skilled nursing, and hospice — most people pay no premium because it's funded through payroll taxes over a working lifetime. Part B covers outpatient care, doctor visits, and preventive services, with a monthly premium (~$185/month in 2025). Part C (Medicare Advantage) allows private insurers to deliver all Part A and B benefits, often with extras. Part D, added in 2003 under the Medicare Modernization Act, covers prescription drugs — a landmark expansion that took years to pass due to its cost implications.

Today Medicare covers approximately 67 million Americans and is one of the largest purchasers of healthcare services in the world, giving it enormous leverage over how providers are paid.

Medicaid — the income-based safety net

Also created in 1965, Medicaid is a *joint federal-state* program for low-income individuals and families. Unlike Medicare, eligibility is based on income (and sometimes assets), not age or work history. Each state administers its own Medicaid program within federal guidelines, which means benefits, eligibility thresholds, and even the name (Florida calls it "Florida Medicaid," California calls it "Medi-Cal") vary widely by state.

Federal funding matches state spending at rates ranging from 50% to over 75% for lower-income states — meaning states have both flexibility and financial incentive to expand or restrict coverage based on political will and budget conditions. Medicaid covers about 90 million Americans today, making it the single largest health insurer in the country by enrollment.

Medicaid expansion under the ACA — the game changer

This is where the biggest coverage shift of the past 20 years happened. Before the ACA, Medicaid eligibility was tightly restricted — in many states, childless adults were ineligible no matter how poor. The ACA's Medicaid expansion, effective 2014, allowed states to cover all adults earning up to 138% of the federal poverty level (~$20,000/year for an individual in 2024), with the federal government covering 90% of the cost for newly eligible enrollees.

The Supreme Court's 2012 ruling in *NFIB v. Sebelius* made expansion optional, not mandatory. This created a patchwork that persists today: 41 states (plus D.C.) have expanded Medicaid, while 10 states — mostly in the South — have not. The coverage gap this creates is stark: in non-expansion states, many low-income adults earn too much to qualify for traditional Medicaid but too little to afford marketplace insurance.

The "dual eligible" population

About 12 million Americans qualify for both Medicare and Medicaid simultaneously — typically elderly or disabled individuals with very low incomes. These "dual eligibles" are among the sickest and most costly patients in the system, often with multiple chronic conditions. Coordinating their care between two programs with different rules, funding streams, and administrative structures has been a persistent challenge, and one the healthcare system is still working to solve.

Medicare drug pricing — the Inflation Reduction Act (2022)

One of the most significant Medicare changes in nearly 20 years came with the 2022 Inflation Reduction Act, which for the first time allowed Medicare to directly negotiate drug prices with pharmaceutical companies. Previously, a provision in the 2003 Medicare Modernization Act had explicitly prohibited this. The IRA also capped out-of-pocket drug costs for Medicare beneficiaries at $2,000/year beginning in 2025 — a major shift for seniors on expensive specialty medications.

Medical is the strongest story — 92% coverage is genuinely impressive by historical U.S. standards, driven by the ACA marketplace, Medicaid expansion, and continued Medicare growth. The 8% uninsured (about 26 million people) is concentrated in non-expansion states and among undocumented immigrants.

Dental is the worst gap — 31% uncovered (~104 million people) reflects that traditional Medicare has no routine dental benefit, adult Medicaid dental coverage varies wildly by state (some offer nothing beyond emergency extractions), and employer plans often cap benefits at $1,500–$2,000/year. The Biden administration proposed adding dental to Medicare; it didn't pass.

Behavioral health has a deceptive coverage picture. Technically, the Mental Health Parity and Addiction Equity Act (2008) and the ACA require commercial and Medicaid plans to cover mental health at the same level as medical. But about 16% of Americans are nominally insured yet have no real access — meaning they live in a mental health professional shortage area, face months-long wait times, or can't find an in-network provider. So the "effective" uncovered rate is closer to 32% when you add nominal-coverage-with-no-access to the truly uninsured.

Pharmacy coverage is the tightest on paper (only ~5% fully uncovered) thanks to Medicare Part D and Medicaid's comprehensive drug benefits. But cost-sharing — deductibles, co-pays, and formulary tiers — causes roughly 29% of insured Americans to skip or ration medications at some point, making effective access much narrower than the numbers suggest. The IRA's $2,000 Medicare Part D out-of-pocket cap (effective 2025) is the most significant pharmacy reform in two decades.

American healthcare spending reached $4.9 trillion in 2024 — approximately 17.6% of GDP, more than any other nation on earth. Behind every dollar of that spending is a transaction: a claim submitted, a payment adjudicated, a member enrolled, a quality measure calculated. Healthcare analytics is the discipline of turning those transactions into decisions. This chapter establishes the conceptual architecture that will frame every query, model, and report in the chapters that follow. **What Is the Healthcare Ecosystem?**

Before writing a single SQL query, an analyst must understand the system that produces the data.

The **healthcare ecosystem** is the network of entities, transactions, regulations, and data flows that determine how care is delivered, paid for, and measured. Every claim, every diagnosis code, every dollar paid exists because of interactions within this system.

At its core, the ecosystem answers four fundamental questions:

- **Who receives care?** → The patient (member)
- **Who provides care?** → The provider (physician, hospital, facility)
- **Who pays for care?** → The payer (insurance company, employer, government)
- **Who regulates care?** → Federal and state agencies

Understanding these roles is not optional—it is the prerequisite for interpreting any dataset correctly.

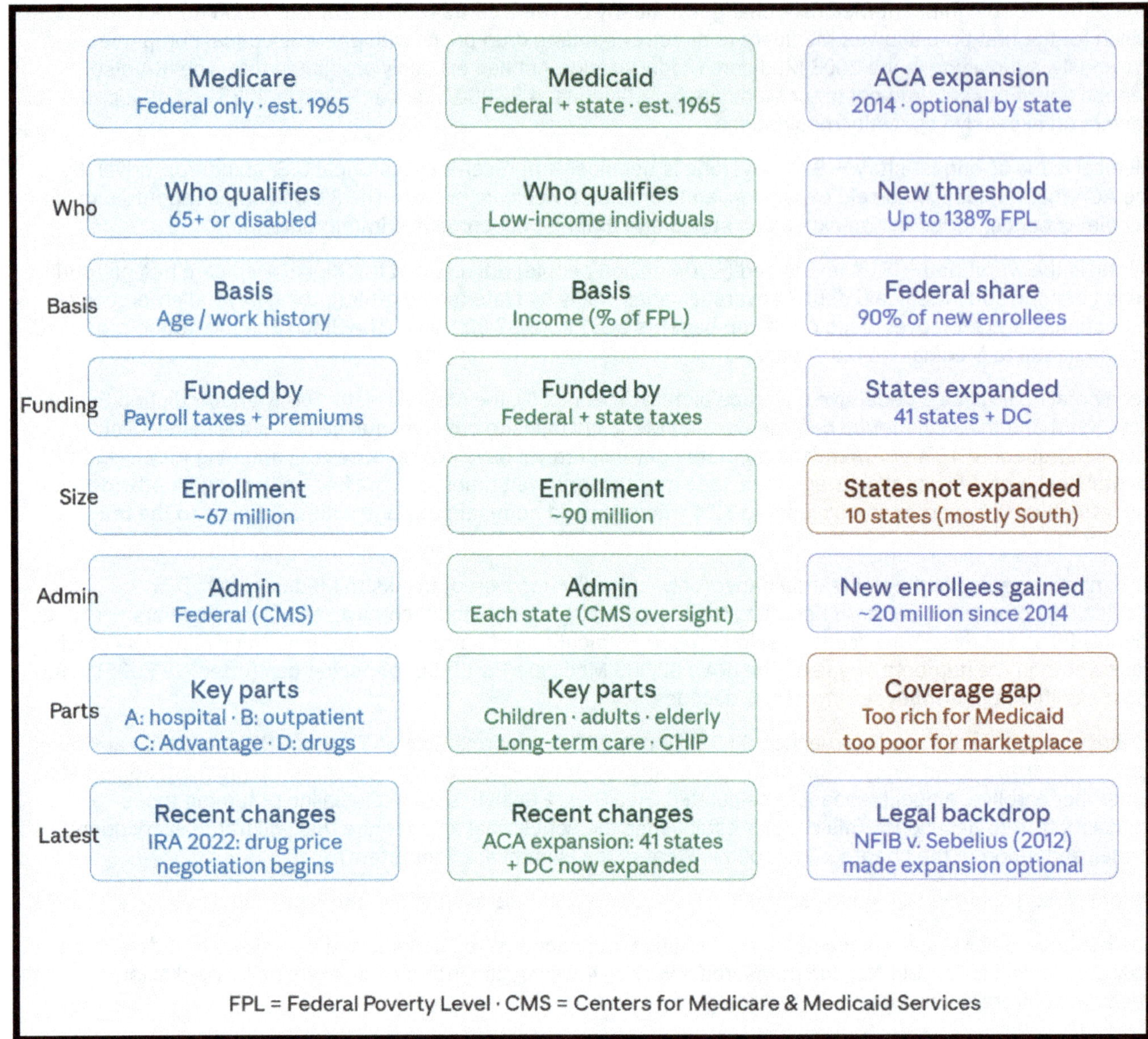

The Four Pillars of the Ecosystem

1. Patients (Members)

The patient is the center of the system. In data, they are referred to as a *member*.

Key attributes:

- Enrollment (coverage start/end dates)
- Demographics (age, gender, geography)
- Clinical history (diagnoses, procedures)
- Utilization patterns (visits, admissions, prescriptions)

👉 Every analysis ultimately traces back to improving patient outcomes or managing patient risk.

2. Providers (Supply Side of Care)

Providers deliver medical services and generate claims.

Types:

- Physicians (primary care, specialists)
- Facilities (hospitals, outpatient centers)
- Ancillary providers (labs, imaging centers, pharmacies)

Key concept:

- **Providers generate the data, but they do not define payment rules.**

3. Payers (Financial Engine)

Payers finance care and adjudicate claims.

Types:

- Commercial insurance (fully insured, self-funded)
- Government programs (Medicare, Medicaid)
- Employer-sponsored plans

Key responsibilities:

- Pricing claims (allowed amount)
- Applying contracts and fee schedules
- Managing risk pools
- Reporting quality metrics (e.g., HEDIS)

👉 Most healthcare analysts work on the **payer side**, where financial and population-level data converge.

4. Regulators (Rules of the System)

Healthcare is one of the most regulated industries in the world.

Examples:

- CMS (Centers for Medicare & Medicaid Services)
- State insurance departments

They define:

- Reporting requirements
- Quality measures
- Payment models

- Compliance standards

☞ Regulations shape the structure of your data more than any database design choice.

How Data Is Created: The Lifecycle of a Claim

Every dataset you analyze is the result of a real-world process.

Step-by-step lifecycle:

1. Patient visits provider
2. Provider documents diagnosis & procedure
3. Claim is generated (ICD, CPT, HCPCS codes)
4. Claim is submitted to payer
5. Payer adjudicates:
    - Applies contract rates
    - Determines allowed amount
    - Assigns member responsibility
6. Claim is paid and stored in the data warehouse

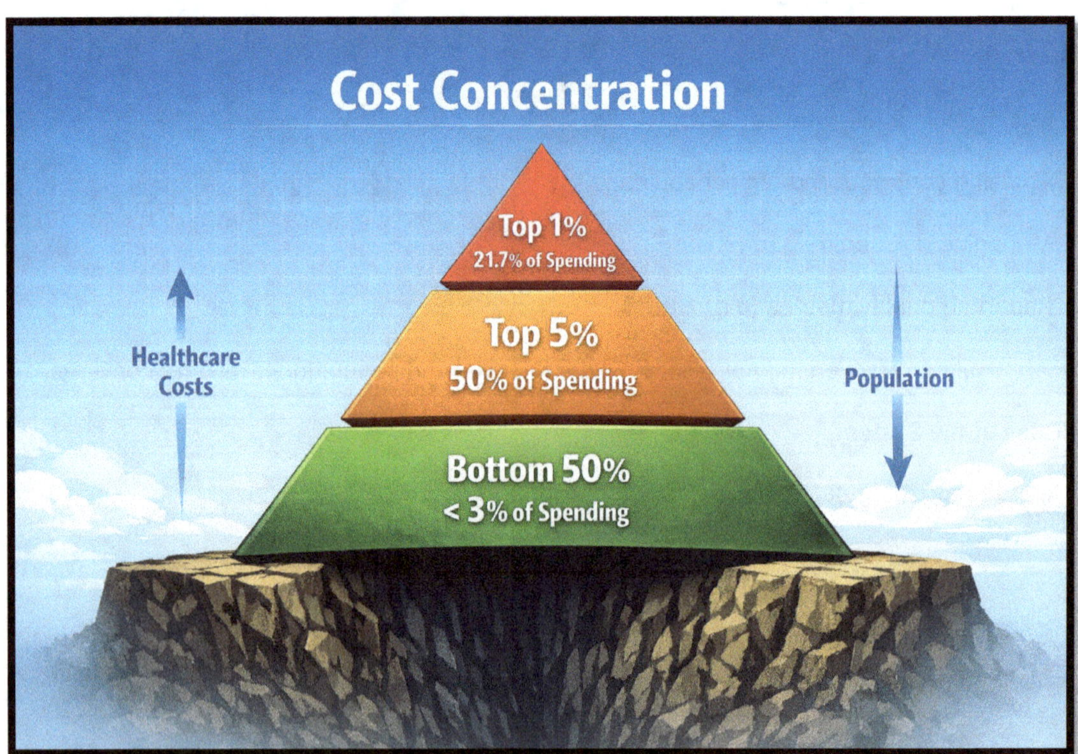

The Analyst as the Bridge

Healthcare analysts are the architects of evidence-based decision-making. By connecting the dots across clinical, operational, and financial data, they detect trends before they escalate, identify threats and opportunities hidden in noise, and generate the predictive intelligence that drives proactive care delivery.

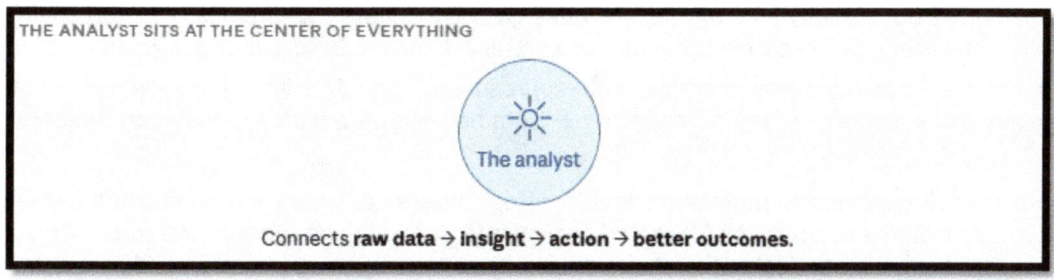

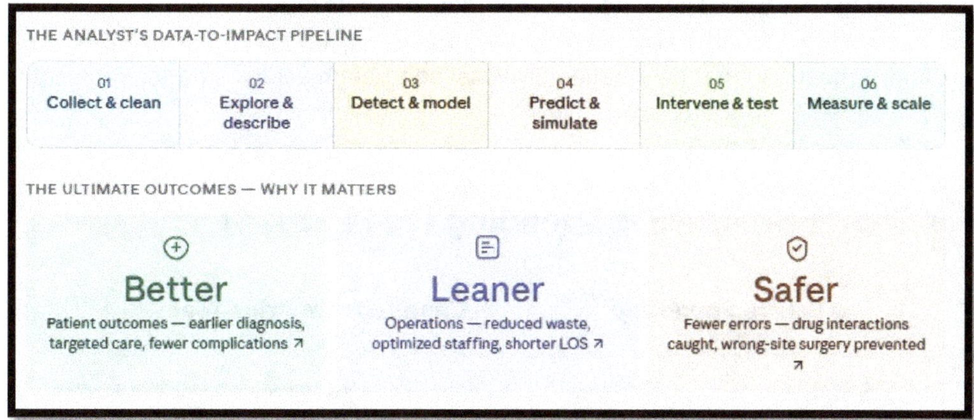

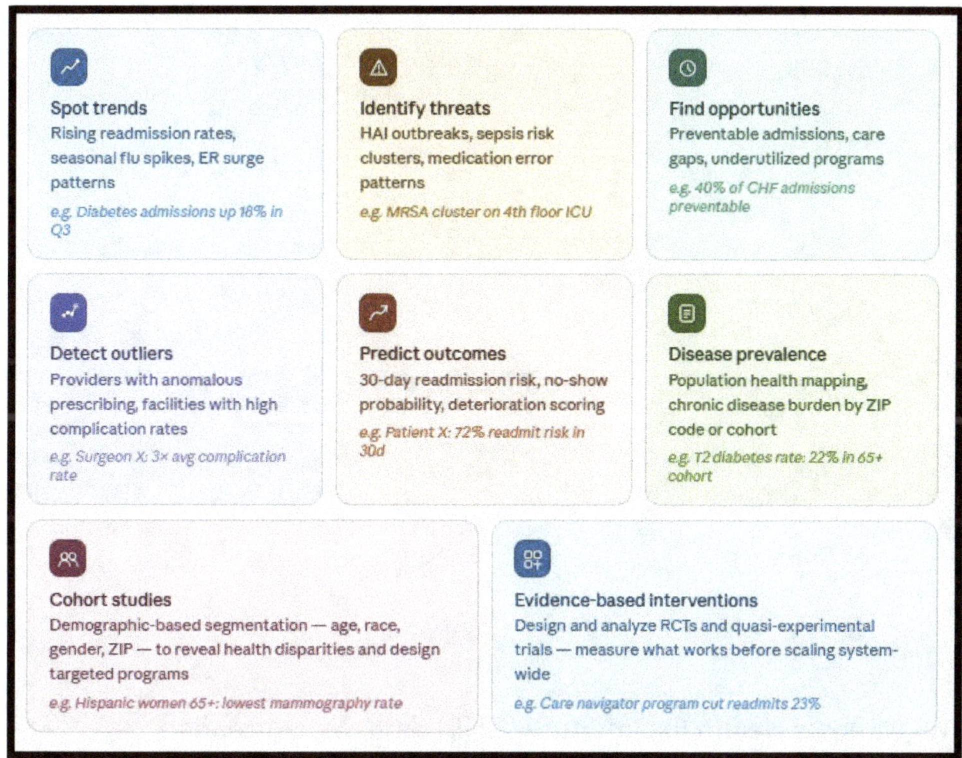

The healthcare analyst is the bridge between what is known and what is done.

The healthcare analyst serves as the critical intelligence layer of a modern health system — transforming vast, fragmented datasets into actionable insight that drives clinical and operational excellence.

Through rigorous trend analysis, outlier detection, and predictive modeling, analysts identify emerging threats before they become crises, uncover opportunities to eliminate preventable utilization, and surface systemic inefficiencies that erode both quality and margin. They design and evaluate evidence-based interventions through controlled trial methodologies, ensuring that programs are proven before they are scaled.

This role is responsible for synthesizing complex, multi-source healthcare data into clear, actionable insights that inform decisions at every level of the organization — from bedside care teams to executive leadership.

Their work spans the full spectrum of population health — from disease prevalence mapping and demographic cohort studies to the design and analysis of targeted clinical interventions and randomized trials. They are equally at home identifying a statistical outlier that signals a quality concern as they are building a risk stratification model that flags a high-risk patient before deterioration sets in.

The impact is measurable and profound: fewer preventable admissions, reduced medical errors, optimized resource allocation, and — most importantly — patient lives saved through earlier, smarter intervention.

📈 U.S. Per Capita Healthcare Spending (2014–2024)

Year	Per Capita Spending	% Change from Prior Year
2024	**$15,474**	+7.2% Centers for Medicare & Medicaid Services
2022	$12,434	+3.6% Macrotrends
2021	$11,999	+2.8%
2020	$11,673	+10.7%
2019	$10,546	+3.6%
2018	$10,185	+4.4%
2017	$9,755	+3.9%
2016	$9,388	+4.3%
2015	$8,998	+5.0%
2014	$8,570	+4.9%

> Source: CMS National Health Expenditure (NHE) data, Macrotrends
> Centers for Medicare & Medicaid Services + 1

Compared with its peers(other developed nations), the U.S. spends dramatically more yet receives far less in terms of quality, access, and outcomes. In short the is a gap in the per capita spending and the patient outcomes.

1.1 The Three Questions Healthcare Analytics Answers

Every healthcare analytics engagement — regardless of the stakeholder, the data source, or the SQL complexity — ultimately serves one of three master questions. Understanding which question you are answering determines the grain of your query, the denominator you choose, and the definition of success.

Cost — What are we spending and why?: PMPM trends, budget variance, service category breakdowns, stop-loss analysis. The financial heartbeat of the plan.

Quality — Are members receiving the right care?: HEDIS measure rates, CMS Star scores, gap-in-care lists, readmission rates. The clinical accountability layer.

Utilization — How is care being consumed?: Admission rates, ED visits per thousand, length of stay, generic dispensing rate. The behavioral pattern layer.

Most production reports answer two or three of these simultaneously — a PMPM dashboard by service category answers cost; adding preventable admission flags adds utilization; layering HEDIS compliance adds quality. Keeping all three in mind prevents the most common analytics error: optimizing for one dimension while unknowingly degrading another.

1.2 The Healthcare Ecosystem — Who the Players Are

Healthcare data is generated by the interaction of three stakeholder groups. Every table in your warehouse traces back to one of these actors.

Stakeholder	Role	What they want from analytics
Payers	Health insurance plans — commercial carriers (UnitedHealth, Anthem, Aetna, BCBS), CMS (Medicare/Medicaid), and self-insured employers.	Predictive risk models, PMPM cost trends, quality measure rates, network performance, fraud detection.
Providers	Hospitals, physician groups, skilled nursing facilities, home health agencies, labs, and pharmacies.	Patient outreach lists, quality scorecards, referral patterns, revenue cycle performance, care gap reports.
Members / Patients	The insured individuals — employees, Medicare beneficiaries, Medicaid recipients.	Cost transparency, care coordination, out-of-pocket estimates, care gap notifications.

The analyst sits at the intersection of all three. A single query might pull enrollment data owned by a payer, claims data generated by a provider, and member demographics from a CMS submission — and join them correctly only if the analyst understands the business logic behind each source.

1.3 The Three Career Pillars of Healthcare Analytics

Healthcare analytics practitioners operate across three distinct career domains. Each pillar uses the same underlying data but asks fundamentally different questions and reports to different organizational stakeholders.

Pillar	Focus	Core deliverables
Financial & Medical Economics	Where is money going? Is cost trend within budget? What is driving variance?	PMPM reports, MLR analysis, budget vs. actual, stop-loss triggers, IBNR triangles.
Clinical & Quality	Are members receiving evidence-based care? Which gaps need to be closed?	HEDIS measure rates, CMS Star gap lists, readmission dashboards, risk stratification.
Network & Provider	Are providers performing efficiently? Is the network adequate and financially sound?	Provider scorecards, fee schedule variance, network adequacy mapping, referral leakage.

1.4 Why Healthcare Data Is Unlike Any Other Industry

If you have worked with data in retail, finance, or technology, healthcare will challenge every assumption you carry in. Four properties make healthcare data fundamentally different — and each one has a direct impact on how you write SQL.

1.4.1 Multi-Format, Multi-System Data

A single member encounter generates data in at least five formats simultaneously: an 837 institutional or professional claim, an 835 remittance advice, an eligibility 834 transaction, potentially an ADT (Admit-Discharge-Transfer) HL7 message from the hospital, and a pharmacy NCPDP claim if drugs were dispensed. Each format has its own grain, its own identifier schema, and its own timing. The analyst's job is to join them correctly — which requires understanding what each source represents before touching the keyboard.

1.4.2 Claims Lag and IBNR

A service rendered today may not appear in your claims warehouse for 30 to 180 days. This phenomenon — Incurred But Not Reported (IBNR) — means that recent months always appear artificially low-cost until claims run out. Every PMPM query must account for claims lag or it will systematically understate recent spending and misidentify false trends. This single issue causes more incorrect executive presentations than any other data problem in the industry.

1.4.3 Regulatory Complexity

Healthcare data is governed by HIPAA (data privacy and security), CMS program rules (Medicare, Medicaid, ACA), NCQA accreditation standards, and state-level insurance regulations — all simultaneously. The analyst must understand which regulatory framework governs each data element, because the business rules embedded in a HEDIS measure or a RAPS submission are not suggestions — they are compliance obligations with financial consequences for non-adherence.

> **Key principle:** In healthcare, the business rule IS the query. You cannot write correct SQL without understanding the regulation that defines the denominator, the exclusion, and the numerator.

1.5 The Essential Code Systems — The Language of Healthcare Data

Healthcare uses multiple parallel coding systems. Each serves a distinct purpose, and a professional healthcare analyst must recognize and navigate all of them without hesitation.

Code System	Purpose	Example
ICD-10-CM	Diagnosis — what condition the patient has	E11.9 = Type 2 diabetes without complications
ICD-10-PCS	Inpatient procedure — what was done surgically	0FB04ZX = Open liver biopsy
CPT / HCPCS	Outpatient procedure & professional services	99214 = Office visit, moderate complexity
DRG	Inpatient hospital payment classification	DRG 470 = Major joint replacement
NDC	Drug identification — what drug, dose, manufacturer	00069-3150-83 = Lipitor 10mg
NPI	Provider identity — unique 10-digit identifier	Every billing provider has one NPI
Revenue Code	Hospital department or service type on UB-04 claim	0450 = Emergency Room services
NUBC TOB	Type of bill — claim type and patient status	131 = Hospital outpatient admit-through-discharge

1.6 How Money Flows Through Healthcare — A Complete Episode

Every data element in your warehouse was created by a step in this payment cycle. Understanding the cycle tells you why the data exists, what it contains, and what can go wrong with each join.

Step	Event	Data generated
1	Member enrolls in a health plan	Enrollment record — member_id, plan_id, coverage_start, line_of_business
2	Member sees a provider	Clinical encounter — diagnosis codes, procedure codes, service date, place of service
3	Provider submits a claim (837)	Professional (837P) or institutional (837I) claim with all codes, charges, and provider NPI
4	Plan adjudicates the claim	Adjudication — paid amount, member liability, CARC/RARC codes, claim status
5	Plan sends remittance (835)	ERA / 835 file — explanation of each payment and adjustment to the provider
6	Plan pays provider	EFT or check — actual dollar disbursement recorded in financial tables
7	CMS or state receives encounter data	Encounter submission — required for risk adjustment and regulatory reporting

1.7 The Analyst's Role — What You Will Build

This book is structured around what analysts actually produce, not around abstract concepts. Every chapter maps to a deliverable that appears in a real health plan, managed care organization, or provider analytics team.

Deliverable	Domain	Covered in
PMPM cost trend by service category	Financial	Ch 3, 14
HEDIS measure rates and gap-in-care lists	Quality	Ch 27
CMS Star Rating simulation	Quality / Regulatory	Ch 29
HCC risk adjustment and RAF scoring	Risk / Revenue	Ch 2, 25
Member month denominator	All domains	Ch 3
Pharmacy PDC drug adherence	Pharmacy	Ch 8
Provider scorecard and leakage report	Network	Ch 16
Fraud, waste & abuse detection	Compliance	Ch 20
Prior authorization compliance	Regulatory	Ch 24
Population risk stratification	Care Management	Ch 22

Chapter 1 Review

Unit Test · Key Takeaways

Answer each question before reading the explanation. Correct answers are highlighted in green with full distractor explanations.

Q1. What are the three master questions every healthcare analytics engagement ultimately answers?

A. Cost, Quality, Access

B. Cost, Quality, Utilization

C. Efficiency, Effectiveness, Equity

D. Financial, Clinical, Operational

Answer: B. *Every deliverable answers Cost (what are we spending and why?), Quality (are members receiving the right care?), or Utilization (how is care being consumed?). Access is an access-to-care concept, not one of the three analytics questions. Efficiency/Effectiveness/Equity and Financial/Clinical/Operational are operational frameworks, not the analytics question set.*

Q2. PMPM is preferred over total paid amount for trend reporting because:

A. PMPM is mandated by NCQA for all quality reporting

B. Total paid is distorted by enrollment size — a plan gaining or losing members shows a misleading cost signal even when per-member efficiency is unchanged. PMPM removes the enrollment effect.

C. PMPM includes pharmacy costs while total paid does not

D. PMPM is easier to calculate in SQL

Answer: B. *A plan losing 10,000 members between Q1 and Q2 will show lower total paid even if per-member cost rose. PMPM divides by member months, isolating the cost-per-member trend independent of enrollment size. NCQA uses PMPM but does not mandate it as the only metric; pharmacy can be included in total paid; the SQL complexity is similar.*

Q3. The denominator for every PMPM calculation must come from:

A. fact_medical_claims — contains all paid services

B. fact_member_months — generated from enrollment; includes every enrolled member regardless of whether they used services

C. dim_members — the member registry

D. ref_procedure_codes — defines the population scope

Answer: B. *Members with no claims in a month are still enrolled and must contribute 1.0 to the denominator. fact_medical_claims excludes healthy members entirely, overstating PMPM. dim_members is a registry with no monthly enrollment structure. ref_procedure_codes is a code reference table.*

Q4. Revenue code 0450 on a UB-04 institutional claim identifies:

A. Room and board — general medical/surgical

B. Emergency Department services

C. Operating room services

D. Intensive care unit services

Answer: B. *0450 = Emergency Room. Revenue codes identify the hospital department on UB-04 claims: 0120 = room and board, 0360 = operating room, 0200 = ICU. These are essential for ED utilization analysis and service-category PMPM breakdowns by site of care.*

Q5. The correct difference between rendering_npi and billing_npi is:

A. They are always the same — both identify the treating physician

B. rendering_npi (Type 1) identifies the individual clinician; billing_npi (Type 2) identifies the organization submitting the claim

C. rendering_npi is for quality measures only; billing_npi is for financial analysis only

D. billing_npi is HIPAA-required; rendering_npi is optional

Answer: B. *A physician employed by a group has their own Type 1 NPI (rendering) while the group holds a Type 2 NPI (billing). For HEDIS and care quality attribution: use rendering_npi. For contract analysis and financial reporting: use billing_npi or billing_tin. Mixing them silently misattributes care and cost.*

Q6. ICD-10-CM code E11.9 — from structure alone, this is:

A. Emergency diagnosis, hospital episode 11, severity index 9

B. **Endocrine/metabolic disease chapter (E); type 2 diabetes mellitus (11); without complications (.9)**
C. External cause chapter (E); injury category 11; body location 9
D. Elective procedure (E); admission type 11; discharge status 9

Answer: B. *ICD-10-CM chapter prefixes identify body systems. E = endocrine, nutritional, and metabolic diseases. 11 = type 2 diabetes mellitus. .9 = without complications. Recognizing chapter prefixes lets analysts identify clinical populations at a glance: C = neoplasms, F = mental/behavioral, I = circulatory, J = respiratory, M = musculoskeletal.*

Q7. Explain the three properties that make healthcare data unique. Give one specific SQL implication for each.

(Short answer)

Sample Answer:
(1) Multi-format, multi-system: a single encounter generates 837 claims, 835 remittance, 834 enrollment, HL7 ADT, and NCPDP pharmacy records — each with different schemas and keys. SQL implication: the same clinical event may exist in multiple tables under different identifiers; cross-table joins require careful key mapping and grain alignment. (2) Claims lag / IBNR: services rendered today may not appear in the warehouse for 30–180 days by claim type. SQL implication: never present recent months as final — add: CASE WHEN svc_month >= DATE_TRUNC('month',CURRENT_DATE) - INTERVAL '3 months' THEN 'INCOMPLETE — IBNR' ELSE 'Final' END AS data_maturity to every trend report. (3) Multi-layered regulatory complexity: HIPAA, CMS program rules, NCQA HEDIS standards, and state law all impose rules that become SQL logic — which claim statuses to include, which diagnosis codes qualify a member, which enrollment windows apply. SQL implication: business rules are not documentation — they are WHERE clauses, CASE WHEN branches, and JOIN conditions that must be coded precisely and audited against the source standard annually.

Q8. A new analyst calculates PMPM using SUM(paid_amount)/COUNT(DISTINCT member_id) from fact_medical_claims. Identify three errors and write the correct SQL pattern.

(Short answer)

Sample Answer:
Error 1 — Wrong denominator source: COUNT(DISTINCT member_id) from claims excludes members with no services. They are still enrolled and must appear in the denominator. Source: fact_member_months. Error 2 — Wrong denominator metric: COUNT(DISTINCT member_id) is unique member count, not member months. A member enrolled all year contributes 12 member months. Dividing by unique members produces cost-per-member, not PMPM. Error 3 — Wrong numerator field: paid_amount is the net cash payment after member cost-sharing. For cost trend analysis use allowed_amount — the contractually allowed amount representing true service cost. Correct pattern: FROM fact_member_months mm LEFT JOIN fact_medical_claims c ON mm.member_id = c.member_id AND mm.membership_year = EXTRACT(YEAR FROM c.service_date) AND mm.membership_month_num = EXTRACT(MONTH FROM c.service_date) AND c.claim_status IN ('PAID','PROCESSED','APPROVED') AND c.claim_type NOT IN ('VOID','REVERSAL') GROUP BY mm.membership_year, mm.membership_month_num — SELECT ROUND(SUM(c.allowed_amount)/NULLIF(SUM(mm.member_months),0),2) AS pmpm.

Q9. Describe the seven-step healthcare money flow and identify one SQL error from misunderstanding each of steps 3, 4, and 5.

(Short answer)

Sample Answer:
Seven steps: (1) Member enrolls — eligibility record created. (2) Member receives service. (3) Provider submits 837 claim — creates a pending record. (4) Payer adjudicates — applies fee schedule, prior auth, COB, deductible. (5) Payer sends 835 remittance — void/replacement cycle may occur. (6) Payer pays provider. (7) Plan submits encounter data to CMS/state. Step 3 error: including pending (submitted but not adjudicated) claims in PMPM. Pending claims have no final paid_amount. Fix: WHERE claim_status IN ('PAID','PROCESSED','APPROVED'). Step 4 error: including denied claims in cost totals. Denied claims were adjudicated but not paid — their allowed_amount should not appear in cost reports. Fix: AND claim_status NOT IN ('DENIED','DENY','D'). Step 5 error: not netting voids and replacements. A void posts a negative transaction; without netting, the original and void together net to zero — but an orphaned void (original missing) creates a phantom negative cost. Fix: GROUP BY original_claim_id, SUM(allowed_amount), HAVING SUM(allowed_amount) > 0.

Q10. Describe the three career pillars of healthcare analytics. For each: name the primary stakeholder, give one deliverable, and name one SQL table central to that pillar.

(Short answer)

Sample Answer:

Pillar 1 — Financial & Medical Economics: Stakeholder: CFO, VP Finance, Actuarial team. Deliverable: 24-month PMPM trend by service category with IBNR flag and YoY variance. Central table: ref_budget_assumptions (plan-filed budget targets by service category — used for variance analysis; quality and network teams rarely use it). Pillar 2 — Clinical & Quality: Stakeholder: CMO, Director of Quality, Stars team. Deliverable: HEDIS gap list ranked by composite Stars priority score, with member contact info for outreach. Central table: ref_star_weights (CMS measure weights by Stars program year — used to score gap closure priority; financial teams rarely need CMS weight coefficients). Pillar 3 — Network & Provider: Stakeholder: VP Network, Contracting, Provider Relations. Deliverable: E&M code distribution vs. peer 95th percentile to flag potential upcoding outliers. Central table: ref_fee_schedule (contracted rates by CPT × provider × effective date — used for unit cost benchmarking; quality teams rarely query contracted rates at claim level).

Key Takeaways

What every analyst must remember from this chapter.

1 Every healthcare analytics deliverable answers one of three master questions: Cost (PMPM trend), Quality (HEDIS/Stars rate), Utilization (admits per 1,000 MM). Define the question before opening the SQL editor — it determines the denominator, metric, and benchmark.

2 PMPM = SUM(allowed_amount) / SUM(member_months). Always use allowed_amount (not paid_amount) for cost trends. Always source the denominator from fact_member_months (not claims). Apply NULLIF(SUM(member_months),0) to every PMPM division to prevent divide-by-zero errors.

3 Healthcare data has three unique properties: multi-format transactions (837/835/834/HL7/NCPDP), claims lag (IBNR — services invisible for 30–180 days by claim type), and multi-layered regulatory rules that become WHERE clauses, CASE WHEN branches, and JOIN conditions in SQL.

4 Revenue code 0450 = Emergency Department. TOB 11X = inpatient acute. DRG classifies the inpatient episode at discharge. CPT/HCPCS identifies the specific procedure on professional claims. These four classifiers are the foundation of every service-category PMPM breakdown.

5 Type 1 NPI = individual rendering provider. Type 2 NPI = billing organization. Use rendering_npi for HEDIS and care quality attribution. Use billing_npi or billing_tin for contract analysis and financial reporting. Mixing them silently misattributes care to the wrong clinician.

6 ICD-10-CM chapter prefixes: C = neoplasms, E = endocrine/metabolic (diabetes E11.x), F = mental/behavioral, I = circulatory (hypertension I10), J = respiratory. Recognizing prefixes lets analysts identify clinical populations from the first letter without memorizing every code.

7 The seven-step money flow (enrollment → service → submission → adjudication → remittance → payment → encounter) defines why each table exists. SQL errors trace to the wrong step: pending claims (step 3), denied claims (step 4), un-netted voids (step 5).

8 Three career pillars — Financial/MedEcon (CFO), Clinical/Quality (CMO), Network/Provider (VP Network) — share the same underlying data but serve different stakeholders and use different reference tables. Identifying the pillar determines every query design decision.

Part I The Healthcare Ecosystem

Chapter 2: Payer Fundamentals & Government Program Analytics

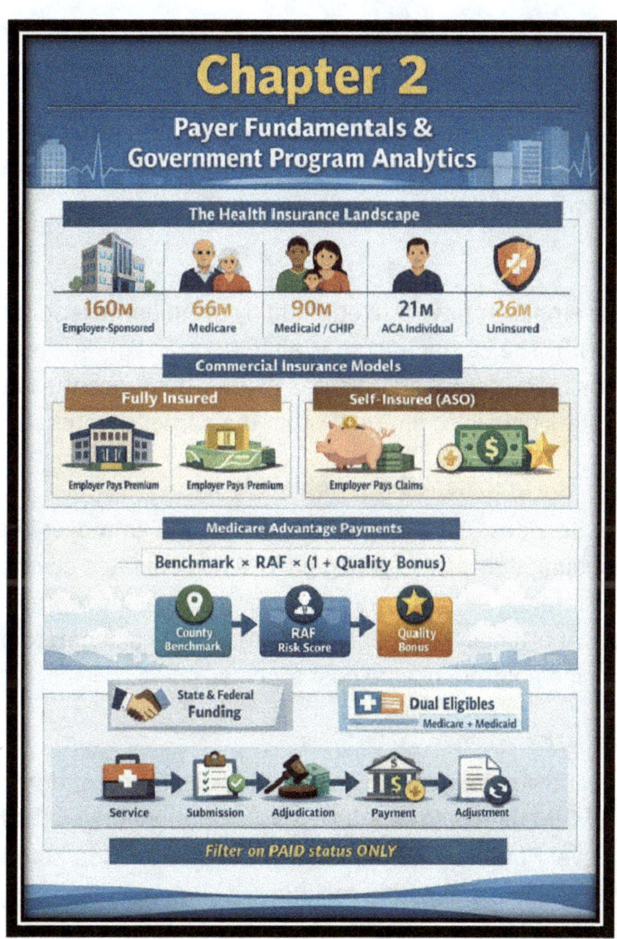

Before writing a single SQL query against healthcare claims, an analyst must understand the financial ecosystem that generated those claims. Who insures the member? Who pays the provider? How much, under what contract, and subject to which regulatory requirements? The answers determine the grain of your denominator, the logic of your status filter, and the validity of every PMPM you will ever calculate. This chapter covers the four major payer types, how each program pays plans and providers, and the complete lifecycle of a claim — from service delivery through adjudication, remittance, and retroactive adjustment.

2.1 The US Health Insurance Landscape — Population Coverage

The United States healthcare system is financed through a mosaic of public programs and private insurance. As of 2024, total national health expenditures exceed $4.9 trillion — approximately 17.6% of GDP. Understanding the relative size and structure of each program is critical because each one generates a different claims format, follows different business rules, and requires different SQL logic.

Program	Population covered	Approx. enrollment	Payer type
Employer-sponsored (commercial)	Working adults and dependents	160M	Private — fully insured or ASO
Medicare	Age 65+, disabled, ESRD	66M	Federal — CMS
Medicaid / CHIP	Low-income adults, children, disabled	90M	Federal/state — managed care
Individual market (ACA)	Self-employed, uninsured adults	21M	Private — ACA-regulated
Uninsured	No coverage	~26M	N/A

2.2 Commercial Insurance & Third-Party Payers

Commercial health insurance covers approximately 160 million Americans through employer-sponsored plans, individually purchased policies, and ACA marketplace plans. Two structural models dominate the commercial market and produce meaningfully different data for the analyst.

2.2.1 Fully Insured Plans

In a fully insured arrangement, the employer pays a fixed monthly premium to a commercial carrier (UnitedHealth, Anthem, Aetna, BCBS). The carrier assumes all financial risk — if claims exceed premium revenue, the carrier absorbs the loss. The carrier adjudicates claims, manages the network, and handles all regulatory filings. Fully insured claims data lives entirely within the carrier's warehouse.

2.2.2 Self-Insured (ASO) Plans — The Dominant Commercial Model

In a self-insured or Administrative Services Only (ASO) arrangement, the employer bears the financial risk. The employer funds a claims bank account; the carrier (acting as TPA) adjudicates claims and draws from that account. The employer pays the carrier an administrative fee only. ASO plans represent over 60% of covered workers in large employer groups. Analytically, ASO data often resides in a separate partition or plan_id range and must be identified before running enterprise-wide cost reports.

2.2.3 Commercial PMPM Benchmarks

Commercial PMPM varies significantly by plan design, geography, and member demographics. As a general benchmark: commercial overall PMPM ranges from $400–$600. Inpatient drives the highest variance — a single large case can move plan-level PMPM by $5–$15 in a small group. Understanding these ranges lets the analyst immediately flag anomalies before presenting results.

2.3 Medicare — Complete 101

Medicare is the federal health insurance program administered by the Centers for Medicare & Medicaid Services (CMS). It serves 66 million Americans — primarily those aged 65 and over, plus individuals with qualifying disabilities and End-Stage Renal Disease (ESRD).

Part	Coverage	How providers are paid
Part A	Inpatient hospital, SNF, hospice, home health	DRG-based prospective payment (IPPS)
Part B	Outpatient, physician services, DME	Fee schedule — Medicare Physician Fee Schedule (MPFS)
Part C	Medicare Advantage — private plans covering A+B	Monthly capitation from CMS to the MA plan
Part D	Prescription drugs	Per-member subsidy to PDP or MA-PD plan

2.3.1 Medicare Advantage Capitation — How MA Plans Get Paid

Medicare Advantage plans receive a risk-adjusted monthly capitation payment from CMS rather than fee-for-service reimbursement. The formula is:

Monthly Capitation = County Benchmark PMPM × RAF Score × (1 + Quality Bonus %)

Where the RAF (Risk Adjustment Factor) score reflects the member's predicted cost relative to an average Medicare beneficiary, derived from submitted HCC (Hierarchical Condition Category) diagnosis codes. A member with multiple chronic conditions may have a RAF of 1.8 — meaning CMS pays 80% more per month for that member than for a healthy average beneficiary.

ANSI SQL — 2.3: MA Capitation Payment Calculation

```
-- PURPOSE: Estimate the monthly capitation payment for each MA member.
-- Formula: County Benchmark × Total RAF × (1 + Quality Bonus %)
-- The plan controls RAF (through CDI and encounter submission)
-- and the quality bonus (through Stars program performance).

SELECT
  m.member_id,
  m.county_fips,                    -- county determines the CMS benchmark
  cb.benchmark_pmpm,                    -- CMS-set county base rate
  m.demo_raf_score,                   -- demographic component (age + sex)
  COALESCE(r.disease_raf, 0)   AS disease_raf,   -- HCC disease component; 0 if no HCCs
  -- Total RAF combines demographic and disease components
  ROUND(m.demo_raf_score
    + COALESCE(r.disease_raf, 0), 4)        AS total_raf,
  qb.quality_bonus_pct,                   -- 0.05 for 4+ Star plans
  -- Monthly capitation = benchmark × RAF × (1 + bonus)
  ROUND(
    cb.benchmark_pmpm
    * (m.demo_raf_score + COALESCE(r.disease_raf, 0))
    * (1 + qb.quality_bonus_pct),
  2)                        AS monthly_capitation
FROM  dim_members        m
JOIN  ref_county_benchmarks cb ON m.county_fips = cb.county_fips
-- LEFT JOIN: members with no HCCs have no row in raf_scores; COALESCE handles NULL
```

```
LEFT JOIN raf_scores        r ON m.member_id   = r.member_id
JOIN  ref_quality_bonus    qb ON m.plan_id     = qb.plan_id
WHERE m.plan_type       = 'MA'
  AND m.coverage_status = 'ACTIVE';  -- active enrollees only
```

2.4 Medicaid — Complete 101

Medicaid is a joint federal-state program providing health coverage to low-income individuals, families, pregnant women, children, and people with disabilities. It is administered by states under broad federal guidelines, which creates significant variation in benefit design, eligibility thresholds, and data formats across state lines.

2.4.1 Federal Medicaid Matching — How States and CMS Share Costs

The federal government matches state Medicaid spending through the Federal Medical Assistance Percentage (FMAP). Poorer states receive a higher federal match. The average FMAP is approximately 57%, meaning CMS covers 57 cents of every dollar a state spends on Medicaid. Analysts working with Medicaid financial data must understand that reported plan costs often reflect only the managed care organization's perspective — the full cost includes federal matching funds not visible in plan-level claims.

2.4.2 Dual Eligible Members — The Bridge Between Programs

Approximately 12 million Americans are eligible for both Medicare and Medicaid simultaneously — known as dual eligibles or duals. These members are among the highest-cost, highest-complexity individuals in any health plan portfolio. In SQL, duals require careful handling: their claims may appear in both Medicare and Medicaid data sets, their liability calculations differ from single-program members, and their enrollment records carry dual-eligibility indicators that must be preserved through all joins.

2.5 How HMOs Get Paid — Capitation Mechanics

Health Maintenance Organizations (HMOs) and other managed care organizations receive capitated payments — a fixed monthly fee per enrolled member regardless of services consumed. This payment model transfers financial risk from the payer to the managed care plan, which then manages utilization and quality to operate within its capitation budget.

The capitation payment flow begins with CMS or a state Medicaid agency sending monthly premium equivalents to the MCO. The MCO may then sub-capitate a portion of that payment to primary care physicians (PCPs) who accept risk for their attributed panels. The analyst's role is to reconcile capitation received against actual medical cost incurred — the surplus or deficit is the plan's operating margin at the provider level.

> **SQL implication:** In capitated plans, member months — not claims — drive the denominator. A member who had no claims in a month still counts as one member month and should appear in your PMPM denominator. Always build denominators from the enrollment table, never from the claims table.

2.6 The Complete Claim Lifecycle — Every State and Status

A claim passes through multiple states between service delivery and final payment. The analyst who does not understand this lifecycle will inadvertently include voided claims, double-count adjustments, or exclude encounters that are still pending — producing materially incorrect cost reports.

Claim Status	Meaning	Include in PMPM?
PAID / PROCESSED	Adjudicated and paid to provider	YES — primary paid population
PENDING / SUSPENSE	Submitted but not yet adjudicated	NO — cost not yet finalized
DENIED	Adjudicated but payment refused	NO — unless tracking denial cost
ADJUSTMENT	Correction to a previously paid claim	YES — use net paid amount
VOID / REVERSAL	Cancellation of a prior payment	NO — must offset original claim
ENCOUNTER	Capitated plan service record (no payment)	YES — for utilization; NO for paid cost

The safe PMPM filter — applied in every production query — is:

```
WHERE claim_status IN ('PAID', 'PROCESSED', 'APPROVED')
  AND claim_type  NOT IN ('VOID', 'REVERSAL', 'ADJUSTMENT_VOID')
  AND service_date BETWEEN :start_date AND :end_date
```

The single most important rule in healthcare SQL: Always filter on claim_status before aggregating paid_amount. A PMPM calculated without this filter will include voids, reversals, and pending claims — producing numbers that are both wrong and different every time the query runs.

ANSI SQL — 2.6: Safe PMPM Claim Status Filter (Fully Annotated)

```
-- PURPOSE: The foundational WHERE clause pattern every PMPM query must use.
-- Including voids, denials, or pending claims distorts allowed_amount totals.

SELECT
   DATE_TRUNC('month', c.service_date)        AS svc_month,
   SUM(c.allowed_amount)                      AS total_allowed,
   -- NULLIF prevents divide-by-zero when a month has zero member months
   ROUND(SUM(c.allowed_amount)
      / NULLIF(SUM(mm.member_months), 0), 2)   AS pmpm
FROM  fact_medical_claims c
JOIN  fact_member_months  mm
  ON c.member_id          = mm.member_id
 AND EXTRACT(YEAR  FROM c.service_date) = mm.membership_year
 AND EXTRACT(MONTH FROM c.service_date) = mm.membership_month_num
-- RULE 1: Only include claims with a final paid adjudication status.
-- Different systems use different status codes -- include all three paid variants.
WHERE c.claim_status IN ('PAID', 'PROCESSED', 'APPROVED')
-- RULE 2: Exclude void and reversal transactions.
-- Voids carry negative dollar amounts; including un-netted voids inflates costs.
 AND c.claim_type NOT IN ('VOID', 'REVERSAL', 'ADJUSTMENT_VOID')
-- RULE 3: Redundant frequency-code safety filter for void transactions.
 AND c.claim_frequency_code <> '8'
GROUP BY 1
ORDER BY 1;
```

Chapter 2 Review

Unit Test · Key Takeaways

Answer each question before reading the explanation.

Q1. An MA plan has a county benchmark of $900. A member's RAF score is 1.75 and the plan earned a 5% quality bonus. Monthly capitation is:

A. $1,575.00
B. $1,653.75
C. $1,620.00
D. $1,417.50

Answer: B. *$900 × 1.75 × (1 + 0.05) = $900 × 1.75 × 1.05 = $1,653.75. The RAF of 1.75 means the plan expects this member to cost 75% more than the average Medicare beneficiary. The quality bonus multiplies the already RAF-adjusted amount — it is not added to the benchmark before the RAF multiplication.*

Q2. The primary analytical difference between fully-insured and ASO (self-insured) commercial plans is:

A. Fully-insured plans always have lower premiums
B. In fully-insured the insurer bears all financial risk; in ASO the employer bears the risk and the plan earns only an admin fee — this changes what PMPM means and who the analytical customer is
C. ASO plans do not use ICD-10 for diagnosis reporting
D. Fully-insured plans always have larger populations

Answer: B. *In fully-insured, claims above premium revenue create a plan financial loss. In ASO, the employer pays claims; the plan earns a per-member admin fee regardless of claims experience. For the analyst, ASO reporting focuses on benchmarks and opportunities for the employer client — not on the plan's own Medical Loss Ratio. Pharmacy data for ASO may flow through a separate PBM with a different data structure.*

Q3. FMAP (Federal Medical Assistance Percentage) is important for Medicaid MCO analysts because:

A. It caps the number of Medicaid members a state can enroll in managed care
B. It determines the federal share of Medicaid costs, creating encounter submission obligations for MCOs — federal funding requires validated encounter data
C. It sets the prior authorization wait-time standard for Medicaid managed care
D. It determines the quality bonus percentage paid to Medicaid MCOs

Answer: B. *FMAP ranges from 50% (wealthiest states) to over 75% (poorest states), calculated annually by HHS. Because federal dollars flow through Medicaid MCO capitation payments, CMS requires complete and timely encounter submission to validate that services were actually delivered. Plans with poor submission rates risk retroactive rate reductions and contract penalties.*

Q4. The correct SQL for PCP panel surplus/(deficit) in a capitation model is:

A. SUM(allowed_amount) - SUM(capitation_pmpm) per PCP
B. SUM(capitation_received) - SUM(paid_amount) per PCP panel — positive = surplus; negative = deficit
C. COUNT(members) × capitation_rate - SUM(claims)
D. SUM(billed_amount) - SUM(capitation_pmpm) per PCP

Answer: B. *Surplus = what the PCP received (capitation) minus what the panel actually cost (paid_amount — net cash, not allowed_amount or billed_amount). Positive = PCP managed within budget (surplus may be shared in risk corridors). Negative = panel exceeded capitation (plan activates stop-loss protection up to the agreed threshold).*

Q5. The safest PMPM claim status filter for multi-system compatibility is:

A. WHERE claim_status = 'PAID'
B. WHERE claim_status IN ('PAID','PROCESSED','APPROVED') AND claim_type NOT IN ('VOID','REVERSAL','ADJUSTMENT_VOID')
C. WHERE claim_status <> 'DENIED'
D. WHERE paid_amount > 0

Answer: B. *Single-status WHERE claim_status = 'PAID' misses legitimate paid claims coded PROCESSED or APPROVED in some systems. WHERE claim_status <> 'DENIED' still includes pending claims not yet adjudicated. WHERE paid_amount > 0 excludes zero-cost preventive encounters needed for utilization analysis. The compound filter in B is the defensive standard.*

Q6. Full dual-eligible members (Medicare + Medicaid) matter disproportionately because:

A. They are the largest enrollment category in most MA plans

B. They are the highest-need, highest-cost segment — RAF scores 1.8–2.5× the non-dual MA average — requiring two-payer COB coordination and D-SNP program tracking

C. They are the only population where HEDIS measures are not required

D. They generate the most prior authorization requests of any member segment

Answer: B. *Full duals are typically 15–20% of MA enrollment but 40–50% of MA costs. Their complexity: two-payer COB coordination, high chronic disease burden driving elevated RAF scores, LTSS covered by Medicaid but not Medicare, and D-SNP eligibility triggering additional CMS reporting. Every MA analytics team needs a dedicated dual-eligible monitoring dashboard.*

Q7. Write the SQL formula for MA monthly capitation. Explain each component and which function controls it.

(Short answer)

Sample Answer:

Formula: ROUND(cb.benchmark_pmpm * (m.demo_raf + COALESCE(r.disease_raf,0)) * (1 + qb.quality_bonus_pct), 2) AS monthly_capitation. Component 1 — benchmark_pmpm: CMS county-level base rate, set annually. The plan has zero control — external input from ref_county_benchmarks. Component 2 — total_raf (demo + disease): the plan drives this indirectly through Clinical Documentation Improvement (CDI) programs and complete, timely encounter submission to CMS. Better diagnosis capture → higher RAF → more monthly revenue. The CDI team and encounter submission operations own this lever. Component 3 — quality_bonus_pct: 5% for 4+ Star plans, 3.5% for some 3.5-Star plans, 0% below that. The Stars program team owns this through HEDIS performance, CAHPS member experience scores, and administrative accuracy measures. Revenue management = RAF + Stars; both require analytics monitoring and improvement programs.

Q8. Explain why claim status filtering is the single most important data quality rule. Describe what happens to PMPM if voids are not excluded. Provide the correct WHERE clause.

(Short answer)

Sample Answer:

Claim status filtering is critical because healthcare claims are not immutable records — they go through submission, adjudication, voiding, and replacement. A void (claim_frequency_code=8) posts a negative transaction canceling a prior payment. A replacement (code=7) posts a corrected amount. In a fully-loaded warehouse the void and original net to zero — correct. But in a warehouse with delayed loads, an orphaned void (original missing) creates a phantom negative cost; an original without its void double-counts the amount. Real-world impact: in a plan processing $50M monthly, 3–5% of volume involves adjustments. Un-netted voids can overstate PMPM by $5–$15, triggering false budget-variance escalations. Correct WHERE clause: WHERE claim_status IN ('PAID','PROCESSED','APPROVED') AND claim_type NOT IN ('VOID','REVERSAL','ADJUSTMENT_VOID') AND claim_frequency_code NOT IN ('8'). Apply in every PMPM query, every HEDIS denominator, and every utilization calculation — no exceptions.

Q9. Explain encounter submission timeliness, why it matters financially for a Medicaid MCO, and what SQL measures it. What is the most common finding by service category?

(Short answer)

Sample Answer:

Encounter submission timeliness = % of Medicaid encounters submitted to the state within defined windows (90, 180, 365 days of service date). Financial importance: (1) States use encounter data for capitation rate-setting — poor submission rates risk retroactive rate reductions. (2) In states with Medicaid risk adjustment, late encounters miss the scoring window, reducing the plan's risk score and next-year capitation. (3) Regulators use encounters for fraud detection — a plan unable to demonstrate services were delivered faces enhanced audit scrutiny. SQL measurement: DATEDIFF('day', service_date, submission_date) per encounter, COUNT(*) within each threshold, divided by total encounters. Group by service_month and service_category to show trends. Most common finding by category: Pharmacy = fastest (NCPDP point-of-sale, >95% within 30 days). Professional = moderate (75–90% within 90 days). Inpatient = slowest (DRG coding + COB resolution: often only 40–60% within 90 days). Action: identify hospital-specific delays and escalate through provider relations before they affect risk scores.

Q10. Describe how the HMO capitation flow runs from CMS to plan to PCP, and provide the SQL join pattern for monitoring PCP panel surplus and deficit.

(Short answer)

Sample Answer:

Flow: (1) CMS pays the MA plan monthly capitation = Benchmark × RAF × Quality Bonus. (2) Plan retains a portion for administration, reinsurance, and profit margin. (3) Plan sub-capitates PCPs a fixed PMPM for each attributed member — the PCP accepts financial risk for their panel's primary care utilization. (4) PCP absorbs deficits up to the stop-loss threshold; plan

> covers the rest. SQL join pattern: FROM dim_pcp_attribution attr JOIN dim_members m ON attr.member_id = m.member_id JOIN fact_provider_capitation cap ON attr.pcp_npi = cap.rendering_npi AND cap.payment_month = :month LEFT JOIN fact_medical_claims c ON m.member_id = c.member_id AND EXTRACT(YEAR FROM c.service_date) = :year AND EXTRACT(MONTH FROM c.service_date) = :month AND c.claim_status IN ('PAID','PROCESSED','APPROVED'). SELECT: SUM(cap.capitation_amount) AS capitation_received, SUM(COALESCE(c.paid_amount,0)) AS panel_actual_cost, SUM(cap.capitation_amount) - SUM(COALESCE(c.paid_amount,0)) AS surplus_deficit. Positive = surplus. Negative = deficit. Monitor monthly — sustained deficit PCPs are candidates for care management partnerships or network review.

Key Takeaways

What every analyst must remember from this chapter.

1 MA capitation = County Benchmark × Total RAF × (1 + Quality Bonus %). Three organizational levers: CMS sets the benchmark (uncontrollable), CDI and encounter submission drive RAF (controllable), Stars program performance drives the quality bonus (controllable).

2 Fully-insured: insurer bears financial risk, MLR is a real financial metric. ASO: employer bears risk, plan earns admin fee only. This distinction changes the analytical deliverable, the stakeholder, and how financial performance is defined and reported.

3 FMAP determines the federal share of Medicaid costs. For the MCO analyst it creates encounter submission obligations — federal co-funding requires validated encounter data, and late or incomplete submission creates financial and audit risk.

4 Safe PMPM claim status filter: WHERE claim_status IN ('PAID','PROCESSED','APPROVED') AND claim_type NOT IN ('VOID','REVERSAL','ADJUSTMENT_VOID'). Apply in every PMPM query, every HEDIS denominator, and every utilization rate — no exceptions.

5 PCP panel surplus/(deficit) = SUM(capitation_received) - SUM(paid_amount). Use paid_amount (net cash), not allowed_amount or billed_amount. Positive = managed within budget. Negative = plan activates stop-loss protection.

6 Full duals (Medicare + Medicaid): 15–20% of MA enrollment but 40–50% of MA costs. RAF scores 1.8–2.5× non-dual average. Two-payer COB coordination. D-SNP program eligibility. Build a dedicated dual-eligible dashboard for every MA plan analytics team.

7 Encounter submission timeliness by claim type: Pharmacy = fastest (>95% within 30 days, NCPDP real-time). Professional = 75–90% within 90 days. Inpatient = slowest (40–60% within 90 days due to DRG coding complexity and COB resolution time).

8 HCC RAF = demographic component + sum of HCC disease coefficients after hierarchy application. Within each disease family, only the highest-severity HCC is counted. Example: DM with acute complications (HCC 17) supersedes DM without complications (HCC 19) — both cannot be counted simultaneously.

PART II: Data Architecture, SQL & Methodology

Rung2 · Chapters 3–4

Part II builds the technical and methodological foundation for everything in this book.

Mastering Part II means you can approach any healthcare analytics problem with a repeatable discipline that produces consistent, defensible, and actionable output.

Part II : Data Architecture, SQL & Methodology

Chapter 3: The Healthcare Data Landscape

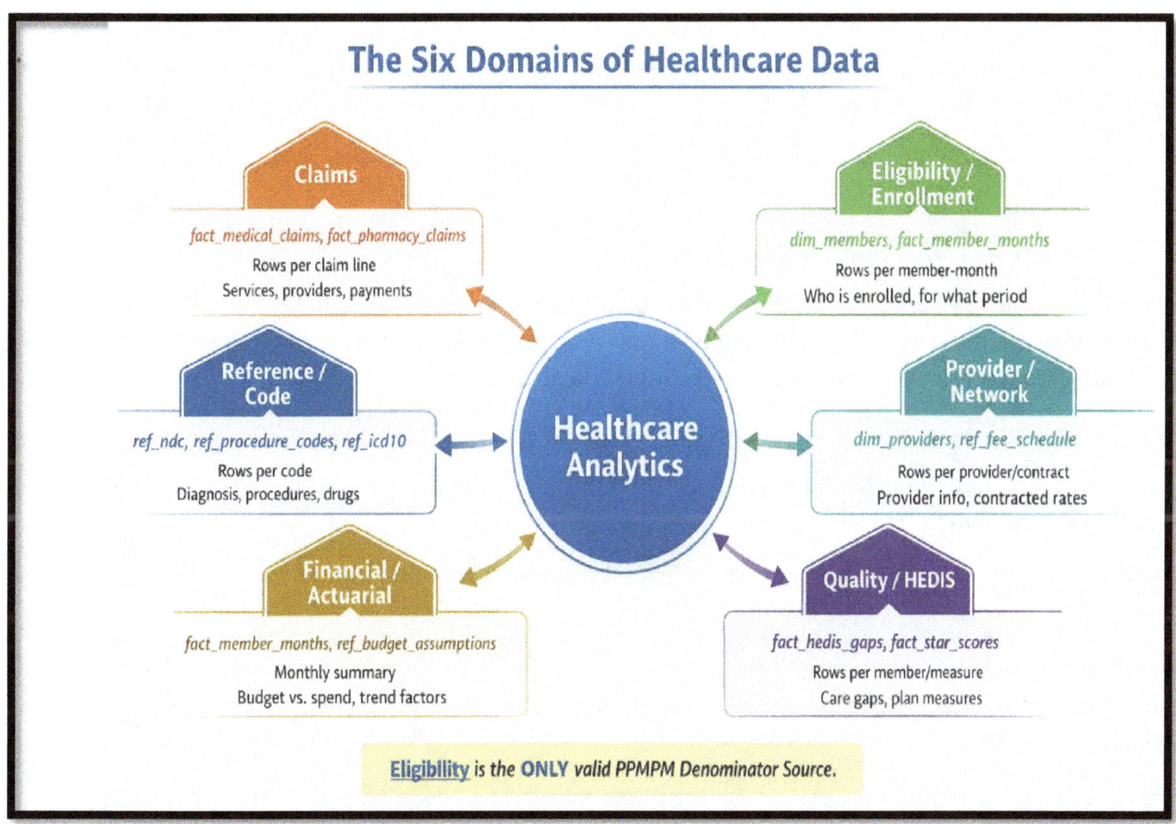

3.0 The Healthcare Data Ecosystem — What Data Exists

A health plan or managed care organization maintains data across six primary domains. Each domain has its own grain, its own update frequency, and its own SQL join logic. Understanding what each domain contains — and what it does not contain — is the prerequisite for correct query design.

Data Domain	Primary Table(s)	Grain	Update Frequency	What it answers
Claims	fact_medical_claims, fact_pharmacy_claims	One row per claim line	Daily / weekly adjudication cycles	What services were rendered, to whom, by whom, and what was paid
Eligibility / Enrollment	dim_members, fact_member_months	One row per enrollment span; one per member-month	Daily 834 file updates	Who is enrolled, in what plan, for what period
Provider / Network	dim_providers, ref_fee_schedule	One row per provider per contract	Contract amendment cycles	Who delivered care, at what contracted rate, in what specialty
Reference / Code	ref_ndc, ref_procedure_codes, ref_icd10	One row per code	Quarterly (ICD-10 Oct; CPT Jan)	What procedure was performed, what diagnosis, what drug
Quality / HEDIS	fact_hedis_gaps, fact_star_scores	One row per member per measure	Annual measurement year cycle	Which members have care gaps, what is the plan measure rate
Financial / Actuarial	fact_member_months, ref_budget_assumptions	Monthly summary grain	Monthly close cycle	What did the plan spend vs. budget, what are trend factors

> **Critical rule:** Claims data is always incomplete for recent months due to claims lag (IBNR). Never use claims as the source of truth for enrollment counts or denominator calculations. Always use the eligibility/enrollment tables for denominators.

3.1 The Star Schema — Healthcare's Data Model

Healthcare data warehouses are almost universally organized as star schemas — a central fact table surrounded by dimension tables. Understanding this architecture is not optional: it determines which tables you join, which grain you query, and how your GROUP BY must be structured.

3.1.1 Fact Tables — The Events

Fact tables record transactions — things that happened. They are wide (many columns), tall (many rows), and numeric-heavy. In healthcare:

fact_medical_claims: One row per claim line. Contains paid_amount, allowed_amount, service_date, claim_status, procedure_code, diagnosis codes, claim_type, member_id, rendering_npi.

fact_pharmacy_claims: One row per pharmacy dispensing. Contains ndc_code, dispensing_date, days_supply, plan_paid_amount, member_id, pharmacy_npi.

fact_member_months: One row per member per calendar month of enrollment. The denominator engine — this is where PMPM denominators come from, not from claims.

3.1.2 Dimension Tables — The Context

Dimension tables provide the descriptive context for each transaction. They are shorter (fewer rows), wider (many descriptive attributes), and text-heavy.

dim_members: Member demographics: birth_date, gender_cd, line_of_business, coverage_start, coverage_end, county_fips, attributed_pcp_npi. Slowly changing — use SCD Type 2 for historical queries.

dim_providers: Provider master: npi, provider_name, specialty_code, billing_tin, network_status, practice_address. Updated when contracts change.

dim_date: Calendar reference: date_key, calendar_year, calendar_month, calendar_quarter, day_of_week. Enables clean fiscal-year and year-over-year joins.

fact_medical_claims	dim_members
claim_id PK	member_id PK
member_id FK → dim_members	line_of_business
service_date FK → dim_date	coverage_start
procedure_code FK → ref_procedure_codes	coverage_end
rendering_npi FK → dim_providers	birth_date / gender_cd
claim_status	county_fips
claim_type	attributed_pcp_npi
paid_amount	**dim_date**
allowed_amount	date_key PK
deductible_applied	calendar_year
copay_amount	calendar_month
member_months (via fact_member_months)	calendar_quarter
	fiscal_year
	ref_procedure_codes
	procedure_code PK
	service_category
	clinical_grouper
	cpt_description

ANSI SQL — 3.1: Star Schema PMPM Query

```
-- PURPOSE: Calculate PMPM broken down by year, month, line of business,
-- and service category using the standard star schema join pattern.
-- One fact table (fact_medical_claims) joined to three dimensions
-- plus the enrollment denominator (fact_member_months).

SELECT
   d.calendar_year,          -- year the service occurred (from dim_date)
   d.calendar_month,         -- month the service occurred
   m.line_of_business,       -- Commercial / MA / Medicaid (from dim_members)
   p.service_category,       -- Inpatient / Outpatient / ED / Professional / Rx
   SUM(c.paid_amount)              AS total_paid,
   SUM(mm.member_months)               AS member_months,
   -- PMPM = total cost divided by enrolled member months.
   -- NULLIF prevents divide-by-zero if a cell has zero enrollment.
   ROUND(SUM(c.paid_amount)
     / NULLIF(SUM(mm.member_months), 0), 2) AS pmpm
FROM  fact_medical_claims  c           -- the central transaction fact table
JOIN  dim_date             d
   ON c.service_date  = d.date_key      -- link claim to calendar attributes
JOIN  dim_members          m
   ON c.member_id     = m.member_id     -- link claim to member demographics
JOIN  ref_procedure_codes  p
   ON c.procedure_code = p.procedure_code -- map procedure to service category
```

3.2 Claim Grain — The Most Important Concept in Healthcare SQL

The single most common cause of incorrect healthcare SQL results is a misunderstanding of claim grain. Healthcare claims have two levels: the claim header and the claim line. Writing a query at the wrong grain produces double-counted paid amounts, inflated utilization counts, or missed episodes.

Grain Level	What it represents	When to use	Duplicate risk
Claim header	One row per claim — total payment, admission date, discharge date, DRG. No procedure code.	Counting admissions, calculating LOS, IP payment analysis	Safe for counting admits; wrong for procedure-level analysis
Claim line	One row per procedure performed. Same claim_id, different line_number. Procedure code present.	Service category classification, procedure-level utilization	SUM(paid_amount) across lines = total claim cost — correct. COUNT(*) of lines ≠ number of claims — wrong for admit counts.
Member month	One row per member per calendar month. No claims. Pure enrollment.	Denominator for all PMPM, rate, and utilization calculations	Never use claims as denominator. Claims are zero for healthy members who had no services.

> **The grain trap:** A hospital inpatient claim may have 40–200 revenue code lines. COUNT(*) on an inpatient claim produces 40–200, not 1 admission. Always COUNT(DISTINCT claim_id) for admission counts. Always use a header-level table or group to claim_id before counting.

3.3 Member Month Generation — The Denominator Engine

Member months are the denominator in every PMPM, every HEDIS rate, and every utilization rate in healthcare analytics. A member month is one member enrolled for one calendar month. A member enrolled January 1 through December 31 contributes 12 member months to the year.

The member month table must be generated from enrollment data — not from claims. A member who had no claims in a given month is still enrolled and must appear in the denominator. If you build your denominator from claims, every member with zero utilization disappears from the calculation, and your PMPM overstates cost because you have divided by too few member months.

ANSI SQL — 3.3: Member Month Generation from Enrollment

```
-- PURPOSE: Generate one row per member per calendar month they were enrolled.
-- This is the correct PMPM denominator source.
-- NEVER use claims as the denominator -- healthy members with no claims
-- are still enrolled and must contribute 1.0 to every month they are active.

-- STEP 1: Create a calendar spine -- one row per month of the measurement year.
-- generate_series produces one timestamp per month; DATE_TRUNC truncates to month start.
WITH calendar AS (
  SELECT DATE_TRUNC('month', seq_date) AS month_start
  FROM  generate_series(
        '2024-01-01'::date,   -- first month of measurement year
        '2024-12-31'::date,   -- last month of measurement year
        '1 month'::interval   -- step: one row per month
     ) AS seq_date
)
```

```
-- STEP 2: Cross each enrolled member against the calendar.
-- The JOIN condition checks that the calendar month falls within the
-- member's coverage window (coverage_start through coverage_end).
-- COALESCE on coverage_end: NULL = still active; treat as far future (2099).
SELECT
  m.member_id,
  m.plan_id,
  m.line_of_business,
  c.month_start                    AS membership_month,
  EXTRACT(YEAR  FROM c.month_start)::INT AS membership_year,
  EXTRACT(MONTH FROM c.month_start)::INT AS membership_month_num,
  1.0                              AS member_months  -- always 1.0 per month row
FROM  dim_members  m
JOIN  calendar     c
  -- Member is enrolled if their coverage window overlaps this calendar month.
  ON c.month_start >= DATE_TRUNC('month', m.coverage_start)
 AND c.month_start <= DATE_TRUNC('month',
       COALESCE(m.coverage_end, '2099-12-31'::date))
WHERE m.plan_id         = :plan_id
 AND m.coverage_status IN ('ACTIVE', 'RETRO_ACTIVE');

-- STEP 3: Use the generated member months as the PMPM denominator.
-- LEFT JOIN: zero-utilization members appear in result with $0 claims.
SELECT
  mm.membership_year,
  mm.membership_month_num,
  SUM(c.allowed_amount)                 AS total_allowed,
  COUNT(DISTINCT mm.member_id)          AS enrolled_members,
  SUM(mm.member_months)                 AS member_months,
  ROUND(SUM(c.allowed_amount)
    / NULLIF(SUM(mm.member_months), 0), 2)  AS pmpm
FROM  fact_member_months mm         -- START from enrollment -- all members
LEFT JOIN fact_medical_claims c     -- LEFT JOIN: keeps zero-utilization members
     ON mm.member_id          = c.member_id
    AND mm.membership_year    = EXTRACT(YEAR  FROM c.service_date)
    AND mm.membership_month_num = EXTRACT(MONTH FROM c.service_date)
    AND c.claim_status        = 'PAID'
    AND c.claim_type NOT IN   ('VOID', 'REVERSAL')
WHERE mm.membership_year = 2024
GROUP BY 1, 2
ORDER BY 1, 2;
```

3.4 SCD Type 2 — Slowly Changing Dimensions

Member attributes change over time. A member may switch from commercial to Medicare Advantage mid-year. A member may move to a different county, change their PCP, or add dependents. If your dimension table overwrites the current value, every historical query will use today's attributes — not the attributes that were true on the date of service.

Slowly Changing Dimension Type 2 (SCD-2) solves this by creating a new row for each attribute change, with effective_date and end_date columns that define when each version was active. A point-in-time join retrieves the version that was active on any given service date.

Column	Type	Description
member_id	FK	Same across all versions for this member
effective_date	DATE	Date this version became active
end_date	DATE / NULL	Date this version ended. NULL = currently active.
line_of_business	VARCHAR	The attribute being tracked — changes trigger new row
plan_id	VARCHAR	Plan identifier for this enrollment span
is_current	BOOLEAN	TRUE for the currently active version only

ANSI SQL — 3.4: SCD-2 Point-in-Time Join

```
-- PURPOSE: Retrieve the line of business (LOB) that was ACTIVE on each
-- claim's service_date -- not the LOB the member holds today.
-- Without SCD-2: a member who switched Commercial → MA on July 1 would
-- have ALL their January–June commercial claims attributed to MA,
-- overstating MA PMPM and understating Commercial PMPM by the full H1 cost.

-- The SCD-2 table has one row per attribute version.
-- effective_date = when this version became active.
-- end_date = when this version was superseded (NULL = still active).
SELECT
    c.claim_id,
    c.member_id,
    c.service_date,
    c.paid_amount,
    m.line_of_business,  -- the LOB that was active ON service_date
    m.plan_id
FROM  fact_medical_claims c
JOIN  dim_members_scd2    m
   ON c.member_id    = m.member_id
  -- service_date must fall WITHIN the version's active window
  AND c.service_date >= m.effective_date
  -- COALESCE: NULL end_date means the version is currently active
  AND c.service_date <  COALESCE(m.end_date, '2099-12-31')
WHERE c.claim_status = 'PAID';

-- VALIDATION: count members with multiple LOB versions this year.
-- These are the members where SCD-2 is required for correct attribution.
SELECT member_id, COUNT(*) AS lob_version_count
FROM   dim_members_scd2
WHERE  effective_date >= '2024-01-01'
GROUP BY member_id
HAVING COUNT(*) > 1
ORDER BY lob_version_count DESC;
```

Why this matters: In a plan with 100,000 members, roughly 2,000–5,000 members will have at least one LOB or plan change in any given year. Without SCD-2 joins, their claims are permanently misattributed — inflating costs in the current LOB and understating costs in the prior LOB. This error compounds in risk adjustment, where incorrect LOB attribution produces wrong RAF scores and incorrect revenue.

3.5 IBNR — Incurred But Not Reported

IBNR is the most consequential data quality issue in healthcare analytics. A service rendered today may not appear in the claims warehouse for 30 to 180 days — or longer for complex institutional claims with coordination of benefits issues. This means the most recent months in any claims query are always artificially low-cost, creating the appearance of favorable trends that do not exist.

The IBNR lag triangle is the actuarial tool for quantifying this incompleteness. It shows what percentage of ultimate claims has been received by each elapsed month after the service date. A completion factor is derived from the triangle and applied to adjust recent months to their estimated ultimate values.

Service Month	Claims received at 1 month	At 3 months	At 6 months	At 12 months	Completion factor at 1 mo
Professional (PB)	55%	85%	96%	99%	1.82×
Outpatient (OP)	45%	80%	93%	98%	2.22×
Inpatient (IP)	30%	70%	88%	97%	3.33×
Pharmacy (Rx)	90%	98%	99%	100%	1.11×

Practical rule: Never present the most recent 2–3 months of claims data as final without applying completion factors. Month 1 inpatient data may be only 30% complete. Showing it raw to executives creates the false impression of a favorable cost trend that will reverse completely when claims run out.

3.6 The Essential Healthcare Code Systems

Healthcare uses multiple parallel coding systems simultaneously. Each claim line may contain an ICD-10 diagnosis code, a CPT procedure code, an NDC drug code (for pharmacy), a revenue code (for institutional claims), and an NPI provider identifier — all on the same transaction. Correct SQL requires understanding what each code system classifies and how codes are maintained.

Code System	What it classifies	Format	Maintained by	SQL table
ICD-10-CM	Diagnosis — what condition the patient has	Letter + 2–7 chars: E11.9	CMS / WHO — updated Oct 1 annually	ref_icd10_cm
ICD-10-PCS	Inpatient procedure — surgical and procedural	7 alphanumeric chars: 0FB04ZX	CMS — updated Oct 1 annually	ref_icd10_pcs
CPT / HCPCS	Outpatient procedure and professional services	5 digits: 99214, G0202	AMA (CPT); CMS (HCPCS) — Jan 1	ref_procedure_codes
DRG	Inpatient payment classification — episode grouping	3 digits: 470, 291	CMS — updated Oct 1	ref_drg
NDC	Drug identification: drug, strength, manufacturer	11 digits: 00069-3150-83	FDA — real-time	ref_ndc
NPI	Provider identity — unique national identifier	10 digits: 1234567890	CMS NPPES — real-time	dim_providers
Revenue Code	Hospital department or service type on UB-04	4 digits: 0450 = ED	NUBC — annual updates	ref_revenue_codes
Type of Bill (TOB)	Claim type and patient status on institutional claim	3–4 digits: 131 = OP	NUBC — annual updates	ref_tob_codes

> **Annual update risk:** ICD-10 adds ~500–1,000 new diagnosis codes each October 1. CPT adds or deletes ~100 codes each January. Any reference table join that uses hard-coded code lists in WHERE clauses will silently miss new codes. Use maintained reference tables — ref_icd10_cm, ref_procedure_codes — and join to them rather than coding values inline.

3.7 How Money Flows — The Complete Episode

Every row in your claims warehouse was created by a specific step in the payment cycle. Understanding the flow tells you why each table exists, what data it contains, and — critically — what can cause a join to fail or produce unexpected results.

Step	Event	Data generated	Common SQL problem
1	Member enrolls	dim_members row with coverage_start, plan_id, LOB	Retroactive enrollment: member_id appears in claims before enrollment row exists
2	Member sees provider	Clinical encounter: diagnosis, procedure, service date, place of service	Service date ≠ claim receipt date — always filter on service_date, not paid_date, for HEDIS
3	Provider submits 837 claim	837P (professional) or 837I (institutional) — raw claim submission	Duplicate submissions: same service submitted twice. Use ROW_NUMBER() to deduplicate
4	Plan adjudicates	claim_status set to PAID/DENIED/PENDING; paid_amount calculated	Pending claims in PMPM: always filter claim_status = 'PAID'
5	Plan sends 835 remittance	CARC/RARC codes explaining adjustments; ERA record	Adjustment claims: original paid + void + replacement — net to correct amount
6	Plan pays provider	EFT disbursement — financial record in AP system	Paid_date lag: payment may post 15–30 days after adjudication
7	Encounter submitted to CMS/state	Encounter record — required for risk adjustment and capitation validation	Encounter ≠ paid claim: encounters may have $0 paid_amount in capitated plans

3.8 The Essential Healthcare Analytics Acronyms

Healthcare is saturated with acronyms that carry precise technical and regulatory meanings. The following table covers the minimum vocabulary required to read a health plan financial report, a quality dashboard, or a network contract.

ACA	Affordable Care Act	**MLR**	Medical Loss Ratio
ACO	Accountable Care Organization	**MSSP**	Medicare Shared Savings Program (ACO)
APM	Alternative Payment Model	**NCQA**	National Committee for Quality Assurance
ASO	Administrative Services Only (self-insured)	**NDC**	National Drug Code
CAHPS	Consumer Assessment of Healthcare Providers and Systems	**NPI**	National Provider Identifier

CARC	Claim Adjustment Reason Code	**OP**	Outpatient (claim type)
CCI	Charlson Comorbidity Index	**PA**	Prior Authorization
COB	Coordination of Benefits	**PB**	Professional Billing (claim type, CMS-1500)
CPT	Current Procedural Terminology	**PBM**	Pharmacy Benefit Manager
DRG	Diagnosis Related Group	**PCP**	Primary Care Physician
ED	Emergency Department	**PDC**	Proportion of Days Covered (adherence metric)
ERA	Electronic Remittance Advice (835)	**PMPM**	Per Member Per Month (cost/utilization unit)
ESRD	End-Stage Renal Disease	**PQI**	Prevention Quality Indicator (avoidable admissions)
FFS	Fee-for-Service	**RAF**	Risk Adjustment Factor (MA capitation)
FMAP	Federal Medical Assistance Percentage (Medicaid matching)	**RAPS**	Risk Adjustment Processing System (CMS)
FWA	Fraud, Waste, and Abuse	**RARC**	Remittance Advice Remark Code
HCC	Hierarchical Condition Category (risk adjustment)	**RCM**	Revenue Cycle Management
HEDIS	Healthcare Effectiveness Data and Information Set (NCQA)	**SCD**	Slowly Changing Dimension (data architecture)
HMO	Health Maintenance Organization	**SDOH**	Social Determinants of Health
HOS	Health Outcomes Survey (Medicare)	**SNF**	Skilled Nursing Facility
IBNR	Incurred But Not Reported (claims lag)	**STAR**	Situation-Task-Action-Result (analytical framework)
IP	Inpatient (claim type)	**TOB**	Type of Bill (institutional claim identifier)
LOB	Line of Business (MA, Commercial, Medicaid)	**TPA**	Third-Party Administrator
MA	Medicare Advantage (Part C)	**UB-04**	Uniform Billing form — institutional claim format
MCO	Managed Care Organization	**VBC**	Value-Based Care

3.9 STAR Scenario — Data Landscape in Practice

The following scenario applies the concepts from this chapter — star schema PMPM, claim status filtering, member month denominator — to a real business question. Notice how the four STAR components force precision before any SQL is written.

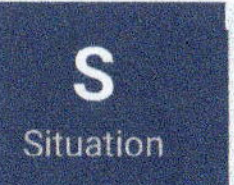

The VP of Finance has asked: "Why is our commercial PMPM showing a 22% drop in October vs. September?" You suspect this is a claims lag artifact, not a real cost reduction. You need to demonstrate this using a budget variance query that exposes the IBNR problem.

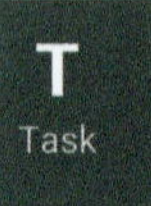

Calculate actual PMPM by service category vs. budget for Q3 2024 commercial paid claims. Show the October anomaly alongside Q3 actuals to make the claims lag visible. Population: commercial fully-insured. Denominator: fact_member_months. Status filter: PAID claims only.

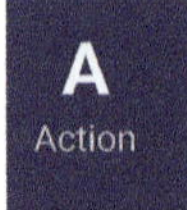

Step 1: Join paid claims to procedure code reference to get service_category. Step 2: Join to member months for denominator. Step 3: Join to budget assumption reference. Step 4: Calculate actual PMPM, budget PMPM, and variance.

ANSI SQL — 3.9: Budget Variance by Service Category

-- PURPOSE: Compare actual PMPM to budget PMPM by service category for Q3.
-- The key feature: flag categories where actual PMPM is more than 15% below
-- budget -- this is almost certainly a claims lag (IBNR) artifact,
-- not a genuine cost improvement.

```
SELECT
   p.service_category,
   -- Actual PMPM: total paid divided by enrolled member months
   ROUND(SUM(c.paid_amount)
      / NULLIF(SUM(mm.member_months), 0), 2)  AS actual_pmpm,
   b.budget_pmpm,                          -- plan-filed budget assumption
   -- Variance: positive = over budget; negative = under budget
   ROUND(SUM(c.allowed_amount) / NULLIF(SUM(mm.member_months), 0)
      - b.budget_pmpm, 2)                  AS variance_pmpm,
   -- IBNR flag: if actual is >15% below budget in a recent month,
   -- the data is likely incomplete due to claims lag.
   CASE
      WHEN SUM(c.allowed_amount) / NULLIF(SUM(mm.member_months),0)
         < b.budget_pmpm * 0.85
      THEN 'CHECK IBNR -- data may be incomplete'
      ELSE 'Within expected range'
   END                          AS ibnr_flag
FROM  fact_medical_claims    c
-- Map each claim's procedure code to a service category
JOIN  ref_procedure_codes    p   ON c.procedure_code   = p.procedure_code
-- Enrollment denominator: Q3 2024 member months
JOIN  fact_member_months     mm  ON c.member_id        = mm.member_id
                  AND mm.membership_year = 2024
                  AND mm.membership_month_num BETWEEN 7 AND 9
-- Budget reference: planned PMPM by service category
JOIN  ref_budget_assumptions  b  ON p.service_category = b.service_category
WHERE c.claim_status     = 'PAID'
  AND c.line_of_business = 'COMMERCIAL'
GROUP BY p.service_category, b.budget_pmpm
ORDER BY ABS(variance_pmpm) DESC; -- largest variances (+ or -) first
```

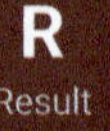

The Q3 actuals show inpatient at budget (+$2 variance) and professional 3% below budget — normal variation. The October numbers show inpatient 22% below budget with the IBNR flag triggered. This is not a cost improvement — it is claims lag. The inpatient completion factor at 1 month is approximately 3.33×, meaning only 30% of October inpatient claims have been received.

Communication to VP Finance: "October's apparent 22% PMPM drop is a claims lag artifact. At 1-month lag, inpatient claims are ~30% complete. Applying a 3.33× completion factor produces an estimated October PMPM of $487 vs. $492 budget — within normal range. Final October actuals will be available in January."

Unit Test · Key Takeaways

Answer each question before reading the explanation.

Q1. What is the "grain" of the fact_medical_claims table and why does it matter most for counting admissions?

A. One row per member — all claims for a member are on a single row

B. One row per claim revenue line — a single inpatient stay may generate 40–200 rows; COUNT(*) gives line count, not admission count

C. One row per paid claim header — voids are stored separately

D. One row per member per month — the same grain as fact_member_months

Answer: B. *Institutional inpatient claims have one row per revenue code line billed. A 5-day stay with room/board, OR, labs, pharmacy, and radiology might generate 80+ rows. COUNT(*) on this table counts lines, not admissions. Always use COUNT(DISTINCT claim_id) for admission or visit counts and SUM(allowed_amount) at header grain for episode cost.*

Q2. In the star schema PMPM query, why is fact_member_months joined rather than using COUNT(DISTINCT member_id) from claims?

A. fact_member_months improves query performance

B. COUNT(DISTINCT member_id) from claims excludes members with no services that month — they are still enrolled and must appear in the denominator. fact_member_months includes all enrolled members regardless of utilization

C. fact_member_months contains demographic data not in claims

D. ANSI SQL requires two fact tables in every join

Answer: B. *A healthy member enrolled for 12 months with zero claims contributes 12 member months to the denominator. Excluding them overstates PMPM by inflating the numerator relative to a smaller denominator. The LEFT JOIN from fact_member_months to fact_medical_claims is the correct pattern — start from enrollment, pull in claims where they exist.*

Q3. SCD Type 2 (Slowly Changing Dimension) solves which specific analytics problem?

A. It speeds up queries by caching the most recent dim_members version

B. It stores one row per attribute version with effective_date and end_date, enabling point-in-time joins that retrieve the value active on any historical date

C. It automatically corrects retroactive eligibility changes in the warehouse

D. It merges member records when a member switches plans mid-year

Answer: B. *Without SCD-2, a query today retrieves only the member's current attribute — attributing all historical claims to the current LOB regardless of what LOB was active when the service occurred. The join condition service_date >= effective_date AND service_date < COALESCE(end_date,'2099-12-31') returns the version that was actually active on the claim date.*

Q4. A plan's October PMPM is 22% below budget. Before presenting this as a favorable trend, the analyst should first check:

A. Whether the plan changed premium rates in October

B. IBNR — October claims may be only 30–50% complete at report time; the low PMPM is a claims lag artifact, not a cost improvement

C. Whether the budget assumption was correct for October

D. Whether member months decreased in October

Answer: B. *IBNR (Incurred But Not Reported) is the most common source of false-positive favorable trends. At 1-month elapsed, inpatient claims are only ~30% complete, outpatient ~45%, professional ~55%. A 22% favorable variance in October with no other explanation is almost certainly incomplete data. Always label recent months: CASE WHEN svc_month >= CURRENT_DATE - INTERVAL '3 months' THEN 'INCOMPLETE — IBNR' ELSE 'Final' END.*

Q5. NULLIF(SUM(member_months), 0) in a PMPM division serves what purpose?

A. It rounds the result to 2 decimal places

B. It converts zero to NULL — dividing by NULL returns NULL instead of a runtime error, preventing divide-by-zero crashes when a service category has no enrollment

C. It filters out zero-value member months from the denominator

D. It converts the result from dollars to PMPM format

Answer: B. *Division by zero in SQL causes a runtime error in most databases. NULLIF(expr, 0) converts 0 to NULL, and any number divided by NULL returns NULL gracefully. Wrap the result in COALESCE if you need 0 instead of NULL in the output: COALESCE(ROUND(SUM(...)/NULLIF(...),2), 0). Apply NULLIF to every division in every PMPM calculation.*

Q6. In the member month generation query, why is the JOIN to the calendar table structured as: c.month_start <= DATE_TRUNC('month', COALESCE(m.coverage_end, '2099-12-31'))?

A. To exclude members who enrolled after December 31

B. COALESCE converts NULL coverage_end (still-active members) to a far-future date so they satisfy the condition for every calendar month through year-end; without it NULL comparisons evaluate to UNKNOWN, silently excluding all currently-active members

C. To cap the enrollment window at December 31 of the measurement year

D. To handle the case where coverage_end is populated with a default date

Answer: B. NULL in SQL comparisons evaluates to UNKNOWN, which is treated as FALSE in WHERE and JOIN conditions. A currently-active member with NULL coverage_end would fail the condition c.month_start <= NULL, meaning they *would appear in zero calendar months — producing zero member months for every active member. COALESCE to 2099-12-31 ensures the active version satisfies every month comparison.*

Q7. Explain what IBNR means, describe the lag completion rate by claim type at 1-month elapsed, and write the SQL CASE WHEN logic that should appear in every monthly trend report.

(Short answer)

> **Sample Answer:**
> IBNR = Incurred But Not Reported. Services are performed today but claims may not reach the warehouse for weeks to months: providers batch submissions, adjudication takes time, COB issues cause delays. The gap between when a service occurs and when the final claim is visible is the IBNR lag. Completion rates at 1-month elapsed (approximate): Pharmacy = 90%+ (NCPDP point-of-sale, near real-time). Professional (CMS-1500) = 55–70%. Outpatient hospital (UB-04) = 45–60%. Inpatient hospital (UB-04) = 25–40% (complex coding + DRG assignment + COB can take 60–120 days). SQL flag for monthly trend reports: CASE WHEN DATE_TRUNC('month', service_date) >= DATE_TRUNC('month', CURRENT_DATE) - INTERVAL '3 months' THEN 'INCOMPLETE — IBNR, apply completion factor' ELSE 'Final' END AS data_maturity. Rule: never present the most recent 2–3 service months as final cost without this label. For executive dashboards, show completed months in solid color and IBNR-impacted months in a lighter shade with a footnote.

Q8. Describe the SCD-2 join condition in plain English. Explain the COALESCE(end_date, '2099-12-31') pattern and give a real financial error that occurs when SCD-2 is not used.

(Short answer)

> **Sample Answer:**
> SCD-2 join plain English: "give me the version of this member's attributes whose active window contains the claim's service_date." The version has two dates: effective_date (when it became active) and end_date (when it was replaced). The condition c.service_date >= effective_date AND c.service_date < end_date selects the row where the service date falls inside the active window. COALESCE(end_date, '2099-12-31'): the currently-active version has NULL for end_date because it has not ended. A NULL in the date comparison evaluates to UNKNOWN, silently excluding the active version. Setting NULL to 2099-12-31 ensures the condition is always satisfied for the currently-active row. Real financial error without SCD-2: a plan has 1,000 members who switched from Commercial FI to MA on July 1. Without SCD-2, all their January–June claims are attributed to MA (the current row). This overstates MA PMPM by the H1 commercial cost of those members: 1,000 × 6 months × ~$350 PMPM = $2.1M misattributed. Commercial PMPM is correspondingly understated. Both LOBs report incorrect financials, and every budget variance report built on this data is wrong.

Q9. Write the complete SQL for a budget variance report that calculates actual vs. budget PMPM, flags IBNR-affected categories, and sorts by absolute variance. Explain each clause.

(Short answer)

> **Sample Answer:**
> SELECT p.service_category, ROUND(SUM(c.allowed_amount)/NULLIF(SUM(mm.member_months),0),2) AS actual_pmpm, b.budget_pmpm, ROUND(SUM(c.allowed_amount)/NULLIF(SUM(mm.member_months),0) - b.budget_pmpm,2) AS variance_pmpm, CASE WHEN SUM(c.allowed_amount)/NULLIF(SUM(mm.member_months),0) < b.budget_pmpm*0.85 THEN 'CHECK IBNR' ELSE 'Reportable' END AS ibnr_flag FROM fact_medical_claims c JOIN ref_procedure_codes p ON c.procedure_code=p.procedure_code JOIN fact_member_months mm ON c.member_id=mm.member_id AND mm.membership_year=2024 AND mm.membership_month_num BETWEEN 7 AND 9 JOIN ref_budget_assumptions b ON p.service_category=b.service_category WHERE c.claim_status='PAID' AND c.line_of_business='COMMERCIAL' GROUP BY p.service_category, b.budget_pmpm ORDER BY ABS(variance_pmpm) DESC. Clause explanations: ref_procedure_codes JOIN maps CPT codes to service categories. fact_member_months JOIN with year and month filters provides the Q3 enrollment denominator. ref_budget_assumptions JOIN links each category to its filed budget. The IBNR CASE WHEN flags categories more than 15% below budget — a threshold suggesting incomplete claims rather than genuine improvement. ABS(variance_pmpm) DESC sorts largest variances (favorable or unfavorable) to the top for executive review.

Q10. The healthcare data ecosystem has six primary domains. Name all six, give one key table from each domain, and explain which domain is the ONLY valid source for PMPM denominators.

(Short answer)

> **Sample Answer:**

Six domains and key tables: (1) Claims — fact_medical_claims (transaction records of all services; primary source for cost and utilization analytics). (2) Eligibility/Enrollment — fact_member_months, fact_eligibility (coverage windows; the ONLY valid source for PMPM denominators). (3) Provider/Network — dim_providers, ref_fee_schedule (provider attributes, contracts, specialties). (4) Reference/Code — ref_icd10_cm, ref_procedure_codes, ref_ndc (code-to-category mappings; updated annually). (5) Quality/HEDIS — fact_hedis_gaps, ref_star_weights (measure-specific gap populations and CMS quality weights). (6) Financial/Actuarial — ref_budget_assumptions, ref_county_benchmarks (plan budget targets and CMS capitation benchmarks). PMPM denominator source: Domain 2, Eligibility/Enrollment, specifically fact_member_months. This is the ONLY valid source because it includes every enrolled member regardless of whether they had any claims. Using any other domain for the denominator systematically excludes zero-utilization members, overstating PMPM.

Key Takeaways

What every analyst must remember from this chapter.

1 The star schema places fact_medical_claims at the center joined to dim_date, dim_members, ref_procedure_codes, and fact_member_months as the enrollment denominator. Every PMPM query follows this pattern: fact → three dimensions → enrollment denominator.

2 Claim grain matters: professional claims are at line grain (one row per CPT line); institutional inpatient claims may have 40–200 revenue code lines per stay. Always use COUNT(DISTINCT claim_id) for admission counts and SUM(allowed_amount) at claim_id grain for episode cost.

3 The PMPM denominator must come from fact_member_months (enrollment), never from claims. The LEFT JOIN pattern — start from enrollment, pull in claims — ensures zero-utilization members appear in the denominator. Members with no claims still contribute 1.0 per enrolled month.

4 NULLIF(expression, 0) converts zero to NULL to prevent divide-by-zero errors in every PMPM calculation. Apply COALESCE around the result if you need 0 instead of NULL: COALESCE(ROUND(SUM(allowed)/NULLIF(SUM(mm),0),2), 0).

5 SCD Type 2 stores one row per attribute version with effective_date and end_date. Join condition: service_date >= effective_date AND service_date < COALESCE(end_date,'2099-12-31'). This retrieves the attribute active on the date of service, not today. Without SCD-2, mid-year LOB changes misattribute millions in claims.

6 IBNR lag by claim type at 1-month elapsed: Pharmacy ≈90% complete, Professional ≈60%, Outpatient ≈50%, Inpatient ≈30%. Always label the most recent 2–3 service months as INCOMPLETE in every trend report. Never present them as final cost without completion factors applied.

7 COALESCE(coverage_end, '2099-12-31') in the member month generation JOIN is required — not optional. NULL coverage_end means the member is still active. NULL in date comparisons evaluates to UNKNOWN (treated as FALSE), silently excluding all currently-active members from the denominator.

8 The six healthcare data domains are: Claims, Eligibility/Enrollment, Provider/Network, Reference/Code, Quality/HEDIS, and Financial/Actuarial. Reference codes (ICD-10, CPT) update annually — always use maintained reference tables, never hard-code diagnosis or procedure values in WHERE clauses.

9 IBNR flag SQL pattern: CASE WHEN SUM(c.allowed_amount)/NULLIF(SUM(mm.member_months),0) < b.budget_pmpm * 0.85 THEN 'CHECK IBNR' ELSE 'Reportable' END. The 15% threshold is conservative — anything more than 15% below budget in a recent month almost always reflects incomplete claims, not genuine cost improvement.

Part II Data Architecture, SQL & Methodology

Chapter 4: The STAR Method —SQL Framework & Worked Examples

STAR is not just a formatting convention — it is a discipline of analytical thinking. The best healthcare SQL analysts do not start from a blank query editor and build outward from syntax. They start from the business situation, define the task precisely, construct the SQL action step-by-step, and interpret the result in terms the stakeholder can act on. This chapter defines that framework and demonstrates it across four complete worked examples drawn from the core analytical domains of this book.

Every STAR scenario in chapters 5 through 31 follows this identical four-component structure. Learning it here once means you will recognize the pattern instantly in every domain — financial, clinical, network, quality, population health — that follows.

4.1 Why This Book Is Built Around the STAR Framework

Healthcare analytics training almost universally starts with the answer — here is a SQL pattern, here is how CTEs work, here is what a window function does. This book starts from the opposite end: here is the business problem, here is why it matters, here is the analytical path from question to output.

The reason is practical. In a real health plan or managed care organization, nobody hands you a query to run. They hand you a problem: "Why did our inpatient PMPM spike 14% in Q1?" or "Which members are most at risk of avoidable hospitalization?" The analyst who can structure a response — who can name the stakeholder, define the metric precisely, decompose the SQL into ordered steps, and then interpret the number — is the analyst who earns trust and influence. The analyst who produces a table of numbers without context is replaced by a report.

STAR provides that structure. It forces four disciplines that separately improve analytical quality and together transform it:

Business context. Who is the stakeholder? What decision depends on this analysis? What data sources apply? What is the measurement window? Situation forces you to understand the problem before touching the keyboard — the single most neglected step in healthcare analytics practice.

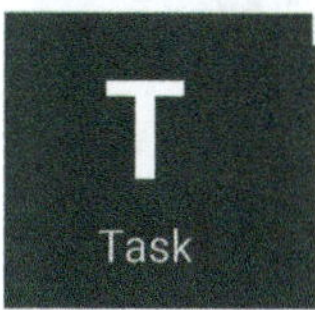

Precise analytical definition. Task forces specificity: "Analyze costs" fails. "Calculate fully-insured commercial PMPM by service category for YTD Q1 2024 vs. Q1 2023, per member per month, at plan level, flagging categories where variance exceeds ±10%" succeeds. A strong Task defines population, metric, time period, grain, and output format.

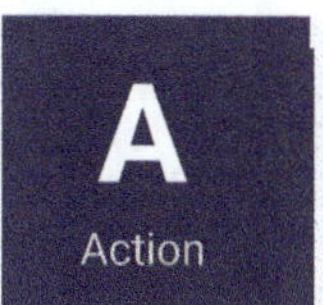

Step-by-step SQL construction plan. Action creates the query architecture before writing syntax — each step identifies a table, a filter, an aggregation, or a business rule. Writing the plan first exposes missing logic, wrong grain assumptions, and join ambiguities before they become runtime errors or silent incorrect results.

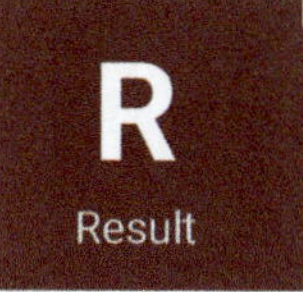

Business interpretation. Result requires translating the output into a stakeholder action — not just "inpatient PMPM is up $18" but "inpatient unit cost increased 11% while utilization held flat, indicating a contracting issue rather than a care management issue — route to the network team." Numbers without interpretation are not analysis.

The order matters: S and T happen before you open the SQL editor. R happens before you open the presentation. The Action (SQL) is the middle step — not the starting point.

4.2 The Four STAR Components — Reference Definition

The following table defines each component precisely. Use this as a checklist before every analysis you produce.

	Component	What it requires	Common failure mode
S	Situation	Stakeholder identity, decision context, data sources, measurement window, regulatory framework	"Analyze costs for the CFO" — no stakeholder specificity, no measurement window, no data source
T	Task	Population filter, metric definition and formula, time period, aggregation grain, output format	"Calculate PMPM" — no LOB filter, no claim status rule, no denominator definition, no grain
A	Action	Ordered SQL steps — each step names a table, filter, business rule, or aggregation. Written before any code.	Writing SQL top-down without a plan — discovers missing joins at runtime, produces silent wrong results
R	Result	Numeric output interpreted in business terms, compared to a benchmark, and translated into a recommended action	"Here is the data" — no interpretation, no benchmark, no next step. Numbers without context are not analysis.

4.3 Worked Examples — Four Complete STAR Scenarios

The following four scenarios are fully worked across all STAR components. Each comes from a different analytical domain, uses a different primary SQL pattern, and produces a different type of deliverable. Read them in order — the complexity builds progressively.

Scenario 4.1 · Financial / Medical Economics

Medical Cost Driver Analysis

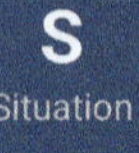

S Situation

The CFO has flagged that fully-insured commercial medical PMPM increased 14% in Q1 2024 vs. Q1 2023. The CMO and VP of Network are in the room and need to know: is this a utilization problem (more services) or a unit cost problem (more expensive services)? The answer determines whether care management or contracting owns the response.

Stakeholder: CFO, CMO, VP Network. | LOB: Fully-insured commercial. | Period: Q1 2024 vs. Q1 2023. | Data: fact_medical_claims, dim_members, dim_date, fact_member_months.

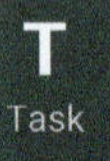

T Task

Calculate PMPM by service category (Inpatient, SNF, ED, Outpatient, Professional) for Q1 2024 and Q1 2023, for fully-insured commercial members only (lob_code = COMM_FI), using paid claims only (claim_status = PAID), with member months as denominator.

Decompose the PMPM variance for each service category into: (a) utilization component — change in claims per member month, and (b) unit cost component — change in allowed amount per claim. Output: executive summary table, one row per service category.

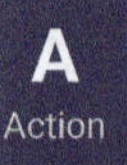

A Action

Step 1: CTE q1_claims — pull paid claims for COMM_FI, Q1 2023 and Q1 2024, classify each claim into service category using claim_type and TOB codes.

Step 2: CTE q1_agg — aggregate total allowed and claim count by service_category × calendar_year × age_band × geography.

Step 3: CTE q1_mm — pull member months from fact_member_months for same population and years.

Step 4: Final SELECT — join aggregates to member months, calculate PMPM = total_allowed / member_months; utilization = claims / member_months; unit_cost = total_allowed / claims. Self-join on prior year to produce side-by-side comparison and variance columns.

ANSI SQL — Scenario 4.1: Medical Cost Driver Analysis

```
-- PURPOSE: Decompose Q1 PMPM variance into two components:
-- (1) Utilization change -- are members using more services per 1,000 MM?
-- (2) Unit cost change -- is each service costing more?
-- This routes the problem: utilization = care management; unit cost = contracting.

-- STEP 1: Pull all Q1 paid claims for commercial FI, classify service category.
-- TOB (Type of Bill) and place_of_service codes identify the care setting.
WITH q1_claims AS (
  SELECT
    CASE
      WHEN c.type_of_bill LIKE '11%'  THEN 'Inpatient'   -- TOB 11x = acute inpatient
      WHEN c.type_of_bill LIKE '21%'  THEN 'SNF'         -- TOB 21x = skilled nursing
      WHEN c.place_of_service = '23'  THEN 'Emergency Dept' -- POS 23 = ER
      WHEN c.type_of_bill LIKE '13%'
       OR c.type_of_bill LIKE '14%'  THEN 'Outpatient'  -- TOB 13x/14x = outpatient hospital
      WHEN c.claim_form_type='CMS1500' THEN 'Professional' -- CMS-1500 = physician billing
      ELSE 'Other'
    END               AS service_category,
    d.calendar_year,
    c.allowed_amount,
    c.claim_id
  FROM  fact_medical_claims  c
  JOIN  dim_date          d  ON c.service_date = d.date_key
  JOIN  dim_plans         pl  ON c.plan_id     = pl.plan_id
  WHERE c.claim_status   = 'PAID'
   AND pl.lob_code       = 'COMM_FI'     -- commercial fully-insured only
   AND d.calendar_quarter = 1            -- Q1 = January through March
   AND d.calendar_year  IN (2023, 2024)  -- both comparison years side by side
```

```
),

-- STEP 2: Aggregate to service_category × year.
-- COUNT(DISTINCT claim_id) avoids double-counting revenue lines.
q1_agg AS (
   SELECT service_category, calendar_year,
         SUM(allowed_amount)       AS total_allowed,
         COUNT(DISTINCT claim_id) AS claim_count
   FROM  q1_claims
   GROUP BY service_category, calendar_year
),

-- STEP 3: Pull Q1 member months for the denominator.
-- Denominator comes from enrollment, not claims.
q1_mm AS (
   SELECT calendar_year, SUM(member_month) AS member_months
   FROM   fact_member_months mm
   JOIN   dim_plans pl ON mm.plan_id = pl.plan_id
   WHERE  pl.lob_code = 'COMM_FI' AND mm.calendar_quarter = 1
    AND  mm.calendar_year IN (2023, 2024)
   GROUP BY calendar_year
)

-- STEP 4: Self-join to put 2023 and 2024 side by side.
-- Calculate PMPM, utilization (claims per 1,000 MM), unit cost ($ per claim).
SELECT
   c24.service_category,
   ROUND(c24.total_allowed / NULLIF(m24.member_months,0), 2)  AS pmpm_2024,
   ROUND(c23.total_allowed / NULLIF(m23.member_months,0), 2)  AS pmpm_2023,
   ROUND(c24.total_allowed/NULLIF(m24.member_months,0)
      - c23.total_allowed/NULLIF(m23.member_months,0), 2)    AS pmpm_variance,
   -- Utilization: claims per 1,000 enrolled member months
   ROUND(1000.0*c24.claim_count/NULLIF(m24.member_months,0),1) AS util_2024_per1k,
   ROUND(1000.0*c23.claim_count/NULLIF(m23.member_months,0),1) AS util_2023_per1k,
   -- Unit cost: average allowed dollars per claim
   ROUND(c24.total_allowed/NULLIF(c24.claim_count,0),0)        AS unit_cost_2024,
   ROUND(c23.total_allowed/NULLIF(c23.claim_count,0),0)        AS unit_cost_2023
-- Self-join: c24 = 2024, c23 = 2023, joined on service_category
FROM  q1_agg c24
JOIN  q1_agg c23  ON c24.service_category = c23.service_category
           AND c23.calendar_year = 2023 AND c24.calendar_year = 2024
JOIN  q1_mm m24   ON m24.calendar_year = 2024
JOIN  q1_mm m23   ON m23.calendar_year = 2023
ORDER BY pmpm_variance DESC;  -- largest unfavorable variances first
```

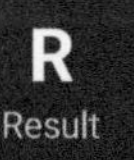

R Result

Inpatient PMPM: +$22 (utilization flat, unit cost +18%) → contracting issue. Route to VP Network for hospital contract review.

ED PMPM: +$6 (utilization +12%, unit cost flat) → care management issue. Route to CMO for avoidable ED intervention program.

Professional PMPM: -$3 (stable) → no action required.

Decomposing into utilization vs. unit cost is not a formatting choice — it routes the problem to the correct organizational owner. A single blended variance number would send everyone to the wrong meeting.

Scenario 4.2 · Quality / Star Ratings

HEDIS Star Rating Gap Closure Prioritization

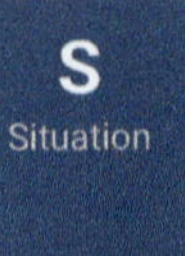

The plan is 0.12 stars below the 4-star cut point in the MA Star Ratings. The quality team has a care gap outreach budget sufficient to contact 2,000 members. The Director of Quality needs a ranked list of which gaps to close first — but "number of open gaps" is the wrong sorting criterion because not all gaps carry the same Star weight or require the same effort to reach the next cut point.

Stakeholder: Director of Quality, VP Stars. | LOB: Medicare Advantage. | Period: Current measurement year. | Data: HEDIS denominator/numerator tables, ref_star_weights, ref_cut_points.

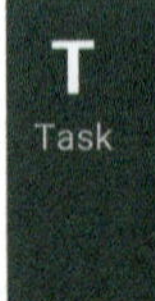

Score each open care gap for each member across all Star-rated HEDIS measures. The scoring formula must account for: (1) the CMS Star weight of the measure (3-star measures worth 3×), (2) the denominator size (impact per gap is higher in smaller denominators), and (3) proximity to the next cut point (gaps in measures already at 4 stars contribute less than gaps in measures that need 2 more percentage points to cross to 5 stars).

Output: member-level gap priority list, sorted by composite score descending, top 2,000 for outreach.

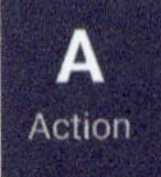

Step 1: CTE measure_gaps — UNION ALL of denominator-minus-numerator for each HEDIS measure, tagged with measure_id.

Step 2: CTE measure_stats — count denominator size, numerator count, and current rate per measure.

Step 3: CTE gap_scores — join to ref_star_weights and ref_cut_points; calculate gaps_to_cut_point = CEIL((next_cut_point - current_rate) × denominator / 100); score = star_weight × (1/denominator_size) × (1/gaps_to_cut_point).

Step 4: Final SELECT — aggregate member-level scores across all measures, join to member demographics, sort descending, limit to 2,000.

ANSI SQL — Scenario 4.2: Star Rating Gap Closure Scoring

```
-- Scenario 4.2: Star Rating Gap Closure Priority Scoring
-- Higher score = closing this gap moves Stars more per unit of outreach effort
WITH measure_gaps AS (
  -- UNION of gap members across all HEDIS Star measures
  SELECT 'BCS' AS measure_id, member_id FROM bcs_denominator
  WHERE  member_id NOT IN (SELECT member_id FROM bcs_numerator)
  UNION ALL
  SELECT 'CBP', member_id FROM cbp_denominator
  WHERE  member_id NOT IN (SELECT member_id FROM cbp_numerator)
  UNION ALL
  SELECT 'CDC_HBA1C', member_id FROM cdc_denominator
  WHERE  member_id NOT IN (SELECT member_id FROM cdc_numerator)
  -- ... repeat for all Star-rated measures
),
measure_stats AS (
  SELECT measure_id,
      COUNT(*)                    AS denominator_size,
      ROUND(100.0 * COUNT(*)
        / SUM(COUNT(*)) OVER(), 1)      AS current_rate
  FROM   measure_gaps
  GROUP BY measure_id
),
gap_scores AS (
  SELECT
    g.member_id,
    g.measure_id,
    w.star_weight,              -- CMS weight (1, 2, or 3)
    ms.denominator_size,
```

```
        ms.current_rate,
        w.next_cut_point,
        – How many gaps does the plan need to close to reach next cut point?
        CEIL((w.next_cut_point - ms.current_rate)
          * ms.denominator_size / 100.0)     AS gaps_to_cut_point,
        – Priority score: weight × (1/denom) × (1/gaps_to_cut)
        – Higher score = higher marginal Star impact per closure
        ROUND(
          w.star_weight
          * (1.0 / NULLIF(ms.denominator_size, 0))
          * (1.0 / NULLIF(
            CEIL((w.next_cut_point - ms.current_rate)
              * ms.denominator_size / 100.0), 0)
          ), 6)                    AS gap_priority_score
    FROM  measure_gaps      g
    JOIN  measure_stats     ms ON g.measure_id  = ms.measure_id
    JOIN  ref_star_weights  w  ON g.measure_id  = w.measure_id
    WHERE ms.current_rate < w.next_cut_point    -- only measures not yet at cut
)
SELECT
    g.member_id,
    m.member_name,
    m.pcp_npi,
    m.phone_number,
    COUNT(DISTINCT g.measure_id)        AS open_gap_count,
    SUM(g.gap_priority_score)           AS composite_priority_score,
    -- List the top measures to address for this member
    STRING_AGG(g.measure_id ORDER BY g.gap_priority_score DESC, ',')
                              AS priority_measures
FROM  gap_scores    g
JOIN  dim_members    m ON g.member_id = m.member_id
GROUP BY g.member_id, m.member_name, m.pcp_npi, m.phone_number
ORDER BY composite_priority_score DESC
LIMIT 2000;
```

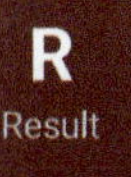

R Result

The top 2,000 members by composite score carry an estimated 3.8× more Star-score impact per outreach contact than a list sorted by raw gap count. Sorting by gaps alone would prioritize members in large-denominator, low-weight measures — the exact opposite of efficient gap closure strategy.

Hand to care management team with phone numbers and PCP NPIs. Track closure rate weekly against the cut-point target. Re-run the scoring query after each 200-member outreach batch to update the ranked list as rates move.

Scenario 4.3 · Clinical / Pharmacy

Pharmacy Adherence Gap Detection — PDC

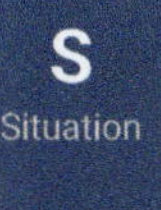

S Situation

The pharmacy team needs to identify members on statin therapy who are non-adherent (PDC < 0.80) and have not been contacted by the medication adherence program in the current measurement year. Non-adherent statin members contribute to both Star Ratings risk (CMC measure) and avoidable cardiovascular events.

Stakeholder: VP Pharmacy, Clinical Pharmacist. | LOB: All commercial + MA. | Period: CY 2024 measurement year. | Data: fact_pharmacy_claims, ref_ndc, fact_cm_contacts.

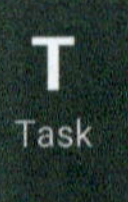

Calculate Proportion of Days Covered (PDC) for each member with at least one statin fill in 2024. PDC = covered days within measurement period ÷ total measurement period days. Measurement period begins 30 days after first statin fill and ends December 31, 2024.

Flag members with PDC < 0.80 who have had no medication adherence contact in CY 2024. Output: intervention list sorted by PDC ascending (lowest adherence first) with fill history summary.

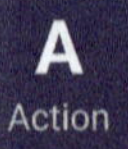

Step 1: CTE statin_fills — pull all paid statin pharmacy claims in 2024, join to ref_ndc to filter by GPI class for statins, calculate fill_end_date = dispensing_date + days_supply - 1.

Step 2: CTE measurement_windows — per member, period_start = MIN(dispensing_date) + 30 days; period_end = Dec 31 2024.

Step 3: CTE adjusted_fills — use LAG() to detect overlapping fills; shift fill start forward using GREATEST(dispensing_date, prior_fill_end + 1). This prevents double-counting days when a member refills early.

Step 4: CTE covered_days — for each fill, calculate days covered within measurement window = MIN(fill_end_date, period_end) - MAX(adjusted_start, period_start) + 1. Sum per member.

Step 5: Final SELECT — calculate PDC = covered_days / period_days; filter PDC < 0.80; left join to fact_cm_contacts to exclude already-contacted members.

ANSI SQL — Scenario 4.3: Statin PDC Calculation

```
-- Scenario 4.3: Statin PDC with Early Refill Overlap Adjustment
WITH statin_fills AS (
  SELECT p.member_id, p.dispensing_date, p.days_supply,
      p.dispensing_date + (p.days_supply - 1) AS fill_end_date
  FROM   fact_pharmacy_claims p
  JOIN   ref_ndc n ON p.ndc_code = n.ndc_code
  WHERE  n.gpi_code BETWEEN '39400010' AND '39400099'  -- statins by GPI
    AND  p.claim_status = 'PAID'
    AND  EXTRACT(YEAR FROM p.dispensing_date) = 2024
),
measurement_windows AS (
  -- Measurement period: 30 days post-first-fill through Dec 31
  SELECT member_id,
      MIN(dispensing_date) + INTERVAL '30' DAY  AS period_start,
      DATE '2024-12-31'                         AS period_end,
      DATEDIFF('day',
        MIN(dispensing_date) + INTERVAL '30' DAY,
        DATE '2024-12-31') + 1                  AS period_days
  FROM   statin_fills
  GROUP BY member_id
  HAVING period_days > 0
),
adjusted_fills AS (
  -- Shift fill start forward if it overlaps the prior fill
  -- Prevents double-counting days when member refills early
  SELECT f.member_id, f.dispensing_date, f.fill_end_date,
      GREATEST(
        f.dispensing_date,
        COALESCE(
          LAG(f.fill_end_date) OVER (
            PARTITION BY f.member_id
            ORDER BY f.dispensing_date
          ) + INTERVAL '1' DAY,
          f.dispensing_date)          -- no prior fill: no shift
      )                               AS adjusted_start
  FROM  statin_fills f
```

```
),
covered_days AS (
  SELECT af.member_id,
      SUM(GREATEST(0,
        DATEDIFF('day',
          GREATEST(af.adjusted_start, mw.period_start),
          LEAST(af.fill_end_date,    mw.period_end)
        ) + 1
      ))                    AS days_covered
  FROM  adjusted_fills af
  JOIN  measurement_windows mw ON af.member_id = mw.member_id
  WHERE af.adjusted_start <= mw.period_end
   AND af.fill_end_date >= mw.period_start
  GROUP BY af.member_id
)
SELECT
  m.member_id, m.member_name, m.pcp_npi, m.phone_number,
  mw.period_days,
  cd.days_covered,
  ROUND(cd.days_covered * 1.0 / NULLIF(mw.period_days,0), 3) AS pdc,
  CASE WHEN cd.days_covered * 1.0 / NULLIF(mw.period_days,0) >= 0.80
     THEN 'Adherent' ELSE 'NON-ADHERENT' END          AS adherence_status
FROM covered_days     cd
JOIN measurement_windows mw ON cd.member_id = mw.member_id
JOIN dim_members      m ON cd.member_id = m.member_id
-- Exclude members already contacted this year
LEFT JOIN fact_cm_contacts cc
    ON cd.member_id  = cc.member_id
   AND cc.contact_type = 'MED_ADHERENCE'
   AND EXTRACT(YEAR FROM cc.contact_date) = 2024
WHERE cd.days_covered * 1.0 / NULLIF(mw.period_days,0) < 0.80
 AND cc.member_id IS NULL       -- not yet contacted
ORDER BY pdc ASC;               -- lowest adherence first
```

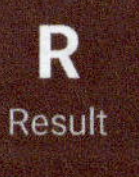

R Result

Output is a ranked intervention list for the clinical pharmacist team. Members with PDC 0.40–0.60 represent the largest gap relative to the 0.80 threshold and are the highest priority for outreach — one or two additional fills would move them to adherent status.

Critical note: without the GREATEST(adjusted_start, prior_fill_end + 1) overlap adjustment in Step 3, members who refill 5–10 days early would have PDC calculated above 1.0 — an impossible result that would silently exclude them from the non-adherent list. The adjustment is not a refinement; it is a correctness requirement.

Scenario 4.4 · Integrity / FWA

Provider E&M Upcoding — Fraud Outlier Detection

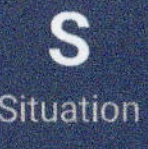

S Situation

The Special Investigations Unit (SIU) has received a tip that a primary care group (TIN: 123456789) may be systematically billing 99215 (highest-complexity office visit) at rates far exceeding peers. A fixed-dollar threshold cannot be used because a high-volume legitimate practice will naturally have higher total billings than a small practice.

Stakeholder: SIU Director, Compliance Officer. | LOB: All. | Period: Rolling 12 months. | Data: fact_medical_claims, dim_providers.

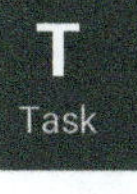

T Task

Calculate the E&M procedure code distribution (% of total E&M claims billed at each CPT code 99202–99215) for the flagged group and compare it to the peer distribution (same specialty, same geography). Flag the group

if its 99215 billing rate exceeds the peer 95th percentile. Peer comparison controls for volume — it compares rates, not dollars.

Output: procedure code distribution table with peer benchmark and flag, plus list of highest-billing individual providers within the group.

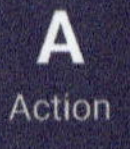

A Action

Step 1: CTE group_claims — pull all E&M claims (CPT 99202–99215) for the flagged TIN in the past 12 months.

Step 2: CTE group_dist — calculate each E&M code as % of total E&M claims for the group.

Step 3: CTE peer_dist — per-provider distribution across all Primary Care / Internal Medicine providers in same geography (excluding the flagged TIN).

Step 4: CTE peer_percentiles — use PERCENTILE_CONT(0.95) to find the 95th percentile billing rate for each E&M code across the peer population.

Step 5: Final SELECT — compare group rate to peer p95; flag where group rate exceeds peer p95.

ANSI SQL — Scenario 4.4: E&M Upcoding Statistical Analysis

```
-- Scenario 4.4: E&M Upcoding Detection — Peer-Adjusted Comparison
WITH group_claims AS (
  SELECT c.procedure_code, COUNT(*) AS claim_count
  FROM   fact_medical_claims c
  JOIN   dim_providers p ON c.rendering_npi = p.npi
  WHERE  p.billing_tin    = '123456789'
   AND c.procedure_code IN ('99202','99203','99204','99205',
                '99211','99212','99213','99214','99215')
   AND c.claim_status    = 'PAID'
   AND c.service_date  >= CURRENT_DATE - INTERVAL '1' YEAR
  GROUP BY c.procedure_code
),
group_totals AS (SELECT SUM(claim_count) AS total_em FROM group_claims),
group_dist AS (
  SELECT gc.procedure_code,
      gc.claim_count,
      -- Rate = this code as % of all E&M for the group
      ROUND(100.0 * gc.claim_count / gt.total_em, 2) AS group_rate_pct
  FROM   group_claims gc CROSS JOIN group_totals gt
),
peer_dist AS (
  -- Per-provider distribution for peer comparison
  -- Using window SUM to get each provider's own total as denominator
  SELECT c.procedure_code, c.rendering_npi,
      ROUND(100.0 * COUNT(*)
        / SUM(COUNT(*)) OVER (PARTITION BY c.rendering_npi),
      2) AS provider_rate_pct
  FROM   fact_medical_claims c
  JOIN   dim_providers p ON c.rendering_npi = p.npi
  WHERE  p.specialty_group IN ('Primary Care','Internal Medicine')
   AND p.billing_tin   <> '123456789'    -- exclude flagged group
   AND c.procedure_code  IN ('99202','99203','99204','99205',
                '99211','99212','99213','99214','99215')
   AND c.claim_status    = 'PAID'
   AND c.service_date   >= CURRENT_DATE - INTERVAL '1' YEAR
  GROUP BY c.procedure_code, c.rendering_npi
),
peer_percentiles AS (
  -- PERCENTILE_CONT: ANSI SQL ordered-set aggregate for percentile calc
  SELECT procedure_code,
```

```
        ROUND(PERCENTILE_CONT(0.50)
          WITHIN GROUP (ORDER BY provider_rate_pct), 2) AS peer_p50,
        ROUND(PERCENTILE_CONT(0.95)
          WITHIN GROUP (ORDER BY provider_rate_pct), 2) AS peer_p95
    FROM   peer_dist
    GROUP BY procedure_code
)
SELECT
    gd.procedure_code,
    gd.claim_count              AS group_claim_count,
    gd.group_rate_pct,
    pp.peer_p50,
    pp.peer_p95,
    ROUND(gd.group_rate_pct - pp.peer_p95, 2) AS variance_vs_p95,
    CASE WHEN gd.group_rate_pct > pp.peer_p95
       THEN 'FLAG — exceeds peer 95th percentile'
       ELSE 'Within normal range' END        AS fraud_flag
FROM  group_dist       gd
JOIN  peer_percentiles pp ON gd.procedure_code = pp.procedure_code
ORDER BY gd.procedure_code;
```

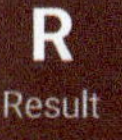
Result

If the group's 99215 rate is 61% of all E&M claims vs. a peer p95 of 38%, this constitutes a statistically significant outlier warranting SIU investigation. The variance_vs_p95 column (+23 percentage points) is the figure cited in the case referral memo.

Peer adjustment is not optional — a fixed dollar threshold would have flagged the group simply for being large. The peer rate comparison controls for volume and isolates the behavioral signal: this group codes at the highest E&M complexity tier at a rate that 95% of similar providers do not approach.

Next step: pull individual provider-level breakdown within the TIN to identify whether the pattern is driven by one or two outlier physicians or is systematic across the group.

4.4 Key Takeaways — The STAR Discipline

1 **STAR is thinking, not formatting.** The four components force you to understand the business problem before writing SQL. The query is the middle step, not the starting point.

2 **A strong Task has five dimensions.** Population (who), metric (what and how calculated), time period (when), aggregation grain (at what level), and output format (what does the deliverable look like). A Task missing any of these will produce a query that answers a different question than the one that was asked.

3 **Decompose before you aggregate.** Blended PMPM variance routes nobody to the right action. Utilization vs. unit cost decomposition routes the problem to contracting or care management. Always ask: what decision does this number enable?

4 **PDC requires overlap adjustment.** GREATEST(dispensing_date, prior_fill_end + 1) is not a refinement — it is a correctness requirement. Without it, early refills double-count covered days and produce PDC > 1.0 or false adherent classifications.

5 **Fraud detection requires peer comparison.** Fixed dollar thresholds penalize volume. Peer-adjusted rate comparison isolates behavioral signal from practice size. PERCENTILE_CONT(0.95) WITHIN GROUP (ORDER BY value) is the ANSI SQL function.

6 **Results require three elements.** What the number means, what it should be compared against, and what action the stakeholder should take. Numbers without all three are not analysis — they are data delivery.

> **What comes next:** Part III applies the STAR framework to its first production domain — Claims, Eligibility, and the Payment Engine. Every scenario in chapters 5, 6, and 7 follows the identical S · T · A · R structure introduced here. The framework does not change. The domain does.

Unit Test · Key Takeaways

Answer each question before reading the explanation.

Q1. What is the primary purpose of the STAR framework in healthcare analytics?

A. To format deliverables in a consistent visual style

B. To enforce four disciplines before writing any SQL: understand the business Situation, define the Task precisely, plan the Action step-by-step, and interpret the Result in business terms — preventing the most common analyst errors

C. To organize SQL CTEs into exactly four steps for every query

D. To provide a template for presenting to senior executives

Answer: B. *STAR is a thinking discipline, not a template. S and T happen before the SQL editor opens. R happens before the presentation opens. The Action (SQL) is the middle step — not the starting point. The framework prevents three common failures: building SQL before understanding the business question, writing queries that answer a vague question, and delivering numbers without business interpretation.*

Q2. In Scenario 4.1, PMPM variance is decomposed into utilization and unit cost. Why is this decomposition essential?

A. It is required by NCQA for all financial reporting

B. A blended PMPM variance routes nobody to the correct action — utilization increase is a care management problem; unit cost increase is a contracting problem

C. It reduces the total variance amount, making results look better

D. SQL cannot calculate variance without separating the components first

Answer: B. *A plan showing inpatient PMPM +$18 has two completely different root causes. If utilization is flat but unit cost rose, the VP of Contracting owns the response. If unit cost is flat but utilization rose, the CMO and care management team own the response. Presenting a combined variance sends everyone to the wrong meeting with no clear owner.*

Q3. Why must early refills be adjusted using GREATEST(dispensing_date, prior_fill_end + 1 day) in the PDC calculation?

A. NCQA requires this adjustment for all HEDIS pharmacy measures

B. Without adjustment a member who refills 10 days early has 10 days of supply counted twice — inflating covered days and potentially producing PDC above 1.0, which is mathematically impossible

C. It is required to handle members who switch pharmacies mid-year

D. The GREATEST function is needed because SQL cannot compare dates directly

Answer: B. *PDC measures days covered, not days of supply purchased. If a member has supply from Jan 1–30 (fill 1) and refills on Jan 25 (fill 2, 30-day supply), without adjustment fill 2 counts Jan 25–Feb 23, double-counting Jan 25–30. With adjustment, fill 2's adjusted_start = Jan 31, extending coverage through Mar 1 — correct and non-overlapping.*

Q4. In the gap scoring formula star_weight × (1/denom_size) × (1/gaps_to_cut_point), what does the 1/gaps_to_cut_point factor represent?

A. The probability a care manager can close any individual gap

B. The marginal Stars impact of closing one more gap — measures where fewer closures are needed to reach the cut point have higher marginal impact per closure

C. The prior year national average rate from HEDIS technical specifications

D. The inverse of denominator size, controlling for population scale

Answer: B. *If a plan needs 5 more BCS closures to reach 4 stars, each closure has impact 1/5 = 0.20. If the plan needs 200 more CBP closures, each closure has impact 1/200 = 0.005. Ranking by raw gap count ignores this critical dimension — a small denominator measure close to its cut point can be worth 40× more per closure than a large denominator measure far from its cut point.*

Q5. In the E&M upcoding query, PERCENTILE_CONT(0.95) WITHIN GROUP (ORDER BY provider_rate_pct) is used instead of a fixed dollar threshold because:

A. PERCENTILE_CONT is required by HIPAA for fraud detection

B. A fixed dollar threshold penalizes high-volume legitimate practices. Peer-adjusted rate comparison controls for volume and specialty mix, isolating the coding behavior pattern regardless of practice size

C. PERCENTILE_CONT is faster than a fixed threshold filter

D. Dollar thresholds are not permitted under ANSI SQL for fraud analysis

Answer: B. *A 15-physician primary care group billing $2M in E&M codes is not comparable to a solo practitioner billing $200K. A fixed $1.5M threshold flags the large legitimate practice and misses the small outlier. Peer rate comparison identifies whether the % of claims billed at the highest E&M codes exceeds 95% of peers — a behavioral signal independent of practice size or volume.*

Q6. A strong STAR Task definition requires five elements. Which set correctly names all five?

A. Population, Metric, Time period, Aggregation grain, Output format
B. Patient, Measure, Year, Table, Chart type
C. Members, Cost, Quarter, Provider, Dashboard
D. LOB, PMPM, Calendar year, Plan, Excel file

Answer: A. *A strong Task specifies: (1) Population — which members with what filters. (2) Metric — what is calculated and how (PMPM using allowed_amount, PDC using NCQA overlap adjustment). (3) Time period — measurement year, quarter, rolling window. (4) Aggregation grain — plan-level, provider-level, member-level. (5) Output format — executive table, member outreach list, ranked report. Missing any one dimension produces a query that answers a different question than was asked.*

Q7. Explain the difference between a weak Task and a strong Task. Rewrite this weak Task as a strong one: "Analyze member utilization."

(Short answer)

Sample Answer:
A weak Task is underspecified along one or more of the five dimensions. "Analyze member utilization" fails on all five: population is undefined, metric is undefined, time period is undefined, grain is undefined, output format is undefined. Strong rewrite: "Calculate inpatient admissions per 1,000 member months (util_per_1k) and average allowed amount per admission (unit_cost) for commercial fully-insured members (lob_code = COMM_FI) in Q1 2024 vs. Q1 2023, at service category × calendar month grain, using paid claims only and member months from fact_member_months as the denominator. Output: Excel table with YoY variance column, sorted by utilization variance descending, emailed to the CFO by Monday." This strong Task tells the developer exactly which tables to query, which filters to apply, what to calculate, at what level to group, and what the deliverable looks like — eliminating ambiguity before the first line of SQL is written.

Q8. The STAR Result for Scenario 4.1 routes inpatient unit cost variance to the contracting team. Describe what the contracting team's next SQL query would look like.

(Short answer)

Sample Answer:
The contracting team needs to identify which hospitals are driving unit cost increases and for which DRGs. Query structure: (1) Pull inpatient claims (TOB LIKE '11%') for Q1 2024 vs. Q1 2023, commercial FI. (2) JOIN to dim_providers on billing_npi to get hospital_name. (3) JOIN to ref_drg on primary_drg to get DRG description. (4) Aggregate to claim_id first (header grain) to avoid double-counting revenue lines. (5) Calculate unit_cost_per_admission = SUM(allowed_amount)/COUNT(DISTINCT claim_id) by hospital × DRG. (6) Self-join to prior year for unit_cost_variance = unit_cost_2024 - unit_cost_2023. (7) JOIN to ref_fee_schedule on billing_npi × DRG to compare actual unit cost against contracted rate. Output: ranked hospital-DRG combinations with largest unit cost increases above contract benchmarks. Findings route to specific hospital contract renegotiation priorities and identify where the plan is paying above the fee schedule — often due to outlier charges that were not caught during adjudication.

Q9. Describe the complete PDC algorithm in plain language — from first fill to adherence flag — and explain what would happen to a member's PDC score if the overlap adjustment were omitted.

(Short answer)

Sample Answer:
PDC algorithm step by step: (1) Collect all paid fills for the drug class (e.g., statins by GPI prefix). (2) Set the measurement period: starts 30 days after the member's first fill (NCQA 30-day grace period for treatment initiation), ends December 31. (3) For each fill, calculate the adjusted_start = GREATEST(dispensing_date, prior_fill_end + 1 day) to prevent early refill overlap. (4) For each fill, calculate covered days within the measurement window: MIN(fill_end, period_end) - MAX(adjusted_start, period_start) + 1, floored at 0. (5) Sum all fill's covered days. (6) PDC = covered_days / period_days. (7) PDC >= 0.80 = adherent (NCQA HEDIS threshold). Impact of omitting overlap adjustment: If a member on 30-day supplies refills 5 days early each time, each fill creates a 5-day overlap with the prior fill. Over 10 fills in a year that is 50 extra days counted. The member's actual covered days might be 280, but without adjustment the query reports 330 — more than the 365-day measurement period. PDC would appear as 330/280 = 1.18 — impossible and incorrect. The member might be classified as adherent when their actual coverage behavior is borderline. The GREATEST function is a correctness requirement, not an optimization.

Q10. Explain why the STAR Result section is the most frequently skipped step and describe what a complete Result section must include for Scenario 4.1.

(Short answer)

Sample Answer:

The Result section is most frequently skipped because analysts conflate delivering data with delivering analysis. Sending a table of numbers to a stakeholder without interpretation forces the stakeholder to do the analytical work — they may misinterpret the numbers, draw wrong conclusions, or take no action. A complete Result section for Scenario 4.1 must include: (1) What the numbers say: "Inpatient PMPM is +$22 vs. prior year Q1. Decomposing variance: utilization is flat (+0.8 admits/1,000 MM, within normal range) while unit cost increased +$780/admission." (2) What benchmark to compare against: "The $780 unit cost increase represents a 12% year-over-year increase vs. a CPI-medical inflation benchmark of 4–6%. This is above normal trend." (3) Root cause hypothesis: "Unit cost increase of this magnitude without a corresponding DRG complexity shift suggests the fee schedule for inpatient services may be underperforming relative to contracted rates." (4) Who owns the action: "Routing to VP of Network for contract review. The contracting team should pull inpatient unit cost by hospital × DRG and compare to fee schedule benchmarks to identify specific contract outliers." (5) Timeline: "Results needed before next hospital contract renewal cycle (Q3 2024)." Without all five elements, the analysis is data delivery, not strategic analytics.

Key Takeaways

What every analyst must remember from this chapter.

1. STAR is a thinking discipline: Situation and Task are defined before the SQL editor opens; Result is interpreted before the presentation opens. The Action (SQL) is the middle step. Never start with SQL.

2. A strong Task has five dimensions: Population (who, with what filters), Metric (what, with what formula), Time period (when), Aggregation grain (at what level), Output format (what does the deliverable look like). A Task missing any dimension produces a query that answers a different question.

3. PMPM variance decomposition: utilization variance (claims per 1,000 MM) → care management team. Unit cost variance (allowed amount per claim) → contracting team. A combined variance number routes nobody. Decompose before presenting.

4. PDC = covered_days / period_days. The measurement period starts 30 days after the first qualifying fill (NCQA). Early refill overlap must be adjusted using GREATEST(dispensing_date, prior_fill_end + 1 day). Without adjustment, PDC can exceed 1.0.

5. The PDC 0.80 threshold is the NCQA HEDIS standard for medication adherence measures (SPC, MAD, MAH). Members with PDC 0.70–0.79 are "near-threshold" — priority outreach targets because one refill can cross them into adherence.

6. Stars gap priority score = star_weight × (1/denom_size) × (1/gaps_to_cut_point). Sorting by raw gap count is wrong — it treats all measures equally. A 3-weight measure needing 5 more closures is worth far more per outreach call than a 1-weight measure needing 300.

7. Peer-adjusted E&M rate comparison (PERCENTILE_CONT at p95) is the correct fraud detection method — not fixed dollar thresholds. Dollar thresholds penalize large legitimate practices. Peer rate comparison isolates coding behavior patterns independent of volume.

8. PERCENTILE_CONT(0.95) WITHIN GROUP (ORDER BY provider_rate_pct) is the ANSI SQL ordered-set aggregate for continuous percentile calculation. It interpolates between values and is available in PostgreSQL, SQL Server (2012+), Oracle, and Snowflake.

9. The STAR Result must include: (1) what the numbers say, (2) what benchmark they compare against, (3) root cause hypothesis, (4) who owns the action, (5) timeline. A table without all five elements is data delivery, not analysis.

PART III: Claims, Eligibility & the Payment Engine

Rung 3 · Chapters 5–7

Part III is the engine room of healthcare analytics. Every PMPM, every quality rate, every risk score ultimately depends on the data generated here — the medical claim, the eligibility record, and the government program enrollment transaction. Chapter 5 dissects the claims lifecycle from submission through void and adjustment, covering the structural differences between professional and institutional claim types and the SQL patterns that handle each correctly. Chapter 6 builds the denominator architecture — eligibility, member months, continuous enrollment, and PCP attribution — without which no rate or average can be trusted. Chapter 7 enters the government program layer: HCC risk adjustment, Medicare Advantage capitation, Medicaid managed care reconciliation, and the regulatory submission cycles that drive hundreds of millions of dollars of plan revenue.

Part III· Claims, Eligibility & the Payment Engine

Chapter 5: Claims Fundamentals

The medical claim is the atomic unit of healthcare finance. Every dollar spent, every diagnosis made, every procedure performed leaves a claim record in the data warehouse. Understanding the claim lifecycle, the structural differences between claim types, and the SQL patterns that correctly handle adjustments and voids is the prerequisite for every financial, quality, and utilization analysis in this book.

5.1 The Claims Lifecycle

A claim does not appear in your database as a finished object. It passes through a lifecycle — from provider submission to adjudication to payment to potential adjustment or void — and each stage creates or modifies records that the analyst must understand to avoid double-counting, missed voids, or incorrect cost totals.

Stage	claim_status value	claim_frequency_code	Include in PMPM?	SQL note
Submitted	SUBMITTED / PENDING	1 = original	NO	Not yet adjudicated — cost not final
Adjudicated — Paid	PAID / PROCESSED	1 = original	YES	Primary paid population
Adjudicated — Denied	DENIED / DENY	1 = original	NO	Unless tracking denial cost separately

Stage	claim_status value	claim_frequency_code	Include in PMPM?	SQL note
Replacement (corrected)	PAID	7 = replacement	YES — net with original	Keep replacement; offset original if still present
Void (cancellation)	VOID / REVERSED	8 = void	NO — offsets prior paid	Negative allowed_amount cancels original payment
Encounter (capitated)	ENCOUNTER	1	NO for $cost; YES for utilization	Capitated plans: $0 paid but service occurred

> **The safe status filter:** Always use: WHERE claim_status IN ('PAID','PROCESSED','APPROVED') AND claim_type NOT IN ('VOID','REVERSAL','ADJUSTMENT_VOID'). This single filter prevents the most common error in healthcare SQL — including voided or pending claims in cost totals.

5.2 Claim Types and Their SQL Signatures

Each claim type has structural differences that require different SQL logic. Mixing claim types without accounting for these differences produces incorrect grain, double-counted costs, and invalid utilization rates.

5.2.1 Professional Claims (CMS-1500)

Professional claims are submitted by individual providers and group practices for outpatient services, office visits, and diagnostic tests. Key SQL characteristics:

Grain: One row per procedure line. A single office visit may generate 2–5 lines (E&M code + labs + injections).

Cost field: Use allowed_amount — never billed_amount. Billed is the chargemaster rate; allowed is what the plan actually pays.

Place of Service (POS): 11=Office, 22=Outpatient Hospital, 23=ED, 31=SNF, 81=Hospice. Critical for site-of-care analysis.

Provider identity: rendering_npi = individual who performed the service; billing_npi = group that submitted the claim. Both needed for network analysis.

Diagnosis hierarchy: primary_diag (position 1) = principal reason for visit. Secondary diagnoses inform HCC capture — include all 12 positions in risk adjustment queries.

5.2.2 Institutional Claims (UB-04)

Institutional claims are submitted by hospitals, SNFs, home health agencies, and hospices for facility-level services. Structurally different from professional claims in every key field:

Type of Bill (TOB): The primary routing field. First digit: facility type (1=hospital, 2=SNF, 3=home health, 8=hospice). Second: classification (1=inpatient, 3=outpatient). Third: frequency (1=admit through discharge, 8=void).

Revenue codes: Identify services within the admission: 0120=room & board, 0360=OR, 0450=ED, 0730=EEG. A single inpatient stay may have 40–200 revenue code lines.

DRG: Diagnosis Related Group — assigned at header level after discharge. The basis of inpatient payment. Use for LOS benchmarking and cost per episode.

Admit date / discharge date: Header-level fields. LOS = DATEDIFF('day', admit_date, discharge_date). Same-day admits have LOS = 0 — valid for same-day surgeries.

Discharge status: 01=home, 02=transfer to another hospital, 03=SNF, 20=expired. Exclude 02 and 20 from readmission index admission denominators.

Field	Professional (CMS-1500)	Institutional (UB-04)	SQL difference
Primary routing	claim_form_type = 'CMS1500'	type_of_bill LIKE '11%' (inpatient)	Always filter claim type before aggregating
Service identifier	procedure_code (CPT/HCPCS)	revenue_code + procedure_code	Revenue code required for IP service classification
Provider identifier	rendering_npi (individual)	billing_npi (facility NPI)	Never mix individual and facility NPIs
Episode grouping	COUNT(DISTINCT claim_id) = visits	COUNT(DISTINCT claim_id) = admissions (header)	IP: filter to header grain before counting
Cost field	allowed_amount per line	allowed_amount at header level	IP: SUM at header to avoid revenue line duplication
Diagnosis location	primary_diag through secondary_diag_12	principal_diag + admit_diag + 24 secondary	Admit diag ≠ principal diag; use principal for DRG/HCC

5.3 Handling Claim Adjustments and Voids

One of the most dangerous mistakes in claims analytics is ignoring the adjustment lifecycle. When a claim is corrected — because of a coding error, a COB update, or a contract rate change — the original claim is not deleted. Instead, a void (frequency code 8, negative amount) cancels the original, and a replacement (frequency code 7) posts the corrected values. Failure to net these three transactions overstates costs by the full amount of every adjusted claim.

ANSI SQL — 5.3: Claim Adjustment Netting

```
-- Net paid amounts across original, void, and replacement claims
-- claim_frequency_code: 1=original, 7=replacement, 8=void (negative)
WITH claim_net AS (
  SELECT
    original_claim_id,          -- links all transactions for one claim
    SUM(allowed_amount)  AS net_allowed,
    SUM(paid_amount)     AS net_paid,
    MAX(service_date)    AS service_date,
    MAX(member_id)       AS member_id,
    MAX(rendering_npi)   AS rendering_npi,
    MAX(primary_diag)    AS primary_diag,
    -- Retain the most recent non-void adjudication status
    MAX(CASE WHEN claim_frequency_code <> '8'
        THEN claim_status END) AS final_status
  FROM  fact_medical_claims
  GROUP BY original_claim_id
  -- Net positive = claim remains paid after adjustments
  HAVING SUM(allowed_amount) > 0
)
SELECT * FROM claim_net
WHERE final_status = 'PAID';

-- Validation: check for un-netted voids (net_paid < 0)
SELECT COUNT(*) AS orphan_voids
FROM  claim_net
WHERE  net_paid < 0;  -- should be 0; any rows = data quality issue
```

Watch for: Some organizations store voids as negative-amount rows sharing the original claim_id. Others use a separate void_claim_id column linking to the original. Confirm your data model convention before building the netting logic — the pattern above assumes a shared original_claim_id.

5.4 Coordination of Benefits (COB)

When a member has coverage under more than one health plan — covered by both their own employer and their spouse's employer, for example — the plans must coordinate to avoid paying more than 100% of the claim. The primary plan pays first; the secondary plan pays a portion of the remaining balance. In SQL, COB affects cost calculations: the plan's net liability is paid_amount minus other_payer_paid.

Field	Description	SQL use
other_payer_paid	Amount paid by the other carrier before this plan	Subtract from allowed_amount for plan net cost
cob_flag	Indicator that COB is active for this claim	Filter: AND cob_flag = 'Y' for COB-specific analysis
payer_sequence	Primary (1) or Secondary (2) payer sequence	Primary plan sees full allowed; secondary sees residual
coordination_method	Maintenance of benefits / non-duplication / birthday rule	Determines how the secondary plan calculates liability

5.5 Claims Scenarios

Each scenario below is fully worked using the STAR framework. Read the S·T·A·R fields before the SQL — the business context defines why the query is structured the way it is.

Scenario 5.1 · Financial / Cost Intelligence

Top 20 Diagnosis Groups by Allowed Cost

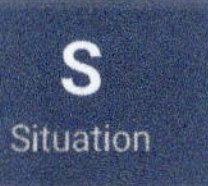

The CMO wants to know where medical spend is concentrated by clinical condition this year — fully-insured commercial. The output will feed the care management prioritization meeting next week.

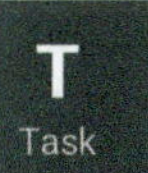

Rank all CCSR diagnosis categories by total allowed amount for the current year, commercial fully-insured paid claims only. Include member count and claim count. Output: top 20 ranked by cost.

ANSI SQL — Scenario 5.1: Top 20 Diagnosis Groups by Allowed Cost

```
-- Top 20 CCSR diagnosis categories by allowed cost — current year, COMM_FI
-- Step 1: Build cost aggregation at diagnosis group level
WITH dx_costs AS (
SELECT
i.ccsr_category, -- Clinical grouping (e.g., MSK, Cardio)
i.ccsr_description, -- Human-readable label for reporting

-- 🔑 Core metric: total cost
SUM(c.allowed_amount) AS total_allowed,
```

```
-- 👥 Unique members impacted (population size)
COUNT(DISTINCT c.member_id) AS member_count,

-- 📄 Total claims (utilization proxy)
COUNT(DISTINCT c.claim_id) AS claim_count,

-- 💰 Cost intensity per member
ROUND(
SUM(c.allowed_amount)
/ NULLIF(COUNT(DISTINCT c.member_id),0)
,0) AS allowed_per_member

FROM fact_medical_claims c

-- 🔗 Map diagnosis → CCSR category
JOIN ref_icd10 i
ON c.primary_diag = i.icd10_code

-- 🔗 Restrict to line of business (Commercial Fully Insured)
JOIN dim_plans pl
ON c.plan_id = pl.plan_id

-- 🔗 Time dimension (ensures clean year filtering)
JOIN dim_date d
ON c.service_date = d.date_key

WHERE
-- ✅ Only financially valid claims
c.claim_status = 'PAID'

-- ✅ Business segment filter
AND pl.lob_code = 'COMM_FI'

-- ✅ Current year only
AND d.calendar_year = EXTRACT(YEAR FROM CURRENT_DATE)

-- 🔑 Aggregate at diagnosis group level
GROUP BY
i.ccsr_category,
i.ccsr_description
)
SELECT
-- 🏆 Rank by cost (highest spend first)
RANK() OVER (ORDER BY total_allowed DESC) AS cost_rank,

ccsr_category,
ccsr_description,

-- 💰 Rounded for executive readability
ROUND(total_allowed,0) AS total_allowed,

member_count,
claim_count,
allowed_per_member,
```

```
-- 📊 % contribution to total spend
ROUND(
100.0 * total_allowed
/ SUM(total_allowed) OVER ()
,1) AS pct_of_total

FROM dx_costs

-- 📈 Sort by highest cost first
ORDER BY cost_rank

-- 🎯 Only top 20 for executive focus
LIMIT 20;
```

R
Result

Common Mistakes This Query Avoids

☑ Uses **allowed_amount (not billed)**
☑ Uses **DISTINCT for members/claims**
☑ Filters to **correct LOB**
☑ Uses **window function for % contribution**

Executive Interpretation (What You Say in a Meeting)

"Medical spend is highly concentrated. The top 3 CCSR categories represent ~45–50% of total cost, primarily driven by musculoskeletal, circulatory, and behavioral health conditions. These should be prioritized for care management programs and cost containment strategies."

Scenario 5.2 · Financial / Trend Analysis

Monthly Claims Volume & Cost Trend

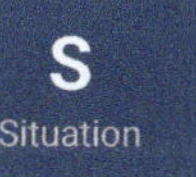

Finance needs a 24-month trailing PMPM trend dashboard for commercial FI. The chart must show both total allowed PMPM and YoY change. IBNR flag required for most recent 3 months.

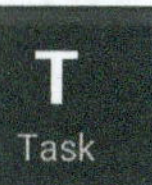

Calculate monthly PMPM and claims-per-1,000-member-months for 24 trailing months, commercial FI. Self-join to prior year same month for YoY%. Flag last 3 months as IBNR-impacted.

ANSI SQL — Scenario 5.2: 24-Month Claims Trend Dashboard

```
ANSI SQL — Scenario 5.2: 24-Month Claims Trend Dashboard
-- 24-month PMPM trend with YoY comparison and IBNR flag
WITH monthly_base AS (
  SELECT
    DATE_TRUNC('month', c.service_date)   AS svc_month,
    SUM(c.allowed_amount)                 AS total_allowed,
    COUNT(DISTINCT c.claim_id)            AS claim_count
  FROM fact_medical_claims c
  JOIN dim_plans       pl ON c.plan_id = pl.plan_id
  WHERE c.claim_status  = 'PAID'
   AND pl.lob_code      = 'COMM_FI'
   AND c.service_date >= CURRENT_DATE - INTERVAL '24' MONTH
  GROUP BY 1
),
```

```
monthly_mm AS (
  SELECT DATE_TRUNC('month', month_start) AS svc_month,
      SUM(member_months) AS member_months
  FROM  fact_member_months mm
  JOIN  dim_plans pl ON mm.plan_id = pl.plan_id
  WHERE  pl.lob_code = 'COMM_FI'
   AND  month_start >= CURRENT_DATE - INTERVAL '24' MONTH
  GROUP BY 1
)
SELECT
  curr.svc_month,
  ROUND(curr.total_allowed / NULLIF(mm.member_months,0),2)  AS pmpm,
  ROUND(1000.0*curr.claim_count / NULLIF(mm.member_months,0),1) AS claims_per_1k,
  -- YoY: same month prior year
  ROUND(prior.total_allowed / NULLIF(pmmm.member_months,0),2) AS prior_yr_pmpm,
  ROUND(100.0*((curr.total_allowed/NULLIF(mm.member_months,0))
    /(NULLIF(prior.total_allowed/NULLIF(pmmm.member_months,0),0))-1),1) AS yoy_pct,
  -- Flag recent months as IBNR-impacted
  CASE WHEN curr.svc_month >= DATE_TRUNC('month',CURRENT_DATE) - INTERVAL '3' MONTH
    THEN 'IBNR — incomplete' ELSE 'Final' END AS data_maturity
FROM  monthly_base curr
JOIN  monthly_mm   mm    ON curr.svc_month = mm.svc_month
LEFT JOIN monthly_base prior ON curr.svc_month = prior.svc_month + INTERVAL '1' YEAR
LEFT JOIN monthly_mm   pmmm   ON prior.svc_month = pmmm.svc_month
ORDER BY curr.svc_month;
```

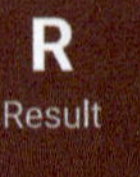

Present the 21 mature months as final; annotate the last 3 with the IBNR flag. YoY% reveals whether current trend is above or below prior year. A sustained positive YoY (e.g., +8%) that exceeds the filed trend assumption (+6%) signals a rate adequacy concern for the next filing cycle.

Scenario 5.3 · Revenue Cycle / Provider Analytics

Claim Denial Rate by Provider Group

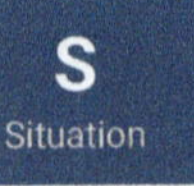

The network team suspects several provider groups have unusually high denial rates, indicating coding or credentialing issues. They need a ranked list of provider TINs by denial rate with the top denial reason codes.

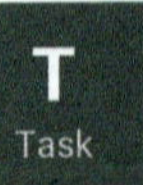

Calculate denial rate (denied claims / total submitted) and top denial reason codes by billing TIN for the current year. Exclude voids. Rank by denial rate descending, minimum 50 submissions for statistical stability.

ANSI SQL — Scenario 5.3: Claim Denial Rate by Provider Group

```
-- Denial rate by billing TIN with top denial reason codes
WITH claim_flags AS (
  SELECT
    c.billing_tin,
    c.claim_id,
    c.allowed_amount,
    CASE WHEN c.claim_status IN ('DENY','DENIED','D')
      THEN 1 ELSE 0 END       AS is_denied,
    c.denial_reason_code
  FROM  fact_medical_claims c
  WHERE EXTRACT(YEAR FROM c.service_date) = EXTRACT(YEAR FROM CURRENT_DATE)
   AND c.claim_frequency_code <> '8'   -- exclude voids
),
tin_summary AS (
  SELECT
    billing_tin,
```

```
        COUNT(*)                        AS total_submitted,
        SUM(is_denied)                  AS total_denied,
        ROUND(100.0*SUM(is_denied)/COUNT(*),2)    AS denial_rate_pct,
        SUM(CASE WHEN is_denied=1 THEN allowed_amount ELSE 0 END) AS denied_value
    FROM  claim_flags
    GROUP BY billing_tin
    HAVING COUNT(*) >= 50    -- minimum volume for statistical validity
),
top_reasons AS (
    SELECT billing_tin, denial_reason_code,
        COUNT(*) AS reason_count,
        ROW_NUMBER() OVER (PARTITION BY billing_tin ORDER BY COUNT(*) DESC) AS rn
    FROM  claim_flags
    WHERE  is_denied = 1 AND denial_reason_code IS NOT NULL
    GROUP BY billing_tin, denial_reason_code
)
SELECT
    ts.billing_tin,
    p.provider_group_name,
    p.specialty_group,
    ts.total_submitted,
    ts.total_denied,
    ts.denial_rate_pct,
    ROUND(ts.denied_value,0)        AS denied_allowed_value,
    tr.denial_reason_code           AS top_denial_reason,
    r.carc_description              AS reason_description
FROM  tin_summary        ts
JOIN  dim_providers      p  ON ts.billing_tin = p.billing_tin
LEFT JOIN top_reasons    tr ON ts.billing_tin = tr.billing_tin AND tr.rn = 1
LEFT JOIN ref_carc_codes  r  ON tr.denial_reason_code = r.carc_code
ORDER BY ts.denial_rate_pct DESC
LIMIT 25;
```

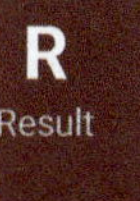

R Result

Flag any TIN with denial rate > 15% (industry benchmark: 5–10% for in-network providers). CARC code 97 (bundling) and CARC 4 (prior authorization missing) are the most common correctable denial reasons – route those to the provider relations team for education. CARC 96 (non-covered service) warrants a credentialing review.

Scenario 5.4 · Clinical / Utilization Management

Inpatient LOS Benchmarking by DRG

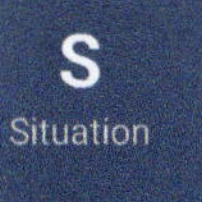

S Situation

The VP of Medical Management needs to identify hospitals with significantly longer-than-expected lengths of stay for the top 10 inpatient DRGs. Outlier hospitals are candidates for case management intervention and contract renegotiation.

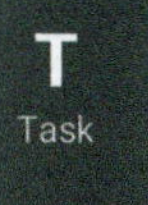

T Task

Calculate average LOS by hospital NPI and DRG for the current year. Compare to the plan-wide average LOS for each DRG. Flag hospitals where actual LOS exceeds plan average by 20%+ with minimum 10 admissions per DRG.

ANSI SQL – Scenario 5.4: Inpatient LOS by Hospital and DRG

```
-- Inpatient LOS benchmark: hospital vs. plan average by DRG
WITH inpatient_admits AS (
    SELECT
        c.billing_npi,
```

```sql
        c.primary_drg,
        c.claim_id,
        c.allowed_amount,
        DATEDIFF('day', c.admit_date, c.discharge_date) AS los_days
    FROM  fact_medical_claims c
    WHERE c.type_of_bill LIKE '11%'  -- inpatient acute
      AND c.claim_status = 'PAID'
      AND EXTRACT(YEAR FROM c.service_date) = EXTRACT(YEAR FROM CURRENT_DATE)
      AND c.admit_date IS NOT NULL AND c.discharge_date IS NOT NULL
      AND c.discharge_status_code NOT IN ('02','20') -- exclude transfers and expired
),
plan_avg AS (
    SELECT primary_drg,
         ROUND(AVG(los_days),2)  AS plan_avg_los,
         COUNT(claim_id)         AS plan_admissions
    FROM  inpatient_admits
    GROUP BY primary_drg
)
SELECT
    ia.billing_npi,
    p.hospital_name,
    ia.primary_drg,
    d.drg_description,
    COUNT(ia.claim_id)           AS hospital_admissions,
    ROUND(AVG(ia.los_days),2)      AS hospital_avg_los,
    pa.plan_avg_los,
    ROUND(AVG(ia.los_days) - pa.plan_avg_los, 2)  AS los_variance,
    ROUND(100.0*(AVG(ia.los_days)-pa.plan_avg_los)
      /NULLIF(pa.plan_avg_los,0),1)              AS variance_pct,
    CASE WHEN AVG(ia.los_days) > pa.plan_avg_los * 1.20
         AND COUNT(ia.claim_id) >= 10
         THEN 'FLAG — outlier LOS'
         ELSE 'Within range' END  AS los_flag
FROM  inpatient_admits ia
JOIN  plan_avg pa        ON ia.primary_drg  = pa.primary_drg
JOIN  dim_providers p    ON ia.billing_npi  = p.npi
JOIN  ref_drg d          ON ia.primary_drg  = d.drg_code
GROUP BY ia.billing_npi, p.hospital_name, ia.primary_drg, d.drg_description, pa.plan_avg_los
HAVING COUNT(ia.claim_id) >= 10
ORDER BY variance_pct DESC;
```

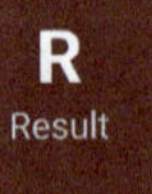

Hospitals with los_flag = 'FLAG' are candidates for concurrent review programs and targeted case management outreach. For contract renegotiation, quantify the cost impact: (hospital_avg_los - plan_avg_los) × average_cost_per_day × admission_count = estimated excess cost per hospital per DRG.

Scenario 5.5 · Clinical / Care Management

ED Utilization by NYU Classification

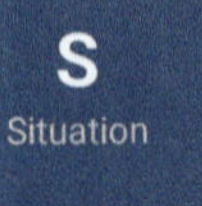

The medical director wants to know what percentage of ED visits are avoidable — treatable in a primary care or urgent care setting. Results will be segmented by attributed PCP to identify which provider panels have the highest avoidable ED rates, informing care management outreach.

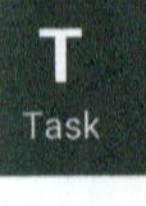

Calculate ED visits per 1,000 member months by NYU ED classification category and attributed PCP. Flag PCPs with avoidable ED rate >150 per 1,000 MM (industry benchmark: <120).

ANSI SQL — Scenario 5.5: ED Utilization by NYU Category and PCP

```
-- ED utilization rate by NYU avoidability classification and attributed PCP
WITH ed_claims AS (
  SELECT
    c.member_id,
    c.service_date,
    COALESCE(n.nyu_category, 'Unclassified') AS nyu_category
  FROM fact_medical_claims c
  LEFT JOIN ref_nyu_ed_algorithm n ON c.primary_diag = n.icd10_code
  WHERE (c.place_of_service = '23'
     OR c.revenue_code BETWEEN '0450' AND '0459')
    AND c.claim_status = 'PAID'
    AND EXTRACT(YEAR FROM c.service_date) = EXTRACT(YEAR FROM CURRENT_DATE)
),
pcp_mm AS (
  SELECT m.attributed_pcp_npi,
      SUM(mm.member_months) AS total_mm
  FROM  fact_member_months mm
  JOIN  dim_members m ON mm.member_id = m.member_id
  WHERE EXTRACT(YEAR FROM mm.month_start) = EXTRACT(YEAR FROM CURRENT_DATE)
  GROUP BY m.attributed_pcp_npi
)
SELECT
  m.attributed_pcp_npi,
  p.provider_full_name,
  pm.total_mm,
  SUM(CASE WHEN e.nyu_category IN ('Non-Emergent','Primary Care Treatable')
       THEN 1 ELSE 0 END)        AS avoidable_ed_visits,
  COUNT(e.member_id)             AS total_ed_visits,
  ROUND(1000.0*COUNT(e.member_id)
    /NULLIF(pm.total_mm,0),1)        AS ed_per_1k_mm,
  ROUND(1000.0*SUM(CASE WHEN e.nyu_category IN
    ('Non-Emergent','Primary Care Treatable') THEN 1 ELSE 0 END)
    /NULLIF(pm.total_mm,0),1)        AS avoidable_per_1k_mm,
  CASE WHEN ROUND(1000.0*SUM(CASE WHEN e.nyu_category IN
    ('Non-Emergent','Primary Care Treatable') THEN 1 ELSE 0 END)
    /NULLIF(pm.total_mm,0),1) > 150
  THEN 'FLAG — high avoidable ED' ELSE 'Within range' END AS ed_flag
FROM ed_claims e
JOIN dim_members m ON e.member_id = m.member_id
JOIN pcp_mm pm   ON m.attributed_pcp_npi = pm.attributed_pcp_npi
JOIN dim_providers p ON m.attributed_pcp_npi = p.npi
GROUP BY m.attributed_pcp_npi, p.provider_full_name, pm.total_mm
ORDER BY avoidable_per_1k_mm DESC;
```

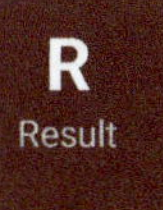

Flagged PCPs receive an outreach package: their avoidable ED rate vs. plan benchmark, the list of members who had avoidable ED visits, and a prompt to assess after-hours coverage. Avoidable ED rate is also a HEDIS-adjacent metric — improvements directly support care quality scores and patient experience.

Chapter 5 Review

Unit Test · Key Takeaways

Answer each question before reading the explanation.

Q1. Claim frequency codes 1, 7, and 8 on institutional claims indicate respectively:

A. Original, corrected, and cancelled

B. Original submission, replacement (corrected), and void (cancellation)

C. First, seventh, and eighth billing attempt

D. Inpatient, outpatient, and professional claim types

Answer: B. *Code 1 = original submission — the first time a claim was sent. Code 7 = replacement — a corrected version of a prior claim; it carries the full corrected dollar amount. Code 8 = void — a cancellation of a prior claim; it carries a negative dollar amount equal to the original. These three codes must be netted by original_claim_id to get the correct net paid amount.*

Q2. The correct SQL pattern to net claim adjustments across original, void, and replacement transactions is:

A. WHERE claim_status = 'PAID' AND claim_frequency_code = '1'

B. GROUP BY original_claim_id, SUM(allowed_amount), HAVING SUM(allowed_amount) > 0 — net positive means payment remains; net zero or negative means fully voided

C. JOIN on claim_id = original_claim_id to link void to original

D. DELETE FROM claims WHERE claim_frequency_code = '8'

Answer: B. *All transactions for one claim share original_claim_id. Grouping by this and summing allowed_amount nets the original (+), void (-), and replacement (+) automatically. HAVING SUM(allowed_amount) > 0 keeps only claims with net positive payment. A net of zero = fully voided. A net negative = orphaned void (data quality issue).*

Q3. The 24-month PMPM trend query flags the most recent 3 months as IBNR-impacted. What is the SQL CASE WHEN condition that identifies these months?

A. CASE WHEN svc_month = CURRENT_DATE THEN 'IBNR'

B. CASE WHEN svc_month >= DATE_TRUNC('month', CURRENT_DATE) - INTERVAL '3 months' THEN 'INCOMPLETE — IBNR'

C. CASE WHEN claim_count < 100 THEN 'IBNR'

D. CASE WHEN total_allowed < budget_pmpm * 0.90 THEN 'IBNR'

Answer: B. *DATE_TRUNC('month', CURRENT_DATE) truncates today's date to the first of the current month. Subtracting 3 months gives the start of the 3-month IBNR window. Months with svc_month >= that date are the most recent three service months and are flagged as incomplete. This pattern must appear in every monthly trend report regardless of the analytics question being answered.*

Q4. The inpatient LOS benchmark query excludes discharge_status_code 02 and 20. Why?

A. Codes 02 and 20 indicate readmission within 30 days

B. Code 02 = transfer to another facility; code 20 = patient expired. Excluding them produces a like-for-like comparison of routine home discharges — transfers have shorter LOS (transferred before clinical resolution) and expired cases have longer LOS (end-of-life patterns)

C. Codes 02 and 20 indicate Medicaid claims that should not be benchmarked against commercial

D. These codes indicate claims that are still pending adjudication

Answer: B. *A hospital that transfers complex patients early will have artificially low LOS. A hospital that manages end-of-life care will have artificially high LOS. Including both in a general LOS benchmark produces misleading comparisons. Excluding codes 02 (transfer) and 20 (expired) isolates routine discharges for a valid like-for-like hospital comparison.*

Q5. In the ED utilization query, NYU categories "Non-Emergent" and "Primary Care Treatable" are combined to calculate the avoidable ED rate. What does this metric represent analytically?

A. The percentage of ED visits that were denied by the plan

B. The rate of ED visits per 1,000 member months for conditions that could have been managed in a primary care setting — a proxy for primary care access barriers and care coordination gaps

C. The percentage of ED visits that resulted in an inpatient admission

D. The rate of ED visits for members without a primary care provider

Answer: B. *NYU avoidability classification divides ED visits into: Emergent (true emergencies), Emergent but Preventable (could have been prevented by better chronic disease management), Primary Care Treatable (should have been seen in primary care), and Non-Emergent (not medically necessary). The avoidable rate (Non-Emergent + Primary Care Treatable) flags PCPs or geographies where members cannot access timely primary care, leading to higher-cost ED substitution.*

Q6. The denial rate query uses HAVING COUNT(*) >= 50 before reporting. What is the purpose of this filter?

A. To ensure the query runs faster by limiting output rows

B. To establish a minimum volume threshold for statistical validity — a provider with 3 claims and 1 denial has a 33% denial rate that is not statistically meaningful and should not be flagged as an outlier

C. To exclude providers who do not submit paper claims

D. To limit results to only the top 50 billing TINs by volume

Answer: B. *A minimum volume threshold prevents false-positive flags on providers with small claim counts. A single denied claim out of 3 submitted produces a 33% denial rate that would rank at the top of any denial analysis. Setting HAVING COUNT(*) >= 50 ensures reported denial rates reflect a pattern of behavior, not statistical noise from small samples.*

Q7. Explain the three-claim transaction set (original, void, replacement) and write the complete SQL for netting them. Describe what HAVING SUM(allowed_amount) > 0 accomplishes.

(Short answer)

Sample Answer:
Three transactions: Original (frequency_code = 1): the initial claim submission with the full allowed_amount. Void (frequency_code = 8): cancels the original, posted with a negative allowed_amount equal to the original. Replacement (frequency_code = 7): a corrected version of the claim with the updated allowed_amount. All three share the same original_claim_id. Net SQL: WITH claim_net AS (SELECT original_claim_id, SUM(allowed_amount) AS net_allowed, SUM(paid_amount) AS net_paid, MAX(service_date) AS service_date, MAX(member_id) AS member_id, MAX(CASE WHEN claim_frequency_code <> '8' THEN claim_status END) AS final_status FROM fact_medical_claims GROUP BY original_claim_id HAVING SUM(allowed_amount) > 0) SELECT * FROM claim_net WHERE final_status = 'PAID'. HAVING SUM(allowed_amount) > 0 filters out claims where the net is zero (original + void = 0, meaning fully voided with no replacement) or negative (orphaned void – the original was not loaded into the warehouse, creating a phantom negative cost). Only claims with net positive allowed_amount represent actual payments that should appear in PMPM calculations.

Q8. Describe the professional vs. institutional claim distinction and give three SQL field names that exist on institutional claims (UB-04) but not on professional claims (CMS-1500).

(Short answer)

Sample Answer:
Professional claims (CMS-1500) are submitted by individual providers or medical groups for physician services. They have: rendering_npi (individual clinician), procedure_code (CPT/HCPCS), place_of_service code, up to 12 diagnosis codes, and no facility-specific fields. Institutional claims (UB-04) are submitted by hospitals, outpatient facilities, SNFs, and other institutional providers for facility services. They contain facility-specific fields including: type_of_bill (TOB) – a 3-digit code identifying the facility type and claim status (e.g., 110 = inpatient admit, 121 = inpatient continuing care, 131 = outpatient); revenue_code – identifies the hospital department or service (0450 = ED, 0120 = room and board, 0360 = OR); admit_date and discharge_date – begin and end of the inpatient stay, used for LOS calculation and COB; discharge_status_code – where the patient went after discharge (01 = home, 02 = transferred, 20 = expired, 30 = still inpatient). None of these fields exist on CMS-1500 professional claims – queries that JOIN both claim types must handle missing fields with COALESCE or conditional logic.

Q9. A plan analyst is asked to build a 24-month PMPM trend with year-over-year comparison. Describe the query structure, explain why prior year data is LEFT JOINed rather than INNER JOINed, and explain what the YoY percentage formula calculates.

(Short answer)

Sample Answer:
Query structure: CTE 1 (monthly_base): GROUP BY DATE_TRUNC('month', service_date) – aggregate total_allowed and claim_count for the last 24 months. CTE 2 (monthly_mm): GROUP BY DATE_TRUNC('month', month_start) – aggregate member months for the same 24-month window. Final SELECT: JOIN current month to its enrollment. LEFT JOIN to prior year cost and enrollment using prior.svc_month = curr.svc_month + INTERVAL '1 YEAR'. Why LEFT JOIN for prior year: the 24-month window starts 24 months ago. The oldest current months (24 months ago) have no prior year data (which would require 36-month history). An INNER JOIN would silently drop these months from the output, truncating the trend to only months where a prior year comparison exists. LEFT JOIN shows all 24 current months and leaves prior_yr_pmpm as NULL where no comparison exists. YoY percentage formula: ROUND(100.0 * ((current_pmpm / NULLIF(prior_pmpm, 0)) - 1), 1). This calculates the percentage increase or decrease: a value of +8.5 means cost rose 8.5% year-over-year. NULLIF prevents divide-by-zero if prior_pmpm is zero. The result is multiplied by 100 to express as a percentage.

Q10. What is the NYU ED Avoidability Classification and how is it used in SQL? Write the WHERE clause that identifies ED claims and the CASE WHEN that classifies each visit.

(Short answer)

Sample Answer:
The NYU ED Avoidability Classification is a diagnosis-based algorithm developed by New York University that classifies emergency department visits into four categories based on the primary diagnosis: (1) Emergent – true emergencies requiring ED care. (2) Emergent but Preventable – emergency presentations that could have been avoided with better chronic disease management. (3) Primary Care Treatable – conditions that should have been managed in a primary care or urgent care setting.

(4) Non-Emergent — visits for conditions that are not medically urgent. The classification is stored in ref_nyu_ed_algorithm keyed to icd10_code. SQL WHERE clause to identify ED claims: WHERE (c.place_of_service = '23' OR c.revenue_code BETWEEN '0450' AND '0459'). The OR handles both professional claims (POS 23) and institutional claims (revenue code 045x). CASE WHEN for avoidability: CASE WHEN e.nyu_category IN ('Non-Emergent','Primary Care Treatable') THEN 'Avoidable' WHEN e.nyu_category IN ('Emergent — Preventable') THEN 'Preventable' WHEN e.nyu_category = 'Emergent' THEN 'True Emergency' ELSE 'Unclassified' END. The avoidable rate (Non-Emergent + Primary Care Treatable per 1,000 MM) by attributed PCP identifies providers whose panels have poor access to timely primary care.

Key Takeaways

What every analyst must remember from this chapter.

1 Claim frequency codes: 1 = original, 7 = replacement (corrected, full dollar amount), 8 = void (cancellation, negative dollar amount). All three share original_claim_id. Always net by original_claim_id using SUM(allowed_amount) — never filter to frequency_code = 1 only.

2 The claim netting pattern: GROUP BY original_claim_id, SUM(allowed_amount), HAVING SUM(allowed_amount) > 0. Net zero = fully voided. Net negative = orphaned void (data quality issue). Net positive = valid paid claim. Run the orphaned void check quarterly.

3 24-month PMPM trend structure: monthly_base CTE (cost) + monthly_mm CTE (enrollment) + LEFT JOIN to prior year. Always LEFT JOIN to prior year — an INNER JOIN silently drops the oldest months where no prior year comparison exists.

4 IBNR flag in trend reports: CASE WHEN svc_month >= DATE_TRUNC('month', CURRENT_DATE) - INTERVAL '3 months' THEN 'INCOMPLETE — IBNR' ELSE 'Final' END. Label every recent month — never present incomplete data as final without this flag visible in the report.

5 Inpatient LOS benchmarking: always exclude discharge_status_code 02 (transfer) and 20 (expired) before comparing hospitals. Transfers have artificially short LOS; expired cases have artificially long LOS. Include only routine home discharges for a valid like-for-like comparison.

6 ED utilization: identify ED claims using (place_of_service = '23' OR revenue_code BETWEEN '0450' AND '0459'). The OR is required — institutional claims use revenue codes; professional claims use POS codes. Using only one identifier misses half the ED population.

7 NYU ED avoidability categories: Non-Emergent and Primary Care Treatable = avoidable ED. Emergent but Preventable = chronic disease management gap. True Emergent = appropriate ED use. Avoidable ED rate > 150 per 1,000 MM by PCP is the flag threshold for access or coordination issues.

8 Minimum volume thresholds in provider analytics: HAVING COUNT(*) >= 50 for denial rate analysis; HAVING COUNT(*) >= 10 for inpatient LOS benchmarking. Without a volume floor, a provider with 2 claims and 1 denial appears to have a 50% denial rate — statistically meaningless.

Chapter 6: Eligibility & Enrollment Analytics

Eligibility data is the denominator of all healthcare analytics. Every rate, every PMPM, every quality measure starts with "who was enrolled and when." A query built on the wrong denominator — or no denominator at all — produces a number that cannot be trusted, compared, or acted upon. This chapter covers the structure of eligibility data, the retroactive eligibility problem that silently distorts denominators, continuous enrollment requirements for quality measures, and the PCP attribution logic that powers care management programs.

6.1 Eligibility Data Architecture

The eligibility table records the contract between the payer and the member: this person is covered, under this plan, from this date to this date. Understanding its structure prevents the most common denominator errors in healthcare SQL.

Column	Type	Description	Common SQL trap
member_id	PK / FK	Unique member identifier	Same person may have multiple member_ids across systems — deduplicate before counting
plan_id	FK	Plan the member is enrolled in	Always filter to specific plan before calculating rates
coverage_start_date	DATE	First day of enrollment	Member may have same-day or retro start — query may not return member if filtering on prior period
coverage_end_date	DATE / NULL	Last day of enrollment. NULL = currently active	Always COALESCE(coverage_end_date, '2099-12-31') in date range filters — NULLs cause active members to be excluded
line_of_business	VARCHAR	Commercial, MA, Medicaid, etc.	One member may have multiple LOB rows — use SCD-2 or date-filtered join, not current-only query
coverage_status	VARCHAR	ACTIVE, TERMINATED, RETRO_ACTIVE	Filter to ACTIVE and RETRO_ACTIVE for enrollment denominators

The NULL trap: Never write WHERE coverage_end_date >= '2024-01-01'. This silently excludes every currently-active member whose coverage_end_date IS NULL. Always write: WHERE COALESCE(coverage_end_date, '2099-12-31') >= '2024-01-01'. This single fix prevents the most common member undercounting error in healthcare SQL.

6.2 Retroactive Eligibility — The Silent Denominator Distorter

Retroactive eligibility changes occur when a member's enrollment start date is backdated after claims have already been processed. A member enrolled on November 1 may have their start date changed to October 1 after a payroll correction. This creates a situation where October claims existed before the enrollment record was created — and any report run before the retro change was loaded will have those claims with no matching member month denominator.

The practical impact: PMPM reports run close to month-end are systematically lower than reports run 30–60 days later, because retro enrollments add member months (increasing the denominator) while the claims were already counted. This creates the appearance of a cost improvement that is purely a denominator artifact.

Retro change type	Impact on PMPM	Impact on HEDIS	Mitigation
Enrollment backdated earlier	Denominator increases → PMPM appears to decrease	Members added to denominator may not meet continuous enrollment — re-run CE flag	Freeze eligibility snapshot at measurement year end for HEDIS; use live data for operational reports
Enrollment backdated later	Members removed from period → denominator decreases → PMPM appears to increase	Members may be removed from HEDIS denominator	Same — frozen snapshot prevents post-measurement changes from affecting submitted rates
Termination backdated earlier	Member removed from months they were counted in	Member may be removed from numerator if qualifying event was during enrollment	Audit retro terminations monthly; alert if >2% of members have retro changes
Plan / LOB change backdated	Claims reclassified to different LOB	HEDIS denominator LOB filter may exclude or include different population	SCD-2 point-in-time joins automatically correct for retroactive LOB changes

6.3 Continuous Enrollment — The Foundation of Quality Measurement

Many healthcare quality measures require continuous enrollment — the member must have been enrolled for a minimum proportion of the measurement year without excessive gaps. The NCQA standard for most administrative HEDIS measures is 11 of 12 months enrolled with no single gap exceeding 45 days.

6.3.1 NCQA Standard Continuous Enrollment Definitions

Measure category	Enrollment requirement	Gap allowance	How to calculate
Most HEDIS administrative measures	11 of 12 months in measurement year	One gap ≤ 45 days allowed	Count distinct calendar months enrolled; flag gaps using LAG() on enrollment spans
Prenatal / Postpartum measures	Specific trimesters — enrollment at delivery + prior period	No gap during delivery hospitalization	Anchor on delivery date; check enrollment window backward
Well-child measures	Enrolled at specific age milestone	No gap around qualifying visit	Filter: coverage_start ≤ birth_date AND COALESCE(coverage_end, '9999-12-31') ≥ age_milestone

Measure category	Enrollment requirement	Gap allowance	How to calculate
Pharmacy PDC measures	Enrolled throughout measurement period	Brief gaps ≤ 30 days depending on measure	Use enrollment-date intersection with measurement window

6.4 Enrollment Scenarios

Scenario 6.1 · Quality / Eligibility

Continuous Enrollment Flag for HEDIS Denominator

🔑 **What "Continuous Enrollment (CE)" Really Means in HEDIS**

In National Committee for Quality Assurance (NCQA) HEDIS:

👉 **Continuous Enrollment = ensuring the member had sufficient coverage to fairly evaluate care quality**

Because:

- You **can't measure care gaps** if the patient wasn't enrolled
- You **don't want to penalize providers** for members who churn in/out

---

🎯 **The Business Rule (Your Scenario)**

For most HEDIS measures:

- ✅ **At least 11 out of 12 months enrolled**
- ✅ **No gap > 45 days**

This is often called:

👉 **"11-of-12 continuous enrollment with allowable gap"**

🧠 **Why This Matters (Strategically)**

Think of CE as a **denominator gatekeeper**:

Without CE	**With CE**
Inflated denominator	Accurate population
False poor performance	True quality signal
Measure instability	Measure reliability

👉 This is why your scenario emphasizes:

"Build once, reuse across 30+ measures"

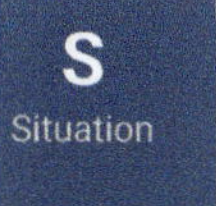

The quality team is building the HEDIS denominator table. Every HEDIS measure that requires 11-of-12 continuous enrollment must be pre-filtered using a CE flag before measure-specific logic is applied. Building this as a reusable table prevents redundant recalculation across 30+ measures.

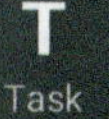

Scalable across measures

Used in:

- Preventive care measures
- Chronic condition adherence
- Utilization-based metrics

🎯 **Objective**

Build a reusable **member-level continuous enrollment table** for measurement year 2024 to support all HEDIS measures requiring:

- ≥ 11 enrolled months
- No single gap > 45 days

ANSI SQL — Scenario 6.1: Continuous Enrollment Flag

```
/* ================================================================
   SCENARIO 6.1 — CONTINUOUS ENROLLMENT FLAG (HEDIS)

   PURPOSE:
   Create a reusable member-level table to determine whether
   a member meets HEDIS continuous enrollment (CE) criteria
   for measurement year 2024.

   OUTPUT:
   - member_id
   - enrolled_month_count (0–12)
   - max_gap_days
   - ce_flag (1 = meets CE, 0 = does not)

   HEDIS RULE:
   - Must be enrolled ≥ 11 months
   - No single enrollment gap > 45 days
   ================================================================ */

WITH clean_spans AS (

    /* ------------------------------------------------------------
       STEP 1: CLEAN & DEDUPLICATE ELIGIBILITY SPANS

       PROBLEM:
       Eligibility data often contains:
       - Duplicate rows
       - Overlapping spans
       - Retroactive updates

       SOLUTION:
       Keep the most reliable version of each coverage span
       using ROW_NUMBER().

       LOGIC:
       - Partition by member + start date
       - Keep the latest record (based on end date + load timestamp)
       - Replace NULL end dates with end of measurement year
       ------------------------------------------------------------ */

    SELECT
        member_id,
        plan_id,
        coverage_start_date,
        COALESCE(coverage_end_date, DATE '2024-12-31') AS coverage_end_date
    FROM (
```

```
        SELECT
            *,
            ROW_NUMBER() OVER (
                PARTITION BY member_id, coverage_start_date
                ORDER BY coverage_end_date DESC NULLS LAST,
                         load_timestamp DESC
            ) AS rn
        FROM fact_eligibility
    ) r
    WHERE rn = 1
),

enrolled_months AS (

    /* --------------------------------------------------------
       STEP 2: CALCULATE ENROLLED MONTHS

       PURPOSE:
       Count how many distinct calendar months a member was enrolled.

       TECHNIQUE:
       - Join to a date dimension table
       - Count only the FIRST day of each month
         → ensures 1 count per month

       WHY THIS WORKS:
       If a member is enrolled on the 1st of the month,
       the entire month is considered covered (HEDIS standard approximation).

       OUTPUT:
       - One row per member
       - enrolled_month_count (0–12)
       -------------------------------------------------------- */

    SELECT
        e.member_id,
        COUNT(DISTINCT EXTRACT(MONTH FROM d.date_key)) AS enrolled_month_count
    FROM clean_spans e
    JOIN dim_date d
      ON d.date_key BETWEEN e.coverage_start_date AND e.coverage_end_date
    WHERE d.calendar_year = 2024
      AND d.calendar_day_of_month = 1   -- ensures one record per month
    GROUP BY e.member_id
),

gap_analysis AS (

    /* --------------------------------------------------------
       STEP 3: IDENTIFY MAXIMUM ENROLLMENT GAP

       PURPOSE:
       Measure the largest break in coverage between consecutive spans.

       LOGIC:
       - Use LAG() to access prior coverage_end_date
       - Compute gap:
           gap_days = (current_start - prior_end - 1)
```

```
   IMPORTANT:
   - Subtract 1 to exclude adjacent days
   - Ignore first span (no prior coverage to compare)

   OUTPUT:
   - One row per member
   - max_gap_days
   ------------------------------------------------------------ */

  SELECT
    member_id,
    MAX(DATEDIFF('day', prior_end, coverage_start_date) - 1) AS max_gap_days
  FROM (
    SELECT
      member_id,
      coverage_start_date,
      LAG(coverage_end_date) OVER (
        PARTITION BY member_id
        ORDER BY coverage_start_date
      ) AS prior_end
    FROM clean_spans
    WHERE coverage_start_date BETWEEN DATE '2024-01-01'
                                  AND DATE '2024-12-31'
  ) g
  WHERE prior_end IS NOT NULL   -- exclude first span
  GROUP BY member_id
)

/* ------------------------------------------------------------
  STEP 4: FINAL CE FLAG ASSIGNMENT

  RULE:
  Member meets continuous enrollment if:
  - enrolled_month_count ≥ 11
  - max_gap_days ≤ 45

  NOTES:
  - COALESCE handles members with no gaps (assume 0 gap)
  - LEFT JOIN ensures all members with enrollment are retained
  ------------------------------------------------------------ */

SELECT
  em.member_id,
  em.enrolled_month_count,
  COALESCE(ga.max_gap_days, 0) AS max_gap_days,

  CASE
    WHEN em.enrolled_month_count >= 11
     AND COALESCE(ga.max_gap_days, 0) <= 45
    THEN 1
    ELSE 0
  END AS ce_flag

FROM enrolled_months em
LEFT JOIN gap_analysis ga
 ON em.member_id = ga.member_id;
```

R
Result

Store result as CE_FLAG_2024. Every HEDIS query then joins: AND ce.ce_flag = 1. Building this once and reusing across 30+ measures eliminates the risk of inconsistent denominator logic between measures — the single most common source of HEDIS rate discrepancies between the quality team and the plan's HEDIS vendor.

The query creates a **member-level table**:

👉 **CE_FLAG_2024**

member_id	enrolled_month_count	max_gap_days	ce_flag
1001	12	0	1
1002	11	30	1
1003	11	60	0
1004	8	10	0

Column Meaning:

- **member_id** → Unique member
- **enrolled_month_count** → How many months enrolled in 2024 (0–12)
- **max_gap_days** → Largest break in coverage
- **ce_flag** →
  - 1 = meets HEDIS continuous enrollment
  - 0 = does NOT qualify

1. 🧱 You've Created a "Denominator Gatekeeper"

Every HEDIS measure has:

- **Denominator** → who is eligible
- **Numerator** → who received the care

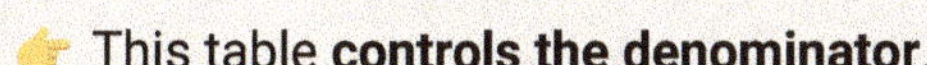

👉 This table **controls the denominator**.

Without it:

- You include ineligible members
- Your rates become unreliable

2. 🔁 Reuse Across 30+ Measures

Examples of measures that depend on this:

- Preventive screenings
- Diabetes care
- Medication adherence
- Utilization metrics

Scenario 6.2 · Care Management / Network

Member Attribution to Primary Care Provider

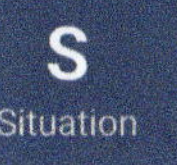

S
Situation

The care management team needs a current PCP attribution table to route gap-in-care outreach to the correct provider. Attribution uses plurality-of-primary-care-visits over the trailing 18 months.

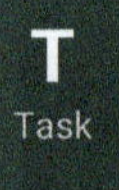

For each member, identify the PCP with the plurality of E&M visits in the trailing 18 months. Break ties by most recent visit date, then by highest allowed amount. Include attribution confidence (attributed visits / total PCP visits).

ANSI SQL — Scenario 6.2: PCP Attribution

```
-- Member-to-PCP attribution: plurality of primary care visits, 18-month window
WITH pcp_visits AS (
  SELECT c.member_id, c.rendering_npi,
      COUNT(DISTINCT c.claim_id)  AS visit_count,
      MAX(c.service_date)         AS most_recent_visit,
      SUM(c.allowed_amount)       AS total_allowed
  FROM  fact_medical_claims c
  JOIN  dim_providers p ON c.rendering_npi = p.npi
  WHERE c.claim_status    = 'PAID'
   AND c.procedure_code  IN ('99202','99203','99204','99205',
               '99211','99212','99213','99214','99215')
   AND p.specialty_group IN ('Primary Care','Internal Medicine',
               'Family Medicine','General Practice')
   AND c.service_date   >= CURRENT_DATE - INTERVAL '18' MONTH
),
member_totals AS (
  SELECT member_id, SUM(visit_count) AS total_pcp_visits
  FROM  pcp_visits GROUP BY member_id
),
ranked AS (
  SELECT pv.*,
      mt.total_pcp_visits,
      ROUND(100.0*pv.visit_count/NULLIF(mt.total_pcp_visits,0),1) AS attribution_pct,
      ROW_NUMBER() OVER (
        PARTITION BY pv.member_id
        -- Plurality: most visits; tie-break: most recent, then highest $
        ORDER BY pv.visit_count DESC, pv.most_recent_visit DESC,
            pv.total_allowed DESC
      ) AS rn
  FROM  pcp_visits pv
  JOIN  member_totals mt ON pv.member_id = mt.member_id
)
SELECT
  r.member_id,
  r.rendering_npi          AS attributed_pcp_npi,
  p.provider_full_name     AS attributed_pcp_name,
  r.visit_count            AS attributed_visits,
  r.total_pcp_visits,
  r.attribution_pct        AS attribution_confidence_pct,
  CASE WHEN r.attribution_pct < 50
    THEN 'LOW — member sees multiple PCPs'
    ELSE 'Strong' END      AS attribution_quality
FROM  ranked r
JOIN  dim_providers p ON r.rendering_npi = p.npi
WHERE r.rn = 1;
```

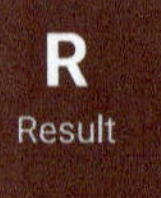

Attribution confidence < 50% flags members who split care across multiple providers — they are the highest-risk for care fragmentation and should be prioritized for PCP assignment in care management programs. Update dim_members.attributed_pcp_npi from this result monthly.

Chapter 6 Review

Unit Test · Key Takeaways

Answer each question before reading the explanation.

Q1. The NCQA standard for continuous enrollment in most HEDIS measures requires:

A. 12 full months of enrollment with no gaps allowed

B. 11 of 12 months enrolled AND no single gap greater than 45 days

C. 10 of 12 months enrolled with no gap greater than 60 days

D. 6 continuous months immediately preceding the measurement end date

Answer: B. *11 of 12 months with no single gap >45 days is the NCQA standard for most HEDIS measures requiring continuous enrollment. The 45-day tolerance accommodates short administrative gaps (e.g., a lapse between jobs). Measures requiring a stricter standard (no gap at all) will specify this explicitly in the technical specifications. Always check the measure-specific spec before coding the denominator.*

Q2. Retroactive eligibility changes create which data quality problem for analytics, and how is it resolved in SQL?

A. Retroactive changes add duplicate rows to dim_members which cause incorrect PMPM

B. Retroactive changes create multiple overlapping coverage spans in fact_eligibility — the same member_id appears with conflicting start/end dates. The fix: ROW_NUMBER() OVER (PARTITION BY member_id, coverage_start_date ORDER BY load_timestamp DESC) to keep the most recently loaded version of each span

C. Retroactive changes update claim statuses from DENIED to PAID, affecting PMPM calculations

D. Retroactive changes cause negative member month counts in fact_member_months

Answer: B. *When a member's eligibility is backdated, the original span and the corrected span both exist in the warehouse. Without deduplication, the member is counted twice in the enrollment denominator, understating PMPM. ROW_NUMBER with ORDER BY load_timestamp DESC NULLS LAST keeps only the most recently loaded version of each coverage_start_date, resolving the duplicate.*

Q3. PCP attribution uses plurality of primary care visits over 18 months. What does "plurality" mean and why is 18 months used instead of 12?

A. Plurality means the majority — over 50% of visits must be to one PCP

B. Plurality means the most visits — even if a PCP accounts for 30% of all primary care visits, they are attributed if no other PCP has more. 18 months is used to capture enough visit history for members who see a PCP infrequently (e.g., once or twice a year)

C. Plurality means the most recent provider — the last PCP seen within 12 months

D. Plurality means the highest-paid provider in the network

Answer: B. *Plurality = the most, not the majority. A member who sees PCP A 3 times and PCP B 2 times is attributed to PCP A (3 > 2) even though PCP A accounts for only 60% of visits. 18 months captures members who have annual or biannual PCP visits — using 12 months would leave a large portion of the population unattributed due to insufficient visit history.*

Q4. The continuous enrollment SQL uses AND d.calendar_day_of_month = 1 in the dim_date join. What is the purpose of this condition?

A. To filter results to show only enrollment data from the first of each month

B. To count each calendar month exactly once — if the member was enrolled on the first of the month they get 1 count for that month, preventing a 31-day month from counting 31 times instead of 1

C. To ensure the query only runs at the beginning of each month

D. To filter to members enrolled on January 1st only

Answer: B. *Without this filter, a member enrolled for 31 days in January would get 31 counts of January in the DATE_TRUNC GROUP BY — meaning COUNT(DISTINCT MONTH) would still work correctly with DATE_TRUNC but the intermediate join produces 31 rows for January. The day_of_month = 1 filter creates exactly one row per month per member, making the COUNT(DISTINCT MONTH) clean and efficient.*

Q5. In the PCP attribution query, ROW_NUMBER() OVER (PARTITION BY member_id ORDER BY visit_count DESC, most_recent_visit DESC, total_allowed DESC) achieves which result?

A. It counts the number of unique PCPs for each member

B. It ranks each member-PCP pair so that rank 1 is the most-visited PCP (primary tie-break: visit count; secondary: most recent visit; tertiary: highest spend) — WHERE rn = 1 then selects only the attributed PCP

C. It calculates the percentage of visits attributed to each PCP

D. It assigns a sequential number to each member for reporting purposes

Answer: B. *ROW_NUMBER assigns rank 1 to the member-PCP pair with the highest visit count. If two PCPs have the same visit count, the tie is broken by most_recent_visit (more recently seen PCP wins). If that also ties, total_allowed breaks the final tie. WHERE rn = 1 in the outer query selects exactly one PCP per member — the attributed provider.*

Q6. A member has attribution_confidence_pct of 38% to PCP A. What does this mean analytically?

A. The attribution algorithm is 38% confident in the assignment and it may be wrong

B. The member distributed their primary care visits across multiple providers — PCP A received 38% of total primary care visits, meaning 62% went to other PCPs. This is a low-confidence attribution that should be flagged for care management review

C. The member has been enrolled for only 38% of the 18-month attribution window

D. Only 38% of the member's claims were classified as primary care E&M visits

Answer: B. *Attribution_confidence_pct = visit_count_to_attributed_pcp / total_pcp_visits × 100. A member with 38% confidence sees multiple PCPs — they may lack a true medical home. These members are candidates for care management outreach to establish a primary care relationship. Plans that pay PCPs based on attributed panel size must monitor attribution confidence to ensure panel assignments reflect real care relationships.*

Q7. Explain continuous enrollment in the context of HEDIS measures. Why does NCQA require it, and what would happen to a HEDIS rate if the CE filter were removed from the denominator?

(Short answer)

Sample Answer:
NCQA requires continuous enrollment (CE) for most HEDIS measures because quality measurement is only valid for members who had consistent access to care throughout the measurement year. A member enrolled for only 2 months cannot reasonably be expected to have completed an annual screening or received a follow-up visit that requires year-round access. CE ensures the denominator includes only members who had a full opportunity to receive the measured service. The 11-of-12 months standard (with a 45-day gap tolerance) balances completeness against excluding members with short administrative gaps. Impact of removing CE filter: the denominator would include members who enrolled mid-year, who transferred between plans, and who had coverage lapses. These members had less opportunity to complete the measured service. Their inclusion in the denominator would dilute the rate — making a plan appear to have lower quality performance than it actually achieved for consistently-enrolled members. The denominator would be larger with the same numerator, producing an artificially lower rate. NCQA would reject data submissions built without the CE filter.

Q8. Describe the retroactive eligibility problem and write the SQL deduplication pattern that resolves it.

(Short answer)

Sample Answer:
Retroactive eligibility (retro-eligibility) occurs when a member's coverage start or end date is changed after the fact — for example, when an employer reports a new hire late, or when a state Medicaid agency backdates eligibility for a newly enrolled member. This creates duplicate coverage spans in fact_eligibility: the original span (with the wrong dates) and the corrected span (with the retroactively applied dates) both exist in the table. If both are used in member month generation or CE calculations, the member may appear enrolled in months they were not, or appear enrolled twice in some months, corrupting the denominator. SQL deduplication pattern: SELECT member_id, plan_id, coverage_start_date, COALESCE(coverage_end_date, DATE '2024-12-31') AS coverage_end_date FROM (SELECT *, ROW_NUMBER() OVER (PARTITION BY member_id, coverage_start_date ORDER BY coverage_end_date DESC NULLS LAST, load_timestamp DESC) AS rn FROM fact_eligibility) r WHERE rn = 1. This keeps the most recently loaded version of each (member_id, coverage_start_date) pair — the most recent load is assumed to be the correct retroactive correction. The clean_spans CTE should be the first step in every eligibility-based query.

Q9. Explain the PCP attribution plurality rule and describe the SQL changes needed to implement a different attribution model: "most recent visit in the last 12 months."

(Short answer)

Sample Answer:
Plurality rule: attribute the member to the PCP who received the most primary care E&M visits in the prior 18 months. If two PCPs tie on visit count, break the tie by most recent visit date, then by total allowed spend. The plurality rule is the most common attribution methodology for commercial plans and is used by CMS for ACO attribution. SQL changes for "most recent visit in 12 months" model: (1) Change the date filter from CURRENT_DATE - INTERVAL '18 months' to CURRENT_DATE - INTERVAL '12 months'. (2) Change the ROW_NUMBER ORDER BY from visit_count DESC, most_recent_visit DESC to most_recent_visit DESC, visit_count DESC. This promotes recency as the primary criterion: the member is attributed to whichever PCP they saw most recently, regardless of how many visits went to other providers. (3) Add AND visit_count >= 1 to the outer WHERE clause to ensure at least one visit exists in the window. Practical consideration: the recency model is more appropriate for attribution programs focused on transitions of care or new patient populations, while the plurality model is

better for established panel management. Both require a minimum attribution window — members with zero primary care visits in the window cannot be attributed to any PCP.

Q10. Write the CE flag SQL logic that implements the NCQA standard and explain each condition. Then describe one HEDIS measure that requires a stricter CE standard than the standard 11/12 months.

(Short answer)

Sample Answer:

CE flag SQL: CASE WHEN em.enrolled_month_count >= 11 AND COALESCE(ga.max_gap_days, 0) <= 45 THEN 1 ELSE 0 END AS ce_flag. Condition 1 — enrolled_month_count >= 11: member must have been enrolled on the first day of at least 11 of the 12 calendar months in the measurement year. A member enrolled January through November meets this (11 months). A member enrolled February through December also meets this (11 months). A member enrolled only January through September does not (9 months). Condition 2 — max_gap_days <= 45: even if enrolled 11 months, the member must not have had any single coverage gap greater than 45 days. A member enrolled January through May, then July through December (June gap = 30 days) would meet both criteria. A member enrolled January through April, then July through December (May-June gap = 61 days) would fail condition 2. COALESCE(ga.max_gap_days, 0): members with no gaps have no row in gap_analysis; COALESCE converts NULL to 0. Stricter CE example: the Diabetes Care measures (CDC-H) in some state Medicaid programs require 12 of 12 months enrolled with no gaps at all — the full-year enrollment standard — because the clinical interventions being measured (HbA1c, eye exam, nephropathy screening) require a full year of access. Check the measure-specific HEDIS technical specification for the exact enrollment requirement.

Key Takeaways

What every analyst must remember from this chapter.

1 NCQA continuous enrollment standard: 11 of 12 months enrolled AND no single gap > 45 days. Always apply CE filter before building HEDIS denominators — failure to do so produces artificially low rates that NCQA will reject.

2 Retroactive eligibility creates duplicate coverage spans. Always deduplicate with ROW_NUMBER() OVER (PARTITION BY member_id, coverage_start_date ORDER BY load_timestamp DESC) as the first CTE in every eligibility-based query.

3 PCP attribution = plurality of primary care E&M visits (99202–99215) in the prior 18 months. Tie-break order: (1) visit count, (2) most recent visit date, (3) highest spend. WHERE rn = 1 in the outer query selects exactly one PCP per member.

4 Attribution confidence = visits to attributed PCP / total primary care visits × 100. Members with < 50% confidence see multiple providers and lack a true medical home. Flag them for care management outreach.

5 The ce_flag = 1 SQL logic: enrolled_month_count >= 11 AND COALESCE(max_gap_days, 0) <= 45. Use this flag as a join filter on every HEDIS denominator query: WHERE ce.ce_flag = 1.

6 LAG() OVER (PARTITION BY member_id ORDER BY coverage_start_date) retrieves the prior coverage span's end date for each member. Using this to calculate gap_days and MAX(gap_days) per member identifies the worst enrollment gap — the field used in the CE gap condition.

7 The calendar_day_of_month = 1 filter in the CE enrolled_month_count CTE ensures exactly one count per calendar month per member. Without it, a 31-day month creates 31 intermediate rows — though COUNT(DISTINCT MONTH) handles this, the filter makes the logic explicit and efficient.

8 Primary care E&M CPT codes for attribution: new patient (99202, 99203, 99204, 99205) and established patient (99211, 99212, 99213, 99214, 99215). Specialty group filter: Primary Care, Internal Medicine, Family Medicine, General Practice. Exclude specialist E&M visits — they are not primary care.

Chapter 7: Medicare & Medicaid Analytics

Government health programs — Medicare and Medicaid — operate under a dense layer of federal and state regulation that shapes every analytical decision. For Medicare Advantage, HCC risk adjustment determines how much CMS pays the plan each month — making accurate diagnosis capture a direct revenue function. For Medicaid managed care, capitation reconciliation protects against both underpayment and overpayment risk. This chapter covers the analytical mechanics of both programs, including the HCC RAF calculation, RADV audit preparation, dual-eligible stratification, and Medicaid capitation reconciliation.

7.1 Medicare Analytics Overview

Medicare is the federal health insurance program for Americans 65 and older, as well as younger individuals with qualifying disabilities and End-Stage Renal Disease. For an MA plan, the analyst's primary financial function is risk adjustment: ensuring that every valid HCC diagnosis code present in the medical record is captured in claims data and submitted to CMS, because each captured HCC increases the plan's monthly revenue.

Program	Coverage	How plan is paid	Analyst's primary focus
Original Medicare (FFS)	All Medicare benefits, no network restriction	CMS pays providers directly — plan is not involved	Not applicable for MA plan analysts
Medicare Advantage (Part C)	A+B benefits via private plan	Monthly capitation = Benchmark × RAF × (1 + Quality Bonus)	HCC capture, RAF accuracy, quality bonus maintenance
Medicare Part D (PDP / MA-PD)	Prescription drug benefit	Per-member subsidy + catastrophic reinsurance	PDC drug adherence, medication therapy management, LIS
Medicare Supplement (Medigap)	Cost-sharing wrap for FFS beneficiaries	Premium-based, pays after Medicare	Claims reconciliation, COB with Original Medicare

7.2 HCC Risk Adjustment — The Financial Engine of Medicare Advantage

The Hierarchical Condition Category (HCC) model is the mechanism CMS uses to adjust monthly payments to MA plans based on member health status. A member with multiple chronic conditions generates a higher RAF score — and therefore higher monthly revenue — than a healthy member. The MA plan's role is to ensure all valid diagnoses present in the medical record are submitted to CMS through claims or encounter data.

For the analyst, HCC risk adjustment involves three sequential steps: collecting all diagnosis codes from claims, mapping those diagnoses to HCC categories using the CMS HCC reference table, applying the hierarchy rules that prevent double-counting within disease families, and then summing the coefficients to calculate the member's RAF score.

ANSI SQL — 7.1 Scenario: HCC RAF Score Calculation from Claims

```
-- HCC RAF Score Calculation — collects all dx from claims, maps to HCC, applies hierarchy
WITH all_diagnoses AS (
  -- Collect all diagnosis positions from each claim (primary + secondary)
  SELECT DISTINCT c.member_id, dx.diag_code
  FROM  fact_medical_claims c
  CROSS JOIN LATERAL (
    VALUES (c.primary_diag),(c.secondary_diag_1),(c.secondary_diag_2),
        (c.secondary_diag_3),(c.secondary_diag_4),(c.secondary_diag_5)
  ) AS dx(diag_code)
  WHERE c.claim_status = 'PAID'
   AND c.plan_type    = 'MA'
   AND EXTRACT(YEAR FROM c.service_date) = EXTRACT(YEAR FROM CURRENT_DATE)
   AND diag_code IS NOT NULL
),
hcc_mapped AS (
  -- Map ICD-10 diagnoses to HCC categories
  SELECT DISTINCT ad.member_id, m.hcc_category
  FROM  all_diagnoses ad
  JOIN  ref_icd10_hcc_mapping m ON ad.diag_code = m.icd10_code
  WHERE m.model_year = EXTRACT(YEAR FROM CURRENT_DATE)
),
hierarchy_applied AS (
  -- Apply hierarchy: within each disease family, keep only highest-severity HCC
  -- e.g., HCC 17 (DM with acute complications) supersedes HCC 19 (DM w/o complications)
  SELECT DISTINCT hm.member_id, hm.hcc_category
  FROM  hcc_mapped hm
  JOIN  ref_hcc h ON hm.hcc_category = h.hcc_category
  WHERE NOT EXISTS (
    -- Exclude if a higher-severity HCC in same family is also present
    SELECT 1 FROM hcc_mapped hm2
    JOIN ref_hcc h2 ON hm2.hcc_category = h2.hcc_category
    WHERE hm2.member_id   = hm.member_id
     AND h2.disease_family = h.disease_family
     AND h2.severity_rank  > h.severity_rank
  )
),
raf_calculation AS (
  SELECT
    ha.member_id,
    -- Sum HCC coefficients across all hierarchy-adjusted HCCs
    SUM(h.hcc_coefficient)  AS disease_raf,
    COUNT(DISTINCT ha.hcc_category) AS hcc_count
  FROM  hierarchy_applied ha
  JOIN  ref_hcc h ON ha.hcc_category = h.hcc_category
  GROUP BY ha.member_id
)
SELECT
  m.member_id,
  m.demo_raf_score,           -- CMS demographic component
  COALESCE(r.disease_raf, 0)   AS disease_raf,
  COALESCE(r.hcc_count, 0)     AS hcc_count,
  -- Total RAF = demographic + disease (simplified — actual model more complex)
  ROUND(m.demo_raf_score + COALESCE(r.disease_raf, 0), 4) AS total_raf_score,
  -- Estimated monthly capitation
```

```
  ROUND(cb.benchmark_pmpm
    * (m.demo_raf_score + COALESCE(r.disease_raf, 0)), 2) AS est_monthly_cap
FROM dim_members        m
LEFT JOIN raf_calculation  r ON m.member_id  = r.member_id
JOIN ref_county_benchmarks cb ON m.county_fips = cb.county_fips
WHERE m.plan_type = 'MA'
 AND m.coverage_status = 'ACTIVE';
```

Revenue implication: A member with RAF 1.0 generates the county benchmark PMPM. A member with RAF 2.0 generates 2× the benchmark. For a plan with 50,000 MA members at a $900 benchmark PMPM, a 0.10 RAF improvement across the population equals $900 × 0.10 × 50,000 = $4.5M annually. HCC capture is not just a data quality function — it is a direct revenue function.

7.3 The RAPS/EDPS Submission Cycle

Medicare Advantage plans submit risk adjustment diagnoses to CMS through two systems: the Risk Adjustment Processing System (RAPS) for historical data and the Encounter Data Processing System (EDPS) for encounter-level submissions. CMS uses these submissions to calculate the plan's risk scores for the following payment year.

System	What is submitted	Submission window	Payment year impact
RAPS (legacy)	Diagnosis clusters: member + HCC category + date of service	January–September of payment year	Feeds risk score calculation for following January payment adjustment
EDPS (encounter data)	Full encounter records: all claims with all diagnoses	Ongoing — 3-year look-back	Primary data source since 2020; RAPS being phased out
RADV (audit)	Medical records validating submitted HCCs	CMS-selected audit year	Invalid HCCs trigger payment recoveries — exposure = coefficient × benchmark × 12 months
ODAG (appeals)	Organization determination appeals and grievances	Ongoing regulatory reporting	Not risk adjustment — separate CMS reporting requirement

7.4 Medicare & Medicaid Scenarios

Scenario 7.1 · Government Programs / Care Management

Dual-Eligible Member Identification & Stratification

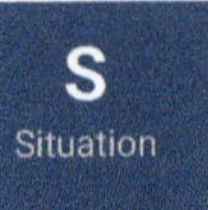

The care management director needs to identify all dual-eligible members (enrolled in both Medicare Advantage and Medicaid) and stratify them by dual status category. Full duals qualify for different care management programs and financial coordination than partial duals.

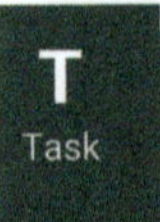

Identify current MA enrollees who also have active Medicaid eligibility. Classify each as Full Dual, Partial Dual (QMB+/SLMB+), QMB Only, or Other Medicaid. Output: stratified list with benefit categories and care management flags.

ANSI SQL — Scenario 7.1: Dual-Eligible Member Identification

```sql
-- Identify and stratify dual-eligible members (MA + Medicaid)
WITH ma_enrolled AS (
  SELECT e.member_id, e.plan_id, m.date_of_birth, m.gender_code
  FROM  fact_eligibility e
  JOIN  dim_members m ON e.member_id = m.member_id
  JOIN  dim_plans  pl ON e.plan_id  = pl.plan_id
  WHERE pl.plan_type = 'MA'
   AND e.coverage_start_date <= CURRENT_DATE
   AND COALESCE(e.coverage_end_date, DATE '9999-12-31') >= CURRENT_DATE
),
medicaid_status AS (
  SELECT me.member_id,
      CASE
        WHEN me.medicaid_benefit_category IN ('A','B','C','D') THEN 'FULL DUAL'
        WHEN me.medicaid_benefit_category IN ('QMB+','SLMB+','QI') THEN 'PARTIAL DUAL'
        WHEN me.medicaid_benefit_category = 'QMB' THEN 'QMB ONLY'
        ELSE 'OTHER MEDICAID'
      END AS dual_status
  FROM  medicaid_eligibility me
  WHERE me.effective_date <= CURRENT_DATE
   AND COALESCE(me.end_date, DATE '9999-12-31') >= CURRENT_DATE
)
SELECT
  ma.member_id,
  ms.dual_status,
  DATEDIFF('year', ma.date_of_birth, CURRENT_DATE) AS age,
  ma.gender_code,
  CASE
    WHEN ms.dual_status = 'FULL DUAL' THEN 'D-SNP Eligible — High Priority'
    WHEN ms.dual_status = 'PARTIAL DUAL' THEN 'Enhanced Benefits Eligible'
    WHEN ms.dual_status = 'QMB ONLY' THEN 'Cost-Sharing Subsidy Only'
    ELSE 'Medicaid Coordination — Review'
  END AS care_management_flag
FROM  ma_enrolled ma
JOIN  medicaid_status ms ON ma.member_id = ms.member_id
ORDER BY ms.dual_status, ma.member_id;
```

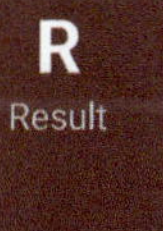

Full duals should be enrolled in the plan's D-SNP (Dual Special Needs Plan) program if available — they qualify for enhanced coordination of Medicare and Medicaid benefits. Full duals typically have RAF scores 1.8–2.5× the non-dual MA average. Any full dual not enrolled in a care management program represents a gap in both clinical and financial risk management.

Scenario 7.2 · Government Programs / Finance

Medicaid Capitation Reconciliation

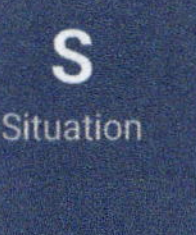

The finance team receives the monthly state Medicaid capitation payment file 5 days before processing. They need to identify discrepancies between the state's payment roster and the plan's eligibility roster before the payment is finalized — catching both overpayments (state pays for members not in the plan) and underpayments (plan has members the state is not paying for).

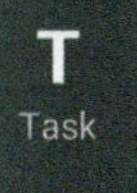

Reconcile the monthly Medicaid capitation payment file against the plan's active Medicaid enrollment. Categorize each discrepancy as PAYMENT_ONLY (overpayment risk), ELIGIBILITY_ONLY (underpayment), or MATCHED. Quantify financial exposure by rate cell.

ANSI SQL — Scenario 7.2: Medicaid Capitation Reconciliation

```
-- Medicaid capitation reconciliation: payment file vs. eligibility roster
-- FULL OUTER JOIN exposes both directions of discrepancy
WITH capitation AS (
  SELECT member_id, capitation_amount, rate_cell_code
  FROM  medicaid_capitation_payment
  WHERE payment_month = EXTRACT(YEAR FROM CURRENT_DATE) * 100
             + EXTRACT(MONTH FROM CURRENT_DATE)
),
mcaid_eligible AS (
  SELECT DISTINCT e.member_id, pl.rate_cell_code
  FROM  fact_eligibility e
  JOIN  dim_plans pl ON e.plan_id = pl.plan_id
  WHERE pl.plan_type = 'MCAID'
   AND e.coverage_start_date <= CURRENT_DATE
   AND COALESCE(e.coverage_end_date, DATE '9999-12-31') >= CURRENT_DATE
)
SELECT
  CASE
    WHEN c.member_id IS NULL  THEN 'ELIGIBILITY_ONLY — potential underpayment'
    WHEN me.member_id IS NULL THEN 'PAYMENT_ONLY — potential overpayment'
    ELSE                      'MATCHED'
  END                         AS reconciliation_status,
  COALESCE(c.rate_cell_code, me.rate_cell_code) AS rate_cell,
  COUNT(*)                      AS member_count,
  SUM(COALESCE(c.capitation_amount, 0))  AS total_capitation,
  CASE
    WHEN c.member_id IS NULL  THEN 'Contact state — missing from payment file'
    WHEN me.member_id IS NULL THEN 'Report to state — not in our eligibility'
    ELSE 'No action required'
  END                         AS action_required
FROM  capitation c
FULL OUTER JOIN mcaid_eligible me ON c.member_id = me.member_id
GROUP BY 1, 2, 5
ORDER BY member_count DESC;
```

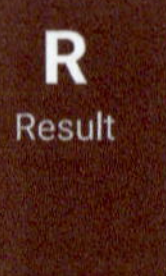

R Result

PAYMENT_ONLY records are the highest priority: the state is paying the plan for members who are not in the plan's eligibility — this is a regulatory compliance issue requiring same-day reporting to the state. ELIGIBILITY_ONLY records are underpayment risk: the plan has enrolled members the state has not included in the payment file. Resolve both categories before the payment processing deadline. MATCHED records require no action.

Chapter 7 Review

Unit Test · Key Takeaways

Answer each question before reading the explanation.

Q1. What is the HCC hierarchy rule and why is it essential for correct RAF calculation?

A. HCCs are ranked alphabetically; only the first HCC in each alphabet group is counted

B. Within each disease family, only the highest-severity HCC is counted. If a member has both HCC 17 (DM with acute complications) and HCC 19 (DM without complications), only HCC 17 is included — HCC 19 is superseded

C. The hierarchy assigns each member a maximum of 5 HCCs regardless of how many conditions they have

D. HCCs are applied hierarchically by data source: claims-based HCCs supersede encounter-based HCCs

Answer: B. *Without hierarchy, a member who has both HCC 17 and HCC 19 documented in their claims would have both coefficients counted — double-counting the diabetes disease burden. The hierarchy rule says: within each disease family group, count only the HCC with the highest severity rank. NOT EXISTS is the SQL pattern: exclude any HCC where a higher-severity sibling in the same disease_family is also present for the same member.*

Q2. The RAPS/EDPS encounter submission cycle matters for MA plan revenue because:

A. RAPS is required for Medicaid encounter submission to state agencies

B. CMS uses RAPS and EDPS encounter data to validate and finalize each member's RAF score — incomplete encounter submission means some HCCs are never validated by CMS, reducing the member's final RAF and therefore the plan's monthly capitation

C. RAPS submission is required only for dual-eligible members

D. EDPS replaces the 837 claim transaction for Medicare Advantage plans

Answer: B. *The RAPS/EDPS cycle: plans submit RAPS (Risk Adjustment Processing System) data to CMS containing the diagnoses from encounters. CMS validates them and uses them in the annual HCC risk adjustment sweep (January final, mid-year prospective). If encounter submission is incomplete, diagnoses are missing, HCC coefficients are lower, RAF scores are lower, and monthly capitation is lower — a direct revenue leak that can be measured and corrected.*

Q3. A dual-eligible member with medicaid_benefit_category = 'QMB' (Qualified Medicare Beneficiary) is classified as:

A. Full Dual — eligible for full Medicaid benefits and D-SNP enrollment

B. QMB Only — Medicaid pays Medicare cost-sharing (premiums, deductibles, copays) but the member does not receive full Medicaid benefits

C. Partial Dual — eligible for some Medicaid benefits but not full Medicaid

D. Medicaid-only — not enrolled in Medicare

Answer: B. *QMB = Qualified Medicare Beneficiary. Medicaid pays the member's Medicare Part A and B premiums, deductibles, and cost-sharing — but the member does not receive full Medicaid benefits (no LTSS, no full Medicaid benefit package). This is different from Full Dual (categories A/B/C/D) who receive both full Medicare and full Medicaid. The dual_status classification drives care management program assignments and D-SNP eligibility screening.*

Q4. In the HCC RAF calculation SQL, CROSS JOIN LATERAL with VALUES() is used to unpivot diagnosis columns. What problem does this solve?

A. It creates one row per claim for efficiency

B. Healthcare claims store diagnoses in multiple columns (primary_diag, secondary_diag_1 through 5) rather than rows. CROSS JOIN LATERAL unpivots these 6 columns into individual rows so each diagnosis can be joined to the HCC mapping table — without it each diagnosis column would require a separate JOIN

C. It prevents duplicate HCCs from being counted twice

D. It filters out NULL diagnosis codes automatically

Answer: B. *Without unpivoting, mapping 6 diagnosis columns to HCCs would require 6 separate LEFT JOINs to ref_icd10_hcc_mapping — once per diagnosis position. CROSS JOIN LATERAL with VALUES() is the ANSI SQL 2003 approach to row-value constructor unpivoting: it produces one row per value in the VALUES list, allowing a single JOIN to handle all 6 positions. The DISTINCT in the outer SELECT then deduplicates member-diag_code pairs that appear in multiple claim positions.*

Q5. The Medicaid capitation reconciliation query uses FULL OUTER JOIN between the capitation payment file and the eligibility roster. What does each direction of mismatch indicate?

A. Left-only = member enrolled but not paid; right-only = member paid but not enrolled

B. Payment-only (capitation row exists, eligibility NULL) = potential overpayment — plan received payment for a member not in their eligibility roster; Eligibility-only (eligibility row exists, capitation NULL) = potential underpayment — member is eligible but the state did not send a capitation payment

C. Both directions indicate data corruption in the ETL pipeline

D. The FULL OUTER JOIN only returns unmatched rows; matched rows are automatically excluded

Answer: B. *FULL OUTER JOIN preserves all rows from both tables. Matched rows (member in both payment file and eligibility) = correct. Payment-only rows (member in capitation but not in eligibility) = the plan received money for a member they should not have — report to state as potential overpayment. Eligibility-only rows (member in eligibility but not in capitation) = the plan served a member without receiving payment — contact state to request the missing capitation.*

Q6. What is the difference between RADV (Risk Adjustment Data Validation) audits and routine HCC submission, and why do they matter for analytics teams?

A. RADV is a different name for the annual HCC submission to CMS; there is no difference

B. RADV is a CMS audit of a sample of MA plan members where CMS requests the medical records to verify that the documented diagnoses supporting claimed HCCs actually appear in clinical documentation. Failing RADV means HCC coefficients are extrapolated downward across the entire plan, creating a revenue repayment obligation

C. RADV is used only for Medicaid plans; HCC submission is used for MA plans
D. RADV audits occur every 5 years; routine HCC submission is annual

Answer: B. *CMS conducts RADV audits annually on a sample of MA plans and members. For each selected member, CMS requests the medical records and verifies that the diagnoses supporting HCC claims are documented by a qualified clinician in the medical record. If a high percentage of HCCs cannot be validated from medical records, CMS extrapolates the error rate across the plan's entire HCC-derived revenue and issues a repayment demand. Analytics teams support RADV by building pre-audit HCC validation queries that identify HCCs with thin documentation before CMS selects the audit sample.*

Q7. Explain the four-step HCC RAF calculation algorithm in plain language and identify the SQL function used for hierarchy application.

(Short answer)

Sample Answer:
Step 1 — Collect diagnoses: pull all diagnosis codes from all claim positions (primary + secondary 1–5) for all paid MA claims in the measurement year. Use CROSS JOIN LATERAL with VALUES() to unpivot 6 diagnosis columns into individual rows. Use SELECT DISTINCT member_id, diag_code to deduplicate. Step 2 — Map to HCC categories: JOIN the diagnosis codes to ref_icd10_hcc_mapping to convert each ICD-10 code to its HCC category. One ICD-10 may map to multiple HCCs. Use SELECT DISTINCT member_id, hcc_category to deduplicate member-HCC pairs. Step 3 — Apply hierarchy: within each disease family, exclude any HCC where a higher-severity sibling is also present for the same member. SQL function: NOT EXISTS subquery that checks for a higher severity_rank HCC in the same disease_family for the same member_id. Step 4 — Sum coefficients: join the hierarchy-applied HCC list to ref_hcc to get each HCC's coefficient. SUM(hcc_coefficient) per member = disease_raf. Total_raf = demo_raf_score + disease_raf. Estimated capitation = county_benchmark × total_raf × (1 + quality_bonus).

Q8. What is the FMAP-driven encounter submission obligation for Medicaid MCOs, and write the SQL that measures monthly encounter timeliness by service month and category?

(Short answer)

Sample Answer:
FMAP creates encounter submission obligations because federal Medicaid dollars require CMS and states to validate that services were actually delivered to enrolled members. MCOs that receive capitation payments are required to submit encounter data within defined windows (typically 90 and 180 days of service date). Plans with poor submission rates face capitation rate adjustments, enhanced audits, and in some states, contract penalties. The encounter submission rate = valid encounters submitted within window / total encounters expected. SQL for monthly timeliness by service month and category: SELECT DATE_TRUNC('month', service_date) AS svc_month, CASE WHEN claim_form_type = 'CMS1500' THEN 'Professional' WHEN type_of_bill LIKE '11%' THEN 'Inpatient' WHEN type_of_bill LIKE '13%' OR type_of_bill LIKE '14%' THEN 'Outpatient' ELSE 'Other' END AS service_category, COUNT(*) AS total_encounters, SUM(CASE WHEN DATEDIFF('day', service_date, submission_date) <= 90 THEN 1 ELSE 0 END) AS submitted_within_90, ROUND(100.0 * SUM(CASE WHEN DATEDIFF('day', service_date, submission_date) <= 90 THEN 1 ELSE 0 END) / NULLIF(COUNT(*),0), 1) AS pct_within_90d FROM medicaid_encounters WHERE service_date >= DATE_TRUNC('month', CURRENT_DATE) - INTERVAL '12 months' GROUP BY 1, 2 ORDER BY 1, 2.

Q9. Explain the dual-eligible classification tiers (Full Dual, Partial Dual, QMB, QMB-Only) and describe the care management implication of each tier.

(Short answer)

Sample Answer:
Dual-eligible classification tiers: Full Dual (medicaid_benefit_category IN ('A','B','C','D')): member receives both full Medicare and full Medicaid benefits. Eligible for D-SNP (Dual Eligible Special Needs Plan) enrollment. Receives LTSS (long-term services and supports), behavioral health services, and personal care services through Medicaid. These are the highest-need members — complex care management, often with multiple chronic conditions and social determinants of health challenges. Care implication: assign to a dedicated high-intensity care management program; D-SNP enrollment triggers additional CMS reporting requirements and quality measures. Partial Dual (SLMB+, QI): Medicaid pays a portion of Medicare cost-sharing but the member does not receive full Medicaid benefits. Care implication: monitor for cost-sharing barriers to care access; eligible for some supplemental benefits under MA plans. QMB Only (QMB without full dual): Medicaid pays Medicare Part A and B premiums, deductibles, and copays only. No full Medicaid benefits. Care implication: providers cannot bill QMB members for Medicare cost-sharing (federal law prohibits it); the plan must ensure provider billing compliance. Other Medicaid: members with Medicaid coverage that does not fit the other categories — review individually for program eligibility. Analytics use: build a monthly dual-status monitoring query that identifies members who became newly dual-eligible and flag them for D-SNP eligibility screening.

Q10. Describe the Medicaid capitation reconciliation query and explain what each FULL OUTER JOIN mismatch type means operationally. What action should an MCO analyst take for each mismatch type?

(Short answer)

> **Sample Answer:**
> The reconciliation query compares the state's monthly capitation payment file against the plan's eligibility roster. FULL OUTER JOIN: all members in either table appear in the output, with NULL in the columns of the table they are missing from. Three result types: (1) MATCHED (member appears in both): capitation received for an eligible member. No action required — this is the expected outcome for all active members. Verify that rate_cell_code matches between the two sources to confirm the correct capitation rate was applied. (2) PAYMENT_ONLY (capitation row exists, eligibility NULL): the plan received capitation for a member who is not in its eligibility roster. Operational meaning: the member may have disenrolled before the payment month, or the state's file contains an error. Action: report to the state as a potential overpayment; if confirmed, the plan must return the funds. Do not use the payment to fund services for this member. (3) ELIGIBILITY_ONLY (eligibility row exists, capitation NULL): the plan has an eligible member but received no capitation payment for them. Operational meaning: the state's payment file missed this member, or the member was added to the roster after the payment file was generated. Action: contact the state's Medicaid agency to request the missing capitation payment. Document the discrepancy for audit purposes. Run this reconciliation every month, first business day after the payment file arrives.

Key Takeaways

What every analyst must remember from this chapter.

1 HCC RAF score = demo_raf_score + SUM(hcc_coefficients) after hierarchy application. Within each disease family, only the highest-severity HCC is counted. SQL pattern: NOT EXISTS subquery to exclude HCCs where a higher severity_rank sibling exists in the same disease_family.

2 The HCC hierarchy application SQL: NOT EXISTS (SELECT 1 FROM hcc_mapped hm2 JOIN ref_hcc h2 ON hm2.hcc_category = h2.hcc_category WHERE hm2.member_id = hm.member_id AND h2.disease_family = h.disease_family AND h2.severity_rank > h.severity_rank). Memorize this pattern — it appears in every MA plan risk adjustment query.

3 CROSS JOIN LATERAL with VALUES() unpivots diagnosis columns into rows, enabling a single JOIN to map all 6 diagnosis positions to HCC categories. Without it, 6 separate LEFT JOINs are required — one per diagnosis position. Always use SELECT DISTINCT after unpivoting to deduplicate member-diagnosis pairs.

4 RAPS/EDPS encounter submission to CMS is a revenue mechanism, not just a compliance obligation. Missing HCCs from incomplete encounter submission = lower RAF scores = lower monthly capitation. Build a monthly HCC capture gap report to identify diagnoses documented in the EHR but missing from submitted encounters.

5 Full dual-eligible (Medicare + Medicaid): highest-need, highest-cost. Eligible for D-SNP. Receives LTSS through Medicaid. QMB Only: Medicaid pays Medicare cost-sharing only — providers cannot bill QMB members for Medicare cost-sharing under federal law.

6 Medicaid capitation reconciliation uses FULL OUTER JOIN. Payment-only rows = potential overpayment → report to state. Eligibility-only rows = potential underpayment → request missing payment from state. Run monthly on the first business day after the capitation payment file arrives.

7 RADV audits: CMS selects a sample of MA members and requests medical records to validate that documented diagnoses appear in clinical documentation. A high error rate extrapolates to a plan-wide revenue repayment. Analytics teams prepare by building pre-audit HCC validation queries that flag HCCs with thin or missing documentation.

8 The dual-status SQL classification: CASE WHEN medicaid_benefit_category IN ('A','B','C','D') THEN 'FULL DUAL' WHEN medicaid_benefit_category IN ('QMB+','SLMB+','QI') THEN 'PARTIAL DUAL' WHEN medicaid_benefit_category = 'QMB' THEN 'QMB ONLY' ELSE 'OTHER MEDICAID' END. Build this classification into every eligibility-based reporting query for MA plans.

PART IV: Pharmacy, PBM & Specialty Cost

Rung 4 · Chapters 8–10

Part IV enters the pharmacy and specialty cost domain — the fastest-growing component of healthcare spend and the most analytically complex. Chapter 8 builds the pharmacy analytics foundation: the NCPDP claim structure, GPI drug classification hierarchies, the PDC adherence calculation with early-refill overlap adjustment, and five production scenarios from MAD adherence to mail-order conversion. Chapter 9 opens the PBM black box — spread pricing detection using NADAC benchmarks, rebate reconciliation against contract terms, formulary tier optimization, and the full STAR scenarios that expose the financial mechanics most health plan analysts never see. Chapter 10 tackles oncology — the highest-cost, highest-complexity specialty domain — covering patient identification from claims, J-code and oral oncolytic classification, site-of-care optimization, chemotherapy regimen identification, and time-to-treatment analysis.

Chapter 8: Pharmacy Analytics & Drug Adherence

Pharmacy spend represents 20–25% of total healthcare costs for most commercial health plans — and it is growing faster than medical spend. Specialty drugs alone account for over 50% of pharmacy costs despite representing less than 2% of prescriptions. Understanding how pharmacy claims are structured, how drug classification systems work, and how to correctly measure medication adherence is essential for every analyst working in a health plan, PBM, or pharmacy benefit consulting environment.

8.1 Pharmacy Claims Data Architecture

The pharmacy claim (NCPDP transaction) is structurally different from the medical claim. It is generated in real time at the point of dispensing — when the pharmacist processes the prescription, the claim is adjudicated and paid within seconds. This produces a high-volume, clean, near-real-time dataset with a different set of analytical pitfalls than medical claims.

Field	Description	Key analytical use
ndc_code	National Drug Code — 11-digit drug identifier (labeler + product + package)	Join to ref_ndc for drug name, GPI class, brand/generic flag, specialty flag
dispensing_date	Date the drug was dispensed at the pharmacy	Use for PDC measurement period; always dispensing_date not service_date
days_supply	Number of days the dispensed quantity should last	Critical for PDC: 30-day supply fills differently than 90-day fills
quantity_dispensed	Number of units dispensed (tablets, mL, etc.)	With nadac_per_unit: calculates actual acquisition cost for spread pricing analysis
plan_paid_amount	Amount the plan paid after member cost-sharing	Use for plan cost analytics; member_cost_share is separate field

Field	Description	Key analytical use
pharmacy_npi	Dispensing pharmacy identifier	Identifies retail vs. mail vs. specialty channel; join to ref_pharmacy_channel
daw_code	Dispense As Written: 0=generic permitted, 1=brand required by prescriber	Key field for generic substitution opportunity analysis
claim_status	PAID, REVERSED, REJECTED	Always filter to PAID; pharmacy reversals are common (member returns drug)

8.2 Drug Classification Hierarchies

Understanding drug classification is essential for pharmacy analytics. Three classification systems are used depending on the analytical question:

System	What it classifies	Grain	Primary analytical use
NDC (National Drug Code)	Specific drug product: drug name, strength, manufacturer, package size	Most granular — one NDC per product/package	Drug-level cost analysis, spread pricing, drug-drug interaction detection
GPI (Generic Product Identifier)	Drug class hierarchy: 14-digit code grouping by therapeutic class → drug group → drug name	Hierarchical — first 2 digits = drug group, 4 = class, 6 = subclass, 14 = specific drug	Therapeutic class analytics, adherence grouping (statins = GPI 3940xxxx), formulary tier analysis
ATC (Anatomical Therapeutic Chemical)	WHO standard: body system → pharmacological effect → chemical group → drug	5-level hierarchy	Cross-payer benchmarking, international drug classification
Formulary tier	Plan-specific: Tier 1=generic, 2=preferred brand, 3=non-preferred brand, 4=specialty	Plan-defined	Member cost-sharing calculation, generic substitution, rebate optimization

> **GPI for HEDIS:** HEDIS medication adherence measures (MAC, MAD, MAH) specify drugs by GPI prefix — not NDC list. Statins (MAH): GPI starts with 3940. ACE inhibitors/ARBs (MAC): GPI 36 or 3610. Antidiabetic agents (MAD): GPI 27. Using GPI prefix queries is more maintainable than NDC lists — new drugs automatically fall into scope as long as they carry the correct GPI prefix.

8.3 Proportion of Days Covered (PDC) — The Gold Standard Adherence Metric

PDC is the NCQA-specified method for measuring medication adherence in HEDIS Medication Adherence measures (MAC, MAD, MAH). It measures the proportion of days in the measurement period during which the member had the drug available. A PDC of 0.80 or higher = adherent.

PDC formula: Covered days within measurement period ÷ Total days in measurement period. The measurement period starts 30 days after the member's first qualifying fill and runs through December 31 of the measurement year. The 30-day delay prevents counting the first fill's days toward the denominator until the member has demonstrated they filled a second time.

Step	What happens	SQL operation	Common error
1. Identify qualifying fills	Pull all paid claims for the drug class by GPI prefix	JOIN to ref_ndc on ndc_code; filter n.gpi_code LIKE '27%' for diabetes	Using NDC list instead of GPI — misses new drugs added mid-year
2. Set measurement window	period_start = first fill + 30 days; period_end = Dec 31	MIN(dispensing_date) + INTERVAL '30 DAY' per member	Using Jan 1 as period_start instead of 30 days after first fill
3. Adjust for early refills	Shift fill start date forward if prior fill overlaps	GREATEST(dispensing_date, LAG(fill_end) + 1 day)	Omitting overlap adjustment — PDC > 1.0 for early refill members
4. Count covered days	Days in measurement window during which drug supply existed	MIN(fill_end, period_end) - MAX(adjusted_start, period_start) + 1 per fill	Counting days outside measurement window — inflates covered days
5. Calculate PDC	Sum covered days ÷ period days	SUM(covered_days) / period_days per member	Dividing by 365 instead of actual period days — incorrect for partial-year members

8.4 Pharmacy Scenarios

Scenario 8.1 · Pharmacy / Quality

PDC for Diabetes (MAD) with Near-Threshold Identification

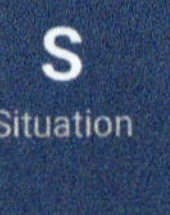

The Stars team needs the MAD (Medication Adherence for Diabetes) PDC for all commercial and MA members. More importantly, they need to identify members with PDC 70–79% — near-threshold members who need just a few additional days of supply to cross the 80% adherence threshold and move to the adherent category.

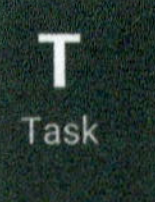

Calculate 2024 MAD PDC for each eligible member using antidiabetic GPI prefix (27xxxx). Apply early-refill overlap adjustment. Identify near-threshold members (PDC 0.70–0.79) and calculate exact days_supply_needed to reach 0.80. Output: member list sorted by PDC ascending with intervention priority flag.

ANSI SQL — Scenario 8.1: MAD PDC Calculation with Near-Threshold Flag

```
-- PURPOSE: Calculate PDC for the HEDIS Medication Adherence for Diabetes (MAD)
-- measure. PDC >= 0.80 = adherent. Members at 0.70–0.79 = near-threshold
-- (one refill closes the gap) and should receive priority outreach.
-- GPI prefix 27 = antidiabetic agents per the NCQA MAD specification.

-- STEP 1: Collect all paid antidiabetic fills for the measurement year.
-- fill_end_raw = last day the supply from this fill lasts.
WITH diabetes_fills AS (
  SELECT p.member_id, p.dispensing_date, p.days_supply,
      p.dispensing_date + (p.days_supply - 1) AS fill_end_raw
  FROM  fact_pharmacy_claims p
  JOIN  ref_ndc n ON p.ndc_code = n.ndc_code
  -- GPI prefix 27 = antidiabetic agents (includes metformin, insulin, GLP-1s, etc.)
  WHERE n.gpi_code LIKE '27%'
   AND p.claim_status = 'PAID'
   AND EXTRACT(YEAR FROM p.dispensing_date) = 2024
),
```

```
-- STEP 2: Set the measurement window.
-- NCQA: period starts 30 days after first fill (treatment initiation grace period).
-- period_days must be > 0 (excludes members whose first fill is in December).
measurement_windows AS (
  SELECT member_id,
      MIN(dispensing_date) + INTERVAL '30' DAY  AS period_start,
      DATE '2024-12-31'                    AS period_end,
      DATEDIFF('day',
        MIN(dispensing_date) + INTERVAL '30' DAY,
        DATE '2024-12-31') + 1             AS period_days
  FROM  diabetes_fills
  GROUP BY member_id
  HAVING DATEDIFF('day',
      MIN(dispensing_date) + INTERVAL '30' DAY,
      DATE '2024-12-31') + 1 > 0
),

-- STEP 3: Adjust each fill start to prevent early-refill overlap.
-- LAG() retrieves the prior fill's end date for the same member.
-- GREATEST picks whichever is later: actual dispensing date or day after prior fill ends.
adjusted_fills AS (
  SELECT f.member_id, f.dispensing_date, f.fill_end_raw,
      GREATEST(f.dispensing_date,
        COALESCE(
          LAG(f.fill_end_raw) OVER (
            PARTITION BY f.member_id ORDER BY f.dispensing_date
          ) + INTERVAL '1' DAY,  -- day after prior fill ends
          f.dispensing_date)    -- no prior fill: use actual date
      ) AS adjusted_start
  FROM  diabetes_fills f
),

-- STEP 4: Count covered days within measurement window per fill.
-- GREATEST(0,...) ensures negative intervals (fill entirely outside window) = 0.
covered_days AS (
  SELECT af.member_id,
      SUM(GREATEST(0,
        DATEDIFF('day',
          GREATEST(af.adjusted_start, mw.period_start),  -- later of two starts
          LEAST(af.fill_end_raw, mw.period_end)         -- earlier of two ends
        ) + 1  -- +1: both endpoints inclusive
      )) AS days_covered
  FROM  adjusted_fills af
  JOIN  measurement_windows mw ON af.member_id = mw.member_id
  WHERE af.adjusted_start <= mw.period_end
   AND af.fill_end_raw  >= mw.period_start
  GROUP BY af.member_id
)

-- STEP 5: Calculate PDC and classify adherence status.
-- near-threshold = 0.70–0.79 = one refill away from HEDIS compliance.
-- days_supply_needed_to_adhere = how many days of supply are needed to cross 80%.
SELECT
  cd.member_id,
  m.member_name, m.pcp_npi, m.phone_number,
  mw.period_days,
  cd.days_covered,
  ROUND(cd.days_covered * 1.0 / NULLIF(mw.period_days, 0), 3) AS pdc,
  CASE
    WHEN cd.days_covered * 1.0 / mw.period_days >= 0.80 THEN 'ADHERENT'
```

```
        WHEN cd.days_covered * 1.0 / mw.period_days >= 0.70 THEN 'NEAR-THRESHOLD -- priority outreach'
        ELSE 'NON-ADHERENT'
    END  AS adherence_status,
    -- Days of supply needed to cross the 0.80 threshold
    CASE WHEN cd.days_covered * 1.0 / mw.period_days < 0.80
        THEN GREATEST(0, CEIL(mw.period_days * 0.80) - cd.days_covered)
        ELSE 0
    END  AS days_supply_needed_to_adhere
FROM  covered_days cd
JOIN  measurement_windows mw ON cd.member_id = mw.member_id
JOIN  dim_members m ON cd.member_id = m.member_id
ORDER BY pdc ASC; -- lowest adherence first = highest outreach priority
```

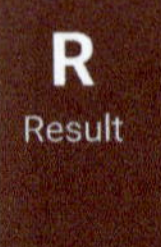

R Result

Near-threshold members (PDC 70–79%) are the highest ROI outreach target — they need only a single additional 30-day fill in most cases to cross the 80% line. The days_supply_needed column tells the pharmacist or care manager exactly what to recommend. One phone call resulting in one additional fill can move a member from non-adherent to adherent, directly improving the plan's HEDIS MAD rate and Star Rating.

Scenario 8.2 · Pharmacy / Financial

Specialty Drug Spend & Trend Analysis

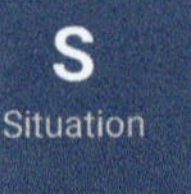

S Situation

The CFO wants to understand which specialty drug therapeutic classes are driving pharmacy cost growth year over year. Specialty drugs (formulary tier 4 or specialty_drug_flag = Y) are growing 15–20% annually and now represent the largest single pharmacy cost category.

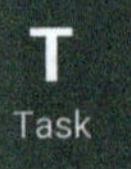

T Task

Compare specialty drug spend by therapeutic class for 2023 vs. 2024. Calculate YoY growth % and PMPM for each class. Identify the top 5 growth drivers. Output: ranked by YoY dollar growth.

ANSI SQL — Scenario 8.2: Specialty Drug Spend by Therapeutic Class

```
-- Specialty drug spend trend: 2023 vs 2024 by therapeutic class
WITH specialty_fills AS (
    SELECT p.member_id, n.therapeutic_class,
           EXTRACT(YEAR FROM p.dispensing_date) AS fill_year,
           p.allowed_amount
    FROM  fact_pharmacy_claims p
    JOIN  ref_ndc n ON p.ndc_code = n.ndc_code
    JOIN  ref_formulary f ON p.ndc_code = f.ndc_code
      AND f.formulary_year = EXTRACT(YEAR FROM p.dispensing_date)
    WHERE (f.formulary_tier = 4 OR n.specialty_drug_flag = 'Y')
      AND p.claim_status = 'PAID'
      AND EXTRACT(YEAR FROM p.dispensing_date) IN (2023, 2024)
),
class_year AS (
    SELECT therapeutic_class, fill_year,
           COUNT(DISTINCT member_id) AS member_count,
           SUM(allowed_amount)       AS total_allowed
    FROM  specialty_fills
    GROUP BY therapeutic_class, fill_year
)
SELECT
    COALESCE(cy24.therapeutic_class, cy23.therapeutic_class) AS therapeutic_class,
    ROUND(COALESCE(cy24.total_allowed,0),0) AS spend_2024,
    ROUND(COALESCE(cy23.total_allowed,0),0) AS spend_2023,
    ROUND(COALESCE(cy24.total_allowed,0) - COALESCE(cy23.total_allowed,0),0) AS yoy_growth,
```

```
    ROUND(100.0*(COALESCE(cy24.total_allowed,0)
      /NULLIF(COALESCE(cy23.total_allowed,0),0)-1),1) AS growth_pct,
    COALESCE(cy24.member_count,0) AS members_2024
FROM  class_year cy24
FULL OUTER JOIN class_year cy23
    ON cy24.therapeutic_class = cy23.therapeutic_class
   AND cy23.fill_year = 2023
WHERE cy24.fill_year = 2024 OR cy24.fill_year IS NULL
ORDER BY yoy_growth DESC
LIMIT 15;
```

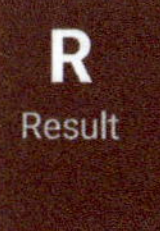

R Result

Immunology (biologics for RA, IBD, psoriasis) and oncology oral agents are typically the top growth drivers. Present to CFO: top 5 classes by dollar growth, with cost-per-member-year for context. Classes with growth_pct > 25% warrant a formulary review cycle — either step therapy requirements, preferred product designation changes, or site-of-care optimization.

Scenario 8.3 · Clinical Safety / Pharmacy

Drug-Drug Interaction Detection

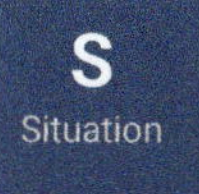

S Situation

The clinical pharmacist team needs a weekly safety report identifying members aged 65+ who have concurrent fills for known high-risk drug pairs. Polypharmacy in elderly members is a leading cause of adverse drug events and avoidable hospitalizations.

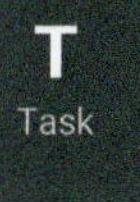

T Task

Identify members 65+ with concurrent fills (overlapping supply dates) for any drug pair listed in ref_ddi_pairs. Calculate overlap days. Output: ranked by DDI severity and overlap duration, for clinical pharmacist review within 48 hours.

ANSI SQL — Scenario 8.3: Drug-Drug Interaction Detection

```
-- Drug-drug interaction: concurrent fills for known high-risk pairs, ages 65+
-- PURPOSE: Identify members age 65+ with concurrent fills of known
-- high-risk drug pairs. "Concurrent" = both fills active at the same time
-- for at least 7 days.

-- STEP 1: Pull all paid fills in the last 90 days for members 65+.
-- fill_end = last day the supply is active.
WITH recent_fills AS (
    SELECT p.member_id, p.ndc_code, n.drug_name, n.gpi_code,
           p.dispensing_date                AS fill_start,
           p.dispensing_date + (p.days_supply - 1) AS fill_end
    FROM  fact_pharmacy_claims p
    JOIN  ref_ndc n ON p.ndc_code = n.ndc_code
    JOIN  dim_members m ON p.member_id = m.member_id
    WHERE p.claim_status  = 'PAID'
      AND p.dispensing_date >= CURRENT_DATE - INTERVAL '90' DAY
      AND m.age_current    >= 65  -- seniors at highest DDI risk
),

-- STEP 2: Find all concurrent drug pairs for each member.
-- Self-join on member_id where fills overlap in time.
-- gpi_a < gpi_b prevents counting (A,B) and (B,A) as two separate pairs.
-- overlap_days = number of days both fills were active simultaneously.
concurrent_pairs AS (
    SELECT
      a.member_id,
```

```
        a.drug_name AS drug_a, a.gpi_code AS gpi_a,
        b.drug_name AS drug_b, b.gpi_code AS gpi_b,
        -- Overlap = from the later start to the earlier end
        DATEDIFF('day',
          GREATEST(a.fill_start, b.fill_start),  -- the later of the two start dates
          LEAST(a.fill_end, b.fill_end)          -- the earlier of the two end dates
        ) + 1  AS overlap_days
    FROM  recent_fills a
    JOIN  recent_fills b
      ON a.member_id = b.member_id
     AND a.gpi_code < b.gpi_code   -- prevent duplicate pairs (A,B) vs (B,A)
     AND a.fill_start <= b.fill_end -- fills overlap: a started before b ended
     AND b.fill_start <= a.fill_end -- fills overlap: b started before a ended
)

-- STEP 3: Join concurrent pairs to the DDI reference table.
-- The OR condition handles both orderings of the drug pair in the reference.
-- Filter to pairs with at least 7 days of concurrent overlap.
SELECT
    cp.member_id, m.member_name, m.pcp_npi, m.phone_number,
    cp.drug_a, cp.drug_b,
    cp.overlap_days,
    ddi.severity_level,           -- HIGH / MODERATE / LOW
    ddi.interaction_description, -- clinical description of the interaction
    ddi.recommended_action       -- what the pharmacist or PCP should do
FROM  concurrent_pairs cp
JOIN  dim_members m ON cp.member_id = m.member_id
JOIN  ref_ddi_pairs ddi
   -- Join on either ordering of the drug pair
   ON (cp.gpi_a = ddi.gpi_drug_1 AND cp.gpi_b = ddi.gpi_drug_2)
   OR (cp.gpi_a = ddi.gpi_drug_2 AND cp.gpi_b = ddi.gpi_drug_1)
WHERE cp.overlap_days >= 7   -- minimum 7 days of concurrent use
ORDER BY ddi.severity_level, cp.overlap_days DESC;
```

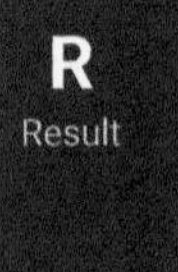

HIGH severity DDIs (e.g., warfarin + NSAID, SSRI + MAOi, ACE inhibitor + potassium-sparing diuretic) require same-day clinical pharmacist outreach and notification to the prescribing PCP. MODERATE severity with overlap > 30 days warrants a medication therapy management (MTM) call. This report directly supports the CMR (Comprehensive Medication Review) Stars measure and reduces avoidable hospitalizations.

Chapter 8 Review

Unit Test · Key Takeaways

Answer each question before reading the explanation.

Q1. In the NCPDP pharmacy claim transaction, the GPI (Generic Product Identifier) is preferred over the NDC for drug classification because:

A. The GPI is shorter and easier to store in a database

B. NDC codes identify a specific manufacturer, package size, and dosage form — the same drug from two manufacturers has two NDC codes. GPI classifies by therapeutic and chemical content regardless of manufacturer, enabling drug class analysis across all NDC variants of the same drug

C. NDC codes are not available for generic drugs

D. GPI codes are updated monthly while NDC codes are static

Answer: B. *NDC (National Drug Code) is an 11-digit code identifying manufacturer (labeler), product, and package. Atorvastatin 40mg from three manufacturers has three different NDCs. GPI (Generic Product Identifier) classifies by therapeutic class,* *chemical entity, and strength — all three atorvastatin NDCs share the same GPI prefix. For formulary tier analysis, adherence measurement, and class-level spend reporting, GPI is the correct key.*

Q2. The MAD PDC near-threshold range (0.70–0.79) is analytically important because:

A. Members in this range are excluded from the HEDIS denominator

B. Members at 0.70–0.79 PDC need only one additional 30-day fill to cross the 0.80 adherence threshold — making them the highest-return outreach targets. A single care management contact can move them from non-adherent to adherent and improve the plan's Stars rate

C. The near-threshold range triggers automatic pharmacy refill reminders

D. PDC of 0.70–0.79 qualifies the member for a medication therapy management (MTM) enrollment

Answer: B. *HEDIS MAD adherence rate = members with PDC >= 0.80 / total denominator. A member at PDC 0.75 is 5 percentage points below threshold. Their period_days × (0.80 - 0.75) = days_supply_needed_to_adhere. Typically one 30-day refill closes the gap. Outreach to near-threshold members produces the highest ROI for Stars improvement programs — they are already mostly adherent and need only a small push.*

Q3. In the drug-drug interaction detection query, AND a.gpi_code < b.gpi_code in the self-join accomplishes what?

A. It sorts drug pairs alphabetically by GPI code

B. It prevents counting the same drug pair twice — without this filter, (Warfarin + Aspirin) and (Aspirin + Warfarin) would both appear as separate rows for the same member interaction

C. It ensures only generic drugs are included in the interaction analysis

D. It limits results to drug pairs where both GPIs begin with the same digit

Answer: B. *A self-join on the same table creates all combinations — for two drugs A and B, it generates rows (A,B) and (B,A) for every member who has both. The gpi_code < gpi_code inequality ensures only one ordering is returned: whichever has the lexically smaller GPI goes in column a, the other in column b. Without it, every DDI would appear twice in the output.*

Q4. The specialty drug trend query uses FULL OUTER JOIN between 2024 and 2023 class-year data. What does a 2024-only row (no 2023 match) indicate?

A. The drug was discontinued in 2023 and reintroduced in 2024

B. A therapeutic class that had fills in 2024 but no fills in 2023 — typically a newly approved specialty drug that entered the formulary during 2024. spend_2023 will be zero; yoy_growth will equal the full 2024 spend

C. A data quality error where the 2023 claims were not loaded

D. A drug class where all 2023 claims were voided and resubmitted in 2024

Answer: B. *FULL OUTER JOIN preserves all rows from both years. A 2024-only row means the therapeutic class had no qualifying fills in 2023. This is the normal pattern for newly FDA-approved specialty drugs (e.g., a new GLP-1 receptor agonist biosimilar). The COALESCE(cy23.total_allowed, 0) produces spend_2023 = 0 and growth_pct shows the full 2024 spend as a percentage increase from zero (handled as NULL or 100% growth depending on the formula).*

Q5. The PDC algorithm uses GREATEST(0, DATEDIFF(...) + 1) to calculate covered days within the measurement window. Why is the +1 required?

A. To convert from zero-based to one-based date counting

B. Because DATEDIFF returns the number of interval boundaries crossed — two dates that are one day apart (Jan 1 and Jan 2) have DATEDIFF = 1, but both days are covered (2 days). Adding +1 converts interval count to day count

C. To account for leap years

D. To add the grace day at the end of the measurement period

Answer: B. *DATEDIFF('day', start, end) counts the number of day boundaries between two dates. Jan 1 to Jan 1 = 0. Jan 1 to Jan 2 = 1. But Jan 1 to Jan 2 covers 2 calendar days of supply. The +1 adjustment converts from "number of boundaries" to "number of inclusive calendar days." Without +1, every fill is short-counted by 1 day, systematically understating PDC across all members.*

Q6. The DAW (Dispense As Written) code on a pharmacy claim indicates:

A. The member's cost-sharing tier for this medication

B. Whether the prescriber authorized a generic substitution: DAW 0 = no restriction (pharmacist may substitute generic); DAW 1 = brand medically necessary (prescriber requires brand); DAW 2 = member requests brand

C. Whether the prescription was filled at a retail or mail-order pharmacy

D. The number of refills authorized on the original prescription

Answer: B. *DAW codes are critical for generic substitution opportunity analysis. DAW 0 = pharmacist discretion (substitutable — the most actionable for plan interventions). DAW 1 = brand medically necessary per prescriber (requires prescriber outreach or prior auth to switch). DAW 2 = member preference (requires member education). A brand fill with DAW 0 is immediately actionable by the pharmacist without prescriber involvement — the lowest-barrier generic substitution opportunity.*

Q7. Describe the five-step MAD PDC algorithm and explain why the measurement period starts 30 days after the first fill rather than on January 1st.

(Short answer)

Sample Answer:
Five-step MAD PDC algorithm: Step 1 — Collect fills: pull all paid antidiabetic pharmacy claims (GPI prefix 27) for the measurement year. Calculate fill_end_date = dispensing_date + (days_supply - 1). Step 2 — Set measurement window: period_start = first_fill_date + 30 days; period_end = December 31. Calculate period_days = period_end - period_start + 1. Step 3 — Adjust for early refills: for each fill, adjusted_start = GREATEST(dispensing_date, prior_fill_end + 1 day) using LAG() over member partition. This prevents overlap double-counting. Step 4 — Calculate covered days: for each fill, covered_days_this_fill = MIN(fill_end, period_end) - MAX(adjusted_start, period_start) + 1, floored at 0. Sum across all fills. Step 5 — Calculate PDC: pdc = total_covered_days / period_days. PDC >= 0.80 = adherent; 0.70–0.79 = near-threshold; < 0.70 = non-adherent. Why 30-day offset: NCQA recognized that patients newly started on a chronic disease medication often have fills delayed during the initiation phase — working with their physician on dose titration, tolerating side effects, or switching formulations. Starting the measurement period 30 days after the first fill excludes this initiation window from the adherence calculation, focusing only on the ongoing therapy maintenance phase where true adherence behavior can be measured.

Q8. Explain the NCPDP pharmacy claim data structure and describe three fields that exist in NCPDP but not in 837 medical claims.

(Short answer)

Sample Answer:
NCPDP (National Council for Prescription Drug Programs) is the transaction standard for pharmacy claims. Unlike 837 professional or institutional claims, NCPDP is transmitted at point of sale from the pharmacy to the PBM in near real-time. The NCPDP transaction contains drug-specific fields not present in medical claims: (1) NDC (National Drug Code): 11-digit code identifying the specific drug product — manufacturer (labeler), product formulation, and package size. Not present on 837 claims; medical claims use CPT/HCPCS procedure codes. (2) days_supply: the number of days of medication the dispensed quantity covers. This is the fundamental unit for PDC calculations and drug utilization reporting. Medical claims have no equivalent field. (3) quantity_dispensed: the number of units (tablets, mL, patches) dispensed. Combined with days_supply and NDC, this allows cost-per-unit and cost-per-day calculations. Not present on medical claims. (4) DAW (Dispense As Written) code: indicates whether a generic substitution is permitted (0), restricted by prescriber (1), or refused by member (2). This field drives generic substitution opportunity analysis. (5) refill_number: sequential refill count for the prescription. Used for medication initiation vs. maintenance analysis. Medical claims have no equivalent.

Q9. Write the SQL to identify specialty drug spend trends by therapeutic class comparing 2023 and 2024. Explain why FULL OUTER JOIN is used and what COALESCE accomplishes in the output.

(Short answer)

Sample Answer:
SQL structure: WITH specialty_fills AS (SELECT n.therapeutic_class, EXTRACT(YEAR FROM p.dispensing_date) AS fill_year, SUM(p.allowed_amount) AS total_allowed, COUNT(DISTINCT p.member_id) AS member_count FROM fact_pharmacy_claims p JOIN ref_ndc n ON p.ndc_code = n.ndc_code JOIN ref_formulary f ON p.ndc_code = f.ndc_code AND f.formulary_year = EXTRACT(YEAR FROM p.dispensing_date) WHERE (f.formulary_tier = 4 OR n.specialty_drug_flag = 'Y') AND p.claim_status = 'PAID' AND EXTRACT(YEAR FROM p.dispensing_date) IN (2023, 2024) GROUP BY 1, 2), cy24 AS (SELECT * FROM specialty_fills WHERE fill_year = 2024), cy23 AS (SELECT * FROM specialty_fills WHERE fill_year = 2023). Final SELECT: COALESCE(cy24.therapeutic_class, cy23.therapeutic_class) AS therapeutic_class, COALESCE(cy24.total_allowed, 0) AS spend_2024, COALESCE(cy23.total_allowed, 0) AS spend_2023, COALESCE(cy24.total_allowed,0) - COALESCE(cy23.total_allowed,0) AS yoy_growth FROM cy24 FULL OUTER JOIN cy23 ON cy24.therapeutic_class = cy23.therapeutic_class ORDER BY yoy_growth DESC LIMIT 15. Why FULL OUTER JOIN: a new specialty drug approved in 2024 exists in cy24 but not in cy23 — INNER JOIN would drop it. A drug class that lost all fills in 2024 (e.g., due to a prior auth policy change) exists in cy23 but not in cy24 — INNER JOIN would drop it too. FULL OUTER JOIN preserves both. COALESCE(value, 0): when one side of the join is NULL (drug class exists in only one year), COALESCE converts NULL to 0 for arithmetic, enabling yoy_growth = spend_2024 - spend_2023 to calculate correctly.

Q10. Describe what the drug-drug interaction detection query identifies, explain the clinical significance of concurrent overlapping fills, and discuss the 7-day minimum overlap threshold.

(Short answer)

Sample Answer:
The DDI detection query identifies members who have concurrent active fills for two drugs known to have a clinically significant interaction. Concurrent = both fills are active at the same time (fill_start_a <= fill_end_b AND fill_start_b <= fill_end_a). The clinical significance of concurrent fills: taking both drugs simultaneously creates a pharmacodynamic or pharmacokinetic interaction. Examples of HIGH-severity interactions: Warfarin + NSAIDs (increased bleeding risk), ACE

inhibitors + potassium-sparing diuretics (hyperkalemia risk), MAO inhibitors + SSRIs (serotonin syndrome risk). Unlike a single prescription review, claims-based DDI detection identifies interactions across multiple prescribers who may not be aware of each other's orders — particularly common in elderly patients (65+) seeing multiple specialists. The 7-day minimum overlap threshold: a single-day overlap could be coincidental (member started a new drug on the last day of an expiring prescription). Seven days of concurrent use indicates a genuine co-prescribing pattern that the patient is actually experiencing both drugs simultaneously. This threshold balances sensitivity (catching real interactions) against specificity (avoiding false positives from brief administrative overlaps). The 7-day threshold is a common analytic convention; some clinical programs use 14 or 30 days for stricter criteria. The severity_level field (HIGH/MODERATE/LOW from ref_ddi_pairs) allows triage: HIGH = immediate clinical outreach; MODERATE = pharmacist review; LOW = documentation only.

Key Takeaways

What every analyst must remember from this chapter.

1 GPI (Generic Product Identifier) is the preferred drug classification key for analytics. NDC identifies manufacturer + package — the same molecule has hundreds of NDCs. GPI classifies by therapeutic class and chemical entity regardless of manufacturer, enabling drug-class PMPM, adherence, and formulary analysis.

2 MAD PDC algorithm: measurement period = first_fill + 30 days through December 31. Overlap adjustment = GREATEST(dispensing_date, prior_fill_end + 1 day). PDC = covered_days / period_days. >= 0.80 = adherent; 0.70–0.79 = near-threshold (priority outreach); < 0.70 = non-adherent.

3 Near-threshold members (PDC 0.70–0.79) are the highest-ROI outreach targets. One 30-day refill can cross them from non-adherent to adherent. Calculate days_supply_needed_to_adhere = CEIL(period_days × 0.80) - days_covered for each non-adherent member.

4 DATEDIFF + 1 is always required when calculating days covered between two inclusive dates. DATEDIFF counts boundaries (Jan 1 to Jan 2 = 1), but two dates one apart cover 2 calendar days. Without +1, every fill is undercounted by 1 day.

5 Drug-drug interaction SQL: self-join recent_fills on member_id with gpi_a < gpi_b (prevents duplicate pairs), fill_start_a <= fill_end_b AND fill_start_b <= fill_end_a (concurrent overlap). Join to ref_ddi_pairs using OR to match both orderings. Filter overlap_days >= 7.

6 DAW codes: 0 = pharmacist may substitute generic (immediately actionable). 1 = brand medically necessary per prescriber (requires prescriber outreach). 2 = member requests brand (requires member education). Focus generic substitution programs on DAW 0 fills first — lowest barrier to intervention.

7 Specialty drug flag criteria: formulary_tier = 4 (specialty tier) OR specialty_drug_flag = 'Y' in ref_ndc. Use both to cast a wide net — not all specialty drugs are on Tier 4 for all plan designs. FULL OUTER JOIN 2024 vs. 2023 to capture newly approved drugs (2024-only rows) and discontinuations (2023-only rows).

8 DDI detection focuses on age >= 65 because polypharmacy is most prevalent in seniors, prescribers are most likely to be unaware of each other's orders, and the clinical consequences of interactions (falls, bleeding, hospitalizations) are most severe. Always include age_current in the DDI member filter.

Chapter 9: PBM Analytics — Rebates, Spread Pricing & Formulary

Between your health plan and every pharmacy counter in America sits an entity most members have never heard of: the Pharmacy Benefit Manager. The PBM adjudicates pharmacy claims in real time, maintains the formulary, negotiates drug prices with manufacturers, contracts with pharmacy networks, and — in most traditional contracts — retains a portion of the financial value it generates as profit. For the healthcare analyst, understanding PBM contract mechanics is not optional: it directly determines whether your pharmacy cost reports reflect reality or a systematic overstatement of net drug cost.

9.1 What Is a PBM and Why Does It Matter?

A Pharmacy Benefit Manager is a third-party administrator that manages prescription drug benefits on behalf of health plans, employers, and government programs. The three largest PBMs — CVS Caremark, Express Scripts (Cigna), and OptumRx (UnitedHealth) — manage pharmacy benefits for approximately 270 million Americans and process over 6 billion claims annually.

PBM function	What they do	Analyst relevance
Claims adjudication	Process pharmacy claims in real time at point of sale	All pharmacy claims data flows through PBM systems — data format and completeness depend on PBM agreement
Formulary management	Decide which drugs are covered, at what tier, with what restrictions	Formulary decisions directly impact drug spend, adherence, and rebate yield — must be analyzed together
Network contracting	Negotiate reimbursement rates with retail, mail, and specialty pharmacies	Spread pricing occurs here — plan pays PBM rate; PBM pays pharmacy less and retains difference
Manufacturer rebates	Negotiate and collect rebates from drug manufacturers for preferred placement	In non-pass-through contracts: rebates stay with PBM, not returned to plan — creates systematic understatement of net cost
Utilization management	Prior authorization, step therapy, quantity limits	PA decisions feed into PA analytics (Ch 24) and MHPAEA parity analysis

9.2 PBM Contract Types — The Most Important Distinction

Before writing a single SQL query against pharmacy data, the analyst must know which type of PBM contract the health plan has. This single variable determines whether your pharmacy cost reports reflect the actual cost of drugs or a systematically inflated number.

Contract type	How rebates flow	Spread pricing	Net cost visibility	Analyst implication
Non-pass-through (traditional)	PBM retains all manufacturer rebates	PBM retains spread — plan pays more than pharmacy receives	plan_paid_amount OVERSTATES true net cost	Never use plan_paid_amount as the final cost metric — subtract estimated rebates and spread

Contract type	How rebates flow	Spread pricing	Net cost visibility	Analyst implication
Partial pass-through	Rebates above a floor returned to plan; spread may be partially returned	Spread partially disclosed	Partial visibility — better than traditional but still incomplete	Adjust costs using rebate remittance data; flag residual hidden spread
Full pass-through	100% of rebates passed to plan	Plan pays actual pharmacy acquisition cost (AWP or NADAC-based)	Most accurate — plan sees actual drug cost	plan_paid_amount is reliable for cost analysis; rebate_remittance adds back gross rebates received
ASO (Administrative Services Only)	Plan manages rebate contracts directly	No spread — plan pays pharmacies directly	Complete transparency	Best analytical environment — all costs visible, no hidden margins

> **Critical implication:** In a non-pass-through contract, every PMPM benchmark, trend analysis, and cost comparison you produce overstates the plan's true net pharmacy cost by an amount equal to the spread retained by the PBM plus the rebates not returned. Industry estimates: spread = \$3–\$15 PMPM for commercial plans; rebates retained = \$8–\$25 PMPM. The analyst must always note the contract type when presenting pharmacy cost data.

9.3 Spread Pricing — SQL Detection

9.3.1 How Spread Pricing Works

Spread pricing is the practice of a PBM charging the health plan a higher amount for a drug than it reimburses the pharmacy, retaining the difference as revenue. Example: the plan's PBM contract sets the reimbursement for generic metformin at \$12. The PBM reimburses the pharmacy \$4 (using its own pharmacy network contracts). The PBM retains the \$8 difference — this is spread.

The NADAC (National Average Drug Acquisition Cost) is a CMS-published weekly benchmark of what pharmacies actually pay to acquire drugs. It is available free at data.medicaid.gov. Comparing plan_paid_amount to NADAC × quantity_dispensed reveals the estimated spread on each claim.

9.3.2 Spread Pricing Detection Query

ANSI SQL — 9.3: Spread Pricing Detection Using NADAC Benchmark

```sql
-- PURPOSE: Compare what the plan paid for each drug to the NADAC
-- (National Average Drug Acquisition Cost) benchmark.
-- Spread = plan_paid - NADAC_cost. High spread = PBM earned a margin
-- by billing the plan more than the pharmacy was actually paid.
-- NADAC is published weekly by CMS at data.medicaid.gov.

-- STEP 1: Pull all paid pharmacy claims for the plan in the last 12 months.
WITH pharmacy_claims AS (
  SELECT p.claim_id, p.ndc_code, p.drug_name, p.days_supply,
      p.quantity_dispensed, p.plan_paid_amount, p.pharmacy_type,
      p.dispensing_date
  FROM  fact_pharmacy_claims p
  WHERE p.claim_status = 'PAID'
   AND p.plan_id = :plan_id
   AND p.dispensing_date >= CURRENT_DATE - INTERVAL '12' MONTH
),
```

```sql
-- STEP 2: Get the NADAC acquisition cost rate effective as of each dispensing date.
-- NADAC is a weekly rate -- find the most recent rate published before the fill date.
-- The correlated subquery MAX(effective_date) WHERE effective_date <= dispensing_date
-- retrieves the NADAC rate that was in effect when the drug was dispensed.
nadac_benchmark AS (
  SELECT DISTINCT n.ndc_code, n.nadac_per_unit, n.effective_date
  FROM  ref_nadac n
),

-- STEP 3: Calculate the spread per claim.
-- spread_amount = plan_paid - (NADAC rate × quantity dispensed)
-- spread_pct = spread as % of plan_paid
spread_analysis AS (
  SELECT
    pc.claim_id, pc.ndc_code, pc.drug_name, pc.pharmacy_type,
    pc.plan_paid_amount,
    -- NADAC cost = per-unit rate × number of units dispensed
    ROUND(nb.nadac_per_unit * pc.quantity_dispensed, 2)   AS nadac_cost,
    -- Spread = what plan paid minus NADAC acquisition cost
    ROUND(pc.plan_paid_amount
      - nb.nadac_per_unit * pc.quantity_dispensed, 2)   AS spread_amount,
    -- Spread as % of plan paid (how much of each dollar is margin?)
    ROUND(100.0 * (pc.plan_paid_amount
      - nb.nadac_per_unit * pc.quantity_dispensed)
      / NULLIF(pc.plan_paid_amount, 0), 1)          AS spread_pct
  FROM  pharmacy_claims pc
  JOIN  nadac_benchmark nb
    ON pc.ndc_code = nb.ndc_code
   -- Get the NADAC rate in effect on the dispensing date
   AND nb.effective_date = (
     SELECT MAX(r2.effective_date) FROM ref_nadac r2
     WHERE r2.ndc_code = pc.ndc_code
      AND r2.effective_date <= pc.dispensing_date)
)

-- STEP 4: Summarize by pharmacy type.
-- Mail order vs. retail vs. specialty pharmacy have different spread patterns.
SELECT
  pharmacy_type,
  COUNT(*)                    AS claims,
  ROUND(SUM(plan_paid_amount), 0)        AS total_plan_paid,
  ROUND(SUM(nadac_cost), 0)          AS total_nadac_benchmark,
  ROUND(SUM(spread_amount), 0)          AS total_estimated_spread,
  ROUND(100.0 * SUM(spread_amount)
    / NULLIF(SUM(plan_paid_amount), 0), 1)  AS spread_pct_of_total
FROM  spread_analysis
GROUP BY pharmacy_type
ORDER BY total_estimated_spread DESC;
```

Spread is highest on generics: Generic drug spread is typically 3–8× higher than brand drug spread as a percentage. Brand drugs have published WAC (Wholesale Acquisition Cost) prices that limit spread opportunity. Generic pricing is opaque — the PBM's network contracts with pharmacies may be far below NADAC, creating large spread on high-volume generic drugs like metformin, lisinopril, and atorvastatin.

9.4 Rebate Reconciliation Analytics

9.4.1 How Rebates Are Calculated

Manufacturer rebates are the largest single financial lever in pharmacy benefit management. A health plan with a pass-through or partial pass-through contract receives quarterly rebate payments from its PBM based on utilization of rebated drugs. The rebate calculation has three components: base utilization rebates (per-claim or per-30-day-equivalent), market share tier bonuses (higher rebate rate when the drug achieves a target share of its therapeutic class), and administrative fees.

ANSI SQL — 9.4: Quarterly Rebate Reconciliation

```
-- PURPOSE: Compare the plan's contract-calculated expected rebate against
-- the rebate amount actually reported by the PBM.
-- Rebate gap = expected_rebate - pbm_reported_rebate.
-- Large gaps trigger contract audits and PBM financial discussions.

-- STEP 1: Aggregate utilization to NDC × quarter × plan.
-- total_30de = 30-day equivalents (standard rebate calculation unit).
-- days_supply / 30.0 converts variable supply lengths to a common unit.
WITH quarterly_utilization AS (
  SELECT p.ndc_code, d.drug_name, d.gpi_2_class, d.gpi_14_drug,
      EXTRACT(YEAR    FROM p.dispensing_date) AS rx_year,
      EXTRACT(QUARTER FROM p.dispensing_date) AS rx_quarter,
      COUNT(*)                      AS total_claims,
      SUM(p.days_supply / 30.0)            AS total_30de  -- 30-day equivalents
  FROM  fact_pharmacy_claims p
  JOIN  ref_drug_master d ON p.ndc_code = d.ndc_code
  WHERE p.claim_status = 'PAID' AND p.plan_id = :plan_id
  GROUP BY 1,2,3,4,5,6
),

-- STEP 2: Calculate market share within each GPI drug class per quarter.
-- Market share determines which rebate tier from the contract applies.
class_totals AS (
  SELECT gpi_2_class, rx_year, rx_quarter,
      SUM(total_30de) AS class_total_30de
  FROM  quarterly_utilization GROUP BY 1,2,3
),
market_share AS (
  SELECT u.*,
      ROUND(100.0 * u.total_30de / NULLIF(ct.class_total_30de, 0), 2)
        AS market_share_pct  -- this drug's % of its class total
  FROM  quarterly_utilization u
  JOIN  class_totals ct USING (gpi_2_class, rx_year, rx_quarter)
),

-- STEP 3: Look up the applicable rebate rate from the contract.
-- Rebate contracts have tiered rates based on market share thresholds.
-- Higher market share = higher rebate rate per 30-day equivalent.
expected_rebates AS (
  SELECT ms.ndc_code, ms.drug_name, ms.rx_year, ms.rx_quarter,
      ms.total_30de, ms.market_share_pct,
      -- Apply the correct tier from the contract based on market share
      CASE
        WHEN ms.market_share_pct >= rc.tier3_threshold THEN rc.tier3_rate_per_30de
        WHEN ms.market_share_pct >= rc.tier2_threshold THEN rc.tier2_rate_per_30de
        ELSE rc.base_rate_per_30de
      END                           AS applicable_rebate_rate,
      -- Expected rebate = rate × volume (in 30-day equivalents)
      ms.total_30de * CASE
        WHEN ms.market_share_pct >= rc.tier3_threshold THEN rc.tier3_rate_per_30de
```

```sql
        WHEN ms.market_share_pct >= rc.tier2_threshold THEN rc.tier2_rate_per_30de
        ELSE rc.base_rate_per_30de
      END                                AS expected_rebate
   FROM  market_share ms
   JOIN  ref_rebate_contracts rc
     ON ms.ndc_code = rc.ndc_code AND rc.contract_year = ms.rx_year
)

-- STEP 4: Compare expected to PBM-reported rebate.
-- LEFT JOIN: some drugs may not appear in pbm_rebate_remittance (PBM omission).
SELECT
   er.drug_name, er.rx_year, er.rx_quarter,
   er.total_30de,
   ROUND(er.market_share_pct, 1)            AS market_share_pct,
   ROUND(er.expected_rebate, 0)             AS expected_rebate,
   COALESCE(pr.rebate_payment, 0)            AS pbm_reported_rebate,
   -- Reconciliation gap: positive = PBM paid less than expected
   ROUND(er.expected_rebate - COALESCE(pr.rebate_payment,0), 0) AS reconciliation_gap,
   -- Flag gaps over $1,000 for investigation
   CASE WHEN ABS(er.expected_rebate - COALESCE(pr.rebate_payment,0)) > 1000
      THEN 'INVESTIGATE' ELSE 'Within tolerance' END   AS flag
FROM  expected_rebates er
LEFT JOIN pbm_rebate_remittance pr
     ON er.ndc_code   = pr.ndc_code
    AND er.rx_year    = pr.payment_year
    AND er.rx_quarter = pr.payment_quarter
WHERE er.expected_rebate > 0  -- only rebate-eligible drugs
ORDER BY ABS(er.expected_rebate - COALESCE(pr.rebate_payment,0)) DESC;
```

9.5 Formulary Analytics — Generic Substitution & Rebate Optimization

ANSI SQL — 9.5: Generic Substitution Opportunity Analysis

```sql
-- Generic substitution opportunity: brand fills where generic equivalent exists
WITH brand_fills AS (
   SELECT p.member_id, d.drug_name AS brand_name, d.gpi_14_drug,
        d.formulary_tier, SUM(p.plan_paid_amount) AS brand_cost_ytd,
        COUNT(*) AS brand_claims_ytd, MAX(p.daw_code) AS daw_code
   FROM  fact_pharmacy_claims p
   JOIN  ref_drug_master d ON p.ndc_code = d.ndc_code
   WHERE p.claim_status = 'PAID'
    AND d.brand_generic_flag = 'BRAND'
    AND d.generic_available_flag = 'Y'
    AND d.formulary_tier IN ('TIER2','TIER3')
    AND EXTRACT(YEAR FROM p.dispensing_date) = EXTRACT(YEAR FROM CURRENT_DATE)
   GROUP BY 1,2,3,4
),
generic_cost AS (
   SELECT d.gpi_14_drug,
        AVG(p.plan_paid_amount / NULLIF(p.days_supply / 30.0, 0))
          AS generic_cost_per_30de
   FROM  fact_pharmacy_claims p
   JOIN  ref_drug_master d ON p.ndc_code = d.ndc_code
   WHERE d.brand_generic_flag = 'GENERIC'
    AND p.claim_status = 'PAID'
    AND EXTRACT(YEAR FROM p.dispensing_date) = EXTRACT(YEAR FROM CURRENT_DATE)
   GROUP BY 1
)
SELECT
```

```
    bf.member_id, m.member_name, m.pcp_npi,
    bf.brand_name, bf.formulary_tier, bf.daw_code,
    ROUND(bf.brand_cost_ytd, 0)          AS brand_cost_ytd,
    ROUND(gc.generic_cost_per_30de
      * bf.brand_claims_ytd * 30, 0)    AS est_generic_cost_ytd,
    ROUND(bf.brand_cost_ytd
      - gc.generic_cost_per_30de * bf.brand_claims_ytd * 30,
      0)                    AS est_annual_savings,
    CASE WHEN bf.daw_code = '0'
      THEN 'Actionable — pharmacist may substitute'
      ELSE 'Requires prescriber change (DAW 1+)'
    END AS intervention_type
  FROM brand_fills bf
  JOIN generic_cost gc ON bf.gpi_14_drug = gc.gpi_14_drug
  JOIN dim_members m ON bf.member_id = m.member_id
  ORDER BY est_annual_savings DESC;
```

Chapter 9 Review

Unit Test · Key Takeaways

Answer each question before reading the explanation.

Q1. What is "spread pricing" in a PBM contract and why is it analytically significant?

A. Spread pricing refers to the formulary tier spread between generic and brand drugs

B. Spread pricing occurs when the PBM bills the plan a higher amount for a drug than it actually reimburses the pharmacy. The spread (plan_paid - pharmacy_reimbursement) is retained by the PBM as additional margin beyond the administrative fee. Plans under non-pass-through contracts are especially vulnerable

C. Spread pricing is a CMS-mandated pricing methodology for Medicare Part D

D. Spread pricing refers to price spreading across therapeutic substitutes in a drug class

Answer: B. *In a non-pass-through PBM contract, the PBM negotiates pharmacy reimbursement rates independently from what it charges the plan. For a generic drug, the PBM might reimburse the pharmacy $8 but bill the plan $15 — keeping $7 as spread. The NADAC benchmark (published weekly by CMS) represents actual pharmacy acquisition costs and serves as the external reference for detecting spread. Plans with pass-through contracts receive the actual ingredient cost plus a transparent fee; non-pass-through plans face spread risk.*

Q2. Rebate contracts use "30-day equivalents" (30DE) as the utilization unit. A fill of 90 days supply represents how many 30DE?

A. 1.0 30DE

B. 3.0 30DE

C. 90.0 30DE

D. 0.33 30DE

Answer: B. *SUM(days_supply / 30.0) converts variable prescription lengths to a common unit. A 90-day supply = 90 / 30 = 3.0 30DE. A 30-day supply = 1.0 30DE. A 14-day supply = 0.47 30DE. Rebate contracts specify rates in dollars per 30DE (e.g., $2.50 per 30DE) so that quarterly utilization volume can be calculated as a consistent unit regardless of whether members fill 30-day or 90-day supplies.*

Q3. The rebate reconciliation query joins to ref_rebate_contracts to determine the applicable rebate tier. What SQL CASE WHEN logic determines the correct tier?

A. CASE WHEN drug_name = 'brand' THEN tier1 ELSE tier2 END

B. CASE WHEN market_share_pct >= tier3_threshold THEN tier3_rate WHEN market_share_pct >= tier2_threshold THEN tier2_rate ELSE base_rate END — rebate tiers are volume-based: higher market share = higher tier = higher rebate rate per 30DE

C. CASE WHEN total_30de > 1000 THEN premium_rate ELSE standard_rate END

D. CASE WHEN formulary_tier IN ('TIER1','TIER2') THEN preferred_rate ELSE standard_rate END

Answer: B. *Rebate contracts are structured with tiered rates based on the drug's market share within its GPI drug class on the plan's formulary. If the plan's utilization of Drug X reaches 20% of the drug class (Tier 2 threshold), the rebate rate jumps from*

$2.00 to $3.50 per 30DE. If it reaches 30% (Tier 3 threshold), the rate jumps to $5.00. This incentivizes plans to prefer formulary positioning that drives market share toward higher-tier drugs — a key lever in PBM contract negotiations.

Q4. The NADAC spread detection query uses a correlated subquery to join NADAC rates. What does MAX(effective_date) WHERE effective_date <= dispensing_date accomplish?

A. It retrieves the highest NADAC rate ever published for each drug

B. It retrieves the most recently published NADAC rate that was in effect on or before the claim's dispensing date — the correct acquisition cost benchmark for that specific fill

C. It filters to NADAC rates that were published within 30 days of the fill

D. It selects the average NADAC rate across all effective dates for the drug

Answer: B. *NADAC is updated weekly, so the rate for a drug changes over time. A fill on March 15 should be compared to the NADAC rate that was in effect on March 15, not the current rate. MAX(effective_date) WHERE effective_date <= dispensing_date finds the most recently published rate that was active on the fill date. This is a point-in-time lookup pattern analogous to the SCD-2 join used for member attributes.*

Q5. In a PBM contract, the difference between a non-pass-through and a pass-through contract arrangement is:

A. Non-pass-through contracts cover only retail pharmacy; pass-through covers retail and mail

B. In non-pass-through (traditional) contracts the PBM retains spread between pharmacy reimbursement and plan billing as additional margin; in pass-through contracts the plan receives the actual ingredient cost plus a transparent administrative fee with no PBM spread

C. Non-pass-through contracts require prior authorization for all specialty drugs

D. Pass-through contracts eliminate rebates; non-pass-through contracts retain rebates

Answer: B. *The financial structure of the PBM contract determines whether the plan can observe the actual ingredient costs the PBM pays pharmacies. In non-pass-through (most common historically), the PBM books spread as additional revenue — the plan cannot see pharmacy reimbursement amounts. In pass-through contracts (growing in prevalence, especially for self-insured employers), the plan can see every ingredient cost, dispensing fee, and rebate — eliminating spread risk but requiring more sophisticated contract management.*

Q6. Generic substitution opportunity analysis filters to brand fills with DAW code 0. Why are DAW 1 fills typically excluded from the actionable opportunity list?

A. DAW 1 fills are for controlled substances and cannot be substituted

B. DAW 1 = brand medically necessary per the prescriber. The pharmacist cannot substitute without a new prescription. The intervention requires prescriber outreach, prior authorization review, or a step therapy protocol — a higher-effort intervention compared to DAW 0 fills where the pharmacist can substitute immediately

C. DAW 1 fills have already been reviewed by the pharmacy and determined to be non-substitutable

D. DAW 1 drugs are not covered by most formularies and therefore do not generate a substitution opportunity

Answer: B. *DAW 0 fills are immediately actionable at the pharmacy counter — the pharmacist can substitute a generic automatically. DAW 1 fills require the prescriber to authorize a new prescription for the generic equivalent or to agree to a therapeutic alternative. This requires a prescriber-facing intervention (phone call, fax, electronic message) — higher effort and lower conversion rate than DAW 0. A mature generic substitution program works both populations but prioritizes DAW 0 for the highest-return interventions first.*

Q7. Explain what NADAC is, why it is used as the spread pricing benchmark, and describe the SQL pattern for looking up the point-in-time NADAC rate for each pharmacy claim.

(Short answer)

> **Sample Answer:**
> NADAC = National Average Drug Acquisition Cost. Published weekly by CMS based on a voluntary survey of independent pharmacies reporting their actual invoice prices for drugs dispensed to Medicaid beneficiaries. NADAC represents a market-average pharmacy acquisition cost — what pharmacies actually pay to purchase drug inventory. Why NADAC is used as the spread benchmark: it is publicly available (data.medicaid.gov), updated weekly, covers virtually all dispensed drugs, and represents a neutral external reference for pharmacy ingredient costs. A plan comparing its PBM-billed amounts to NADAC estimates the PBM's gross margin (spread) on each claim. Spread > 20–30% on generic drugs is a red flag for non-pass-through PBM pricing. Point-in-time NADAC lookup pattern: JOIN ref_nadac nb ON pc.ndc_code = nb.ndc_code AND nb.effective_date = (SELECT MAX(r2.effective_date) FROM ref_nadac r2 WHERE r2.ndc_code = pc.ndc_code AND r2.effective_date <= pc.dispensing_date). This correlated subquery finds the most recently published NADAC rate that was in effect on or before the claim's dispensing date — the correct acquisition cost benchmark for that specific fill. This is the same point-in-time lookup pattern as the SCD-2 date range join.

Q8. Describe the quarterly rebate reconciliation process. What is the plan's analytical role in this process and what does a large reconciliation_gap indicate?

(Short answer)

Sample Answer:

Rebate reconciliation process: Quarterly, after the PBM submits its rebate remittance statement, the plan's analytics team independently calculates expected rebates based on (1) actual drug utilization data (total_30de per NDC per quarter from fact_pharmacy_claims), (2) calculated market share within each GPI drug class (total_30de / class_total_30de × 100), and (3) the applicable rebate rate from the contract's tiered rate schedule (CASE WHEN market_share_pct >= tier thresholds). The expected rebate is then compared to the PBM's reported rebate payment in pbm_rebate_remittance. The plan's analytical role: independently verify that (a) utilization volumes used by the PBM to calculate rebates match the plan's own claims data, (b) market share calculations are consistent with the contract methodology, and (c) the correct tier rate was applied based on achieved market share. A large reconciliation_gap (expected > reported) can indicate: (1) PBM used incorrect utilization volumes — possibly due to claim exclusions not specified in the contract. (2) PBM applied a lower tier rate than the market share warranted — an underpayment requiring repayment. (3) Market share threshold was just below the tier cutoff — an opportunity to identify formulary positioning changes that would push into a higher tier next quarter. (4) A new drug class was added to the formulary mid-quarter but not captured in the PBM's rebate calculation — a contract amendment issue.

Q9. Describe the three PBM contract types and explain which one creates the highest analytics visibility into pharmacy costs.

(Short answer)

Sample Answer:

Three PBM contract types: (1) Non-Pass-Through (Traditional): the PBM negotiates separate rates with pharmacies and charges the plan a different (higher) rate — retaining the spread as margin. The plan sees only the amount billed by the PBM, not the pharmacy reimbursement. Rebates may be partially retained by the PBM. Analytics visibility: LOW. The plan cannot distinguish ingredient costs from PBM margin. (2) Partial Pass-Through: the PBM passes through some pharmacy costs transparently (typically for specialty drugs where the spread risk is highest) but retains spread on retail generic claims. Analytics visibility: MODERATE for specialty, LOW for retail generics. (3) Full Pass-Through (Administrative Services Only): the plan pays actual pharmacy ingredient costs (transparent) plus a fixed per-claim administrative fee to the PBM. All rebates are passed through to the plan net of a contracted retention percentage. Analytics visibility: HIGH. The plan can see every ingredient cost, dispensing fee, and rebate — enabling NADAC comparison, spread monitoring, and complete financial audit. Highest analytics visibility: Full Pass-Through / ASO contracts. These are increasingly common for large self-insured employers who have the analytics sophistication to audit pharmacy costs independently.

Q10. Write the generic substitution opportunity SQL and explain what each calculated field reveals to the care management or pharmacy team.

(Short answer)

Sample Answer:

SQL: WITH brand_fills AS (SELECT p.member_id, d.drug_name AS brand_name, d.gpi_14_drug, d.formulary_tier, SUM(p.plan_paid_amount) AS brand_cost_ytd, COUNT(*) AS brand_claims_ytd, MAX(p.daw_code) AS daw_code FROM fact_pharmacy_claims p JOIN ref_drug_master d ON p.ndc_code = d.ndc_code WHERE p.claim_status = 'PAID' AND d.brand_generic_flag = 'BRAND' AND d.generic_available_flag = 'Y' AND d.formulary_tier IN ('TIER2','TIER3') AND EXTRACT(YEAR FROM p.dispensing_date) = EXTRACT(YEAR FROM CURRENT_DATE) GROUP BY 1,2,3,4), generic_cost AS (SELECT d.gpi_14_drug, AVG(p.plan_paid_amount / NULLIF(p.days_supply/30.0,0)) AS generic_cost_per_30de FROM fact_pharmacy_claims p JOIN ref_drug_master d ON p.ndc_code = d.ndc_code WHERE d.brand_generic_flag = 'GENERIC' AND p.claim_status = 'PAID' GROUP BY 1). Final SELECT: brand_cost_ytd (total plan cost this year for brand fills), est_generic_cost_ytd = generic_cost_per_30de × brand_claims_ytd × 30 (what the same volume would cost as generic), est_annual_savings = brand_cost_ytd - est_generic_cost_ytd (opportunity size), daw_code (0 = pharmacist can substitute immediately; 1+ = requires prescriber), intervention_type ('Actionable -- pharmacist may substitute' for DAW 0; 'Requires prescriber change' for DAW 1+). The pharmacy team uses est_annual_savings sorted descending to prioritize outreach to the members and prescribers with the highest savings potential.

Key Takeaways

What every analyst must remember from this chapter.

1 Spread pricing = PBM bills the plan more than it reimburses the pharmacy. Spread = plan_paid - NADAC_cost. NADAC (published weekly by CMS) is the standard acquisition cost benchmark. High spread % on generic drugs (>20%) signals non-pass-through PBM margin.

2 NADAC point-in-time lookup: JOIN ref_nadac ON ndc_code AND effective_date = (SELECT MAX(effective_date) FROM ref_nadac WHERE ndc_code = claim.ndc_code AND effective_date <= claim.dispensing_date). This is the same point-in-time lookup pattern as SCD-2 date range joins.

3 Rebate reconciliation: expected_rebate = total_30de × applicable_rate_from_contract. applicable_rate = CASE WHEN market_share_pct >= tier3_threshold THEN tier3_rate WHEN >= tier2_threshold THEN tier2_rate ELSE base_rate END. Compare to PBM-reported rebate. reconciliation_gap > $1,000 triggers investigation.

4 30-day equivalents (30DE) = SUM(days_supply / 30.0). This normalizes variable fill lengths for rebate calculations. A 90-day supply = 3.0 30DE. Rebate contracts specify rates in dollars per 30DE.

5 PBM contract types by analytics visibility: Non-pass-through (LOW — plan cannot see pharmacy costs), Partial pass-through (MODERATE), Full pass-through/ASO (HIGH — plan sees every ingredient cost, dispensing fee, and rebate). Always know your contract type before interpreting pharmacy cost data.

6 Generic substitution priority: DAW 0 (pharmacist may substitute immediately) = lowest-barrier intervention. DAW 1 (brand medically necessary per prescriber) = requires prescriber outreach. Sort by est_annual_savings descending to prioritize highest-value substitution opportunities.

7 Market share within GPI drug class determines rebate tier. market_share_pct = total_30de / class_total_30de × 100. Classes where the plan is just below a tier threshold are formulary positioning opportunities — a preferred formulary placement that drives 2–3% more market share can jump to a higher rebate tier worth hundreds of thousands of dollars annually.

8 The 30DE unit standardizes rebate calculations across 30-day and 90-day prescriptions. Without it, plans that encourage 90-day mail-order fills would appear to have the same rebate volume per claim as retail 30-day fills — understating the true rebate-generating utilization by 3×.

Chapter 10: Oncology Analytics

Oncology is the fastest-growing cost category in healthcare — driven by high-cost biologics, immunotherapies, and complex multi-drug regimens that can exceed $500,000 per member per year. Understanding oncology analytics requires integrating three separate data streams: medical claims for IV infusion (J-codes), pharmacy claims for oral oncolytics, and institutional claims for radiation therapy. No single data source captures the complete oncology episode.

10.1 The Oncology Data Landscape

Oncology care generates claims across multiple settings simultaneously. A member receiving chemotherapy may have claims from the oncologist's office (professional J-code claim), the infusion center or hospital outpatient department (institutional revenue code 0331 = chemotherapy), and the oral specialty pharmacy (NCPDP pharmacy claim for oral oncolytics). Complete oncology analytics must integrate all three.

Care setting	Claim type	Primary code field	Drug identification	Cost driver
Physician office infusion	Professional (CMS-1500)	J-code CPT (J9000–J9999)	procedure_code = J-code (e.g., J9355 = trastuzumab)	Drug cost embedded in allowed_amount per unit
Hospital outpatient infusion	Institutional (UB-04)	Revenue code 0331 + J-code	procedure_code on revenue line with rev code 0331	Facility fee + drug fee — both in allowed_amount
Oral oncolytic pharmacy	NCPDP pharmacy claim	NDC code	ndc_code joined to ref_ndc where oncology_drug_flag = Y	Full drug cost in plan_paid_amount
Radiation therapy	Professional or institutional	CPT 77xxx (professional) or revenue code 0330 (institutional)	procedure_code range 77000–77799	Cost per fraction × number of fractions = course cost

10.2 Oncology Patient Identification

Identifying the oncology population from claims requires careful diagnosis code logic. The ICD-10-CM chapter for neoplasms (C00–C96) covers malignant neoplasms. A single claim with a C-code may represent a rule-out scenario — the physician coded for a possible cancer that was later excluded. Using 2+ claims with cancer diagnosis on different service dates significantly reduces false positives.

ANSI SQL — 10.2: Oncology Patient Identification

```
-- PURPOSE: Identify members with confirmed oncology diagnoses.
-- Requiring 2+ claims with primary cancer dx on DIFFERENT dates
-- reduces false positives from rule-out coding
-- (where a physician orders tests to rule out cancer, codes the suspected dx,
-- but the member never had cancer).
```

```
SELECT DISTINCT member_id
FROM (
  SELECT member_id,
      -- Count the number of distinct service dates with a primary cancer diagnosis
      COUNT(DISTINCT service_date) AS dx_date_count
  FROM  fact_medical_claims
  -- ICD-10-CM C00-C96.9 = malignant neoplasms (all cancer types)
  WHERE primary_diag BETWEEN 'C00' AND 'C96.9'
   AND claim_status = 'PAID'
   AND EXTRACT(YEAR FROM service_date) = EXTRACT(YEAR FROM CURRENT_DATE)
  GROUP BY member_id
) cancer_dx
-- Require at least 2 distinct dates to confirm the diagnosis pattern
WHERE dx_date_count >= 2;

-- CANCER TYPE CLASSIFICATION for downstream stratification:
-- Breast:    C50.x   Lung:     C34.x   Colorectal: C18-C20
-- Prostate:  C61     Lymphoma: C81-C85 Leukemia:   C91-C95
-- Melanoma:  C43.x   Pancreatic: C25.x Ovarian:    C56.x
-- Hematologic: C81-C96  (broad hematology group)
```

10.3 Oncology Drug Classification

Oncology drugs are identified through multiple code systems depending on the route of administration. Analysts must query both medical and pharmacy claims to capture the full drug spend for oncology members.

Drug type	Code system	Code range / filter	Claim table
IV chemotherapy (infusion)	HCPCS J-codes	J9000–J9999 = antineoplastic drugs	fact_medical_claims WHERE procedure_code BETWEEN 'J9000' AND 'J9999'
Supportive care drugs (infusion)	HCPCS J-codes	J0640=leucovorin, J9999=misc onco	fact_medical_claims — must use ref_oncology_drugs to identify oncology-specific
Oral oncolytics	NDC + GPI	NDC joined to ref_ndc WHERE oncology_drug_flag = 'Y'	fact_pharmacy_claims
Biosimilars	HCPCS Q-codes or NDC	Q5xxx = biosimilar codes; check ref_ndc for biosimilar_flag	Both medical and pharmacy claims
Radiation therapy	CPT 77xxx	77373/77435=SBRT, 77520-77525=Proton, 77385-77387=IMRT	fact_medical_claims WHERE procedure_code BETWEEN '77000' AND '77799'

10.4 Oncology Scenarios

Scenario 10.1 · Oncology / Financial

Oncology Total Cost by Cancer Type and Site of Care

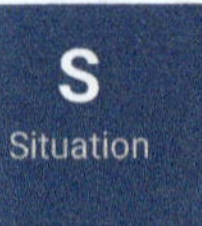

The VP of Medical Management needs a full oncology cost breakdown by cancer type and care setting for the year-end financial review. Oncology costs have grown 19% YoY and the plan needs to identify which cancer types and which care settings are driving the increase.

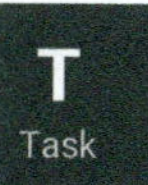

For identified oncology members (2+ C-code dates), calculate total medical + pharmacy cost by cancer type and site of care for 2023 and 2024. Identify YoY cost drivers. Decompose into drug cost vs. non-drug cost.

ANSI SQL — Scenario 10.1: Oncology Cost by Cancer Type and Site

```
-- PURPOSE: Break down oncology costs by cancer type and care site
-- to identify which combinations drive the highest per-member spend.
-- Combines medical claims (IV drugs, inpatient, outpatient, office)
-- with pharmacy claims (oral oncolytics) using UNION ALL.

-- STEP 1: Identify oncology members and their cancer type.
-- HAVING >= 2 dates applies the same 2+ visit confirmation as the ID query.
WITH oncology_members AS (
  SELECT c.member_id,
      EXTRACT(YEAR FROM c.service_date) AS service_year,
      CASE
        WHEN c.primary_diag LIKE 'C50%'         THEN 'Breast'
        WHEN c.primary_diag LIKE 'C34%'         THEN 'Lung'
        WHEN c.primary_diag BETWEEN 'C18' AND 'C20.9' THEN 'Colorectal'
        WHEN c.primary_diag BETWEEN 'C81' AND 'C96.9' THEN 'Hematologic'
        WHEN c.primary_diag = 'C61'           THEN 'Prostate'
        ELSE 'Other Oncology'
      END AS cancer_type
  FROM  fact_medical_claims c
  WHERE c.primary_diag BETWEEN 'C00' AND 'C96.9'
   AND c.claim_status = 'PAID'
   AND EXTRACT(YEAR FROM c.service_date) IN (2023, 2024)
  GROUP BY 1, 2, 3
  HAVING COUNT(DISTINCT c.service_date) >= 2  -- confirmed oncology patient
),

-- STEP 2: Pull medical claims for confirmed oncology members.
-- Classify each claim by care site using procedure codes and place-of-service.
oncology_claims AS (
  SELECT c.member_id, om.cancer_type, om.service_year,
      CASE
        -- J9000-J9999 = chemotherapy IV drugs billed on medical claim
        WHEN c.procedure_code BETWEEN 'J9000' AND 'J9999' THEN 'IV Drug (J-code)'
        WHEN c.type_of_bill LIKE '11%'          THEN 'Inpatient'
        -- Revenue codes 0330-0339 = radiation therapy
        WHEN c.revenue_code BETWEEN '0330' AND '0339' THEN 'Radiation'
        WHEN c.place_of_service = '11'          THEN 'Physician Office'
        WHEN c.place_of_service = '22'          THEN 'Outpatient Hospital'
        ELSE 'Other'
      END AS care_site,
      c.allowed_amount,
      -- Isolate drug cost within medical claims (J-codes only)
      CASE WHEN c.procedure_code BETWEEN 'J9000' AND 'J9999'
        THEN c.allowed_amount ELSE 0 END AS drug_cost
  FROM  fact_medical_claims c
  JOIN  oncology_members om
    ON c.member_id = om.member_id
   AND EXTRACT(YEAR FROM c.service_date) = om.service_year
  WHERE c.claim_status = 'PAID'
  UNION ALL
  -- Add oral oncolytic pharmacy claims (same members, same measurement years)
  SELECT p.member_id, om.cancer_type, om.service_year,
      'Oral Oncolytic (Pharmacy)' AS care_site,
      p.plan_paid_amount,
```

```
        p.plan_paid_amount AS drug_cost  -- all pharmacy cost = drug cost
    FROM  fact_pharmacy_claims p
    JOIN  ref_ndc n ON p.ndc_code = n.ndc_code
    JOIN  oncology_members om
      ON p.member_id = om.member_id
     AND EXTRACT(YEAR FROM p.dispensing_date) = om.service_year
    WHERE p.claim_status = 'PAID' AND n.oncology_drug_flag = 'Y'
)

-- STEP 3: Aggregate by cancer type, care site, and year.
SELECT
    cancer_type, care_site, service_year,
    COUNT(DISTINCT member_id)            AS members,
    ROUND(SUM(allowed_amount), 0)        AS total_cost,
    ROUND(SUM(drug_cost), 0)             AS drug_cost,
    ROUND(SUM(allowed_amount)-SUM(drug_cost),0) AS non_drug_cost,
    -- Per-member cost for cross-cancer-type comparison
    ROUND(SUM(allowed_amount)/NULLIF(COUNT(DISTINCT member_id),0),0) AS cost_per_member
FROM  oncology_claims
GROUP BY cancer_type, care_site, service_year
ORDER BY service_year DESC, total_cost DESC;
```

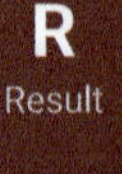

R Result

Focus the financial review on the top 3 cancer types by YoY dollar growth and the care site breakdown within each. The most actionable finding is typically site-of-care: if a cancer type shows high-cost outpatient hospital infusion, a site-of-care optimization program redirecting to physician office infusion (same drug, same clinical outcome, 20–40% lower cost) can generate immediate savings. Present cost_per_member alongside total_cost — a high cost-per-member with few members is a utilization management target; high total cost with moderate cost-per-member is a network contracting target.

Scenario 10.2 · Oncology / Quality

Oncology Time-to-Treatment Analysis

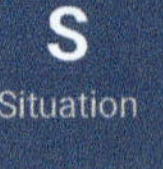

S Situation

The quality team is building an oncology access measure: how quickly are members receiving treatment after a new cancer diagnosis? Delays in treatment initiation are a clinical quality issue and a potential HEDIS-adjacent measure. The benchmark: treatment within 60 days of first diagnosis for most solid tumor types.

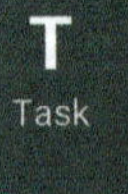

T Task

For new oncology diagnoses in the current year (no cancer claims in prior 24 months), calculate days from first diagnosis to first treatment (chemotherapy, radiation, or surgery). Flag members exceeding 60 days with their PCP and oncologist NPIs. Population: all commercial and MA oncology members.

ANSI SQL — Scenario 10.2: Oncology Time-to-Treatment

```
-- PURPOSE: Measure how many days pass between a new cancer diagnosis
-- and the first treatment (chemotherapy, radiation, or surgery).
-- Benchmark: < 60 days. FLAG > 60 days as a care access concern.

-- STEP 1: Identify NEW diagnoses (no prior cancer claims in 24-month lookback).
-- "New" = first time we see a cancer diagnosis for this member.
-- NOT EXISTS ensures we are not capturing a recurrence or ongoing care.
WITH new_diagnoses AS (
    SELECT c.member_id,
        MIN(c.service_date) AS first_dx_date,  -- earliest cancer diagnosis this year
        CASE
          WHEN MIN(c.primary_diag) LIKE 'C50%'      THEN 'Breast'
          WHEN MIN(c.primary_diag) LIKE 'C34%'      THEN 'Lung'
```

```
            WHEN MIN(c.primary_diag) BETWEEN 'C18' AND 'C21' THEN 'Colorectal'
            WHEN MIN(c.primary_diag) = 'C61'            THEN 'Prostate'
            ELSE 'Other'
        END AS cancer_type
    FROM  fact_medical_claims c
    WHERE c.primary_diag BETWEEN 'C00' AND 'C96.9'
     AND c.claim_status = 'PAID'
     AND EXTRACT(YEAR FROM c.service_date) = EXTRACT(YEAR FROM CURRENT_DATE)
     -- NOT EXISTS: exclude members who had cancer claims in the 24-month lookback
     -- This confirms the diagnosis is new, not ongoing follow-up care
     AND NOT EXISTS (
        SELECT 1 FROM fact_medical_claims h
        WHERE h.member_id    = c.member_id
         AND h.primary_diag BETWEEN 'C00' AND 'C96.9'
         AND h.claim_status = 'PAID'
         -- Prior 24 months: before the current service date
         AND h.service_date < c.service_date
         AND h.service_date >= c.service_date - INTERVAL '24' MONTH
     )
    GROUP BY c.member_id
),

-- STEP 2: Find the date of first treatment after diagnosis.
-- Treatment = chemotherapy J-code, radiation code range, or cancer surgery code.
first_treatments AS (
    SELECT nd.member_id,
        MIN(CASE
            WHEN c.procedure_code BETWEEN 'J9000' AND 'J9999' -- chemotherapy IV
             OR c.procedure_code BETWEEN '77000' AND '77799' -- radiation therapy
             OR c.procedure_code BETWEEN '19100' AND '19499' -- breast surgery
             OR c.procedure_code BETWEEN '32440' AND '32491' -- lung surgery
            THEN c.service_date END) AS first_treatment_date
    FROM  new_diagnoses nd
    JOIN  fact_medical_claims c
      ON nd.member_id = c.member_id
     AND c.service_date > nd.first_dx_date  -- treatment must be AFTER diagnosis
     AND c.claim_status = 'PAID'
    GROUP BY nd.member_id
)

-- STEP 3: Calculate days from diagnosis to first treatment.
-- LEFT JOIN: some members may not yet have a first treatment date.
SELECT
    nd.member_id, m.member_name,
    nd.cancer_type,
    nd.first_dx_date,
    ft.first_treatment_date,
    DATEDIFF('day', nd.first_dx_date, ft.first_treatment_date) AS days_to_treatment,
    m.attributed_pcp_npi,
    CASE
      WHEN DATEDIFF('day', nd.first_dx_date, ft.first_treatment_date) > 60
      THEN 'FLAG -- >60 days to treatment'
      WHEN ft.first_treatment_date IS NULL
      THEN 'FLAG -- no treatment recorded'
      ELSE 'Within benchmark'
    END AS access_flag
FROM  new_diagnoses nd
LEFT JOIN first_treatments ft ON nd.member_id = ft.member_id
JOIN  dim_members m ON nd.member_id = m.member_id
ORDER BY days_to_treatment DESC NULLS FIRST;  -- longest delays at top
```

```
  ROUND(SUM(allowed_amount)/NULLIF(COUNT(DISTINCT member_id),0),0) AS cost_per_member
FROM  oncology_claims
GROUP BY cancer_type, care_site, service_year
ORDER BY service_year DESC, total_cost DESC;
  SELECT c.member_id,
       MIN(c.service_date) AS first_dx_date,
       CASE
          WHEN MIN(c.primary_diag) LIKE 'C50%' THEN 'Breast'
          WHEN MIN(c.primary_diag) LIKE 'C34%' THEN 'Lung'
          WHEN MIN(c.primary_diag) BETWEEN 'C18' AND 'C21' THEN 'Colorectal'
          WHEN MIN(c.primary_diag) = 'C61' THEN 'Prostate'
          ELSE 'Other'
       END AS cancer_type
  FROM  fact_medical_claims c
  WHERE c.primary_diag BETWEEN 'C00' AND 'C96.9'
   AND c.claim_status = 'PAID'
   AND EXTRACT(YEAR FROM c.service_date) = EXTRACT(YEAR FROM CURRENT_DATE)
   -- New diagnosis: no prior cancer claims in 24-month lookback
   AND NOT EXISTS (
      SELECT 1 FROM fact_medical_claims h
      WHERE h.member_id    = c.member_id
       AND h.primary_diag BETWEEN 'C00' AND 'C96.9'
       AND h.claim_status = 'PAID'
       AND h.service_date < c.service_date
       AND h.service_date >= c.service_date - INTERVAL '24' MONTH
   )
  GROUP BY c.member_id
),
first_treatments AS (
  -- First chemotherapy, radiation, or surgery after diagnosis
  SELECT nd.member_id,
       MIN(CASE WHEN c.procedure_code BETWEEN 'J9000' AND 'J9999'
          OR c.procedure_code BETWEEN '77000' AND '77799'
          OR c.procedure_code BETWEEN '19100' AND '19499'  -- breast surgery
          OR c.procedure_code BETWEEN '32440' AND '32491'  -- lung surgery
          THEN c.service_date END) AS first_treatment_date
  FROM  new_diagnoses nd
  JOIN  fact_medical_claims c ON nd.member_id = c.member_id
     AND c.service_date > nd.first_dx_date
     AND c.claim_status = 'PAID'
  GROUP BY nd.member_id
)
SELECT
  nd.member_id, m.member_name,
  nd.cancer_type,
  nd.first_dx_date,
  ft.first_treatment_date,
  DATEDIFF('day', nd.first_dx_date,
        ft.first_treatment_date) AS days_to_treatment,
  m.attributed_pcp_npi,
  CASE WHEN DATEDIFF('day', nd.first_dx_date,
              ft.first_treatment_date) > 60
     THEN 'FLAG — >60 days to treatment'
     WHEN ft.first_treatment_date IS NULL
     THEN 'FLAG — no treatment recorded'
     ELSE 'Within benchmark'
  END AS access_flag
FROM  new_diagnoses nd
LEFT JOIN first_treatments ft ON nd.member_id = ft.member_id
JOIN  dim_members m ON nd.member_id = m.member_id
```

```
ORDER BY days_to_treatment DESC NULLS FIRST;
```

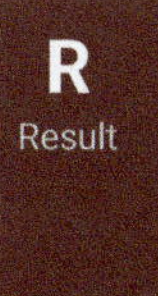

Members with FLAG — no treatment recorded require immediate clinical review — they may have received treatment outside the network, be in watchful waiting, or represent a care coordination failure. Members exceeding 60 days should be reviewed with the oncology navigation team. This report also feeds population health reporting: average days-to-treatment by cancer type and by attributed PCP is a network quality indicator that can be incorporated into provider scorecards.

Chapter 10 Review

Unit Test · Key Takeaways

Answer each question before reading the explanation.

Q1. Why does the oncology patient identification query require 2+ claims with primary cancer diagnosis on DIFFERENT service dates rather than any single claim?

A. CMS requires 2 claims to qualify for oncology risk adjustment

B. A single claim may represent rule-out coding — a clinician ordered cancer tests and coded the suspected diagnosis, but the member does not actually have cancer. Two separate dates of service suggest the clinician is continuing to treat an established cancer, reducing false positives

C. Two claims are required to capture both the inpatient and outpatient components of cancer care

D. Single claims are excluded from analytics reports due to statistical instability

Answer: B. *ICD-10-CM allows "possible" or "suspected" diagnoses on outpatient claims when a condition is being evaluated. A new patient seeing an oncologist for a suspicious finding might have C50.x coded on the referral evaluation visit before a biopsy confirms the diagnosis. Requiring 2+ dates of service with C00–C96 as primary diagnosis dramatically reduces these false positives. DATE_COUNT >= 2 is the standard filter used by most health plan oncology analytics programs.*

Q2. In the oncology cost decomposition query, UNION ALL combines medical and pharmacy claims. Why is UNION ALL used instead of UNION?

A. UNION ALL is faster because it does not sort the results

B. UNION removes duplicate rows — but the same member legitimately appears in both medical claims (for an IV chemotherapy J-code infusion) and pharmacy claims (for an oral oncolytic). UNION would incorrectly drop one of these real and distinct rows. UNION ALL preserves all rows from both sources

C. UNION ALL is required when combining claims with different schemas

D. UNION does not work across tables with different numbers of columns

Answer: B. *A member receiving concurrent IV chemotherapy (billed via a J-code on a medical claim) AND an oral targeted therapy (billed via a pharmacy claim) has real, non-duplicate cost in both datasets. UNION would identify these as "duplicates" based on member_id matching and drop one record. UNION ALL preserves both, ensuring the full picture of oncology cost is captured across both medical and pharmacy channels.*

Q3. J-codes (J9000–J9999) on a medical claim identify which type of oncology cost?

A. Inpatient chemotherapy administered during a hospital stay

B. Physician-administered or hospital-administered injectable and infusion chemotherapy drugs — these are billed on medical claims (not pharmacy claims) because a clinician administers them in an office, infusion center, or hospital outpatient setting

C. Oral chemotherapy drugs dispensed at a specialty pharmacy

D. Radiation therapy procedures performed in a radiation oncology facility

Answer: B. *J9000–J9999 are HCPCS Level II codes for injectable and infused oncology drugs administered by a clinician. They appear on CMS-1500 or UB-04 medical claims. Examples: J9070 = cyclophosphamide, J9355 = trastuzumab (Herceptin). Oral oncolytics (e.g., imatinib/Gleevec, lenalidomide/Revlimid) are dispensed at specialty pharmacies and appear in fact_pharmacy_claims. The distinction matters for both analytics (cost by care site) and utilization management (J-codes require prior auth from the medical benefit; oral drugs from the pharmacy benefit).*

Q4. The time-to-treatment query uses NOT EXISTS to confirm a new diagnosis. What does this subquery check?

A. That the member has not previously received chemotherapy

B. That the member has no prior cancer claims in the 24 months before the current service date — confirming this is a new diagnosis rather than follow-up care for an existing cancer

C. That the member's insurance was active for the full 24 months before diagnosis

D. That no other member with the same diagnosis has been treated within 24 months

Answer: B. *NOT EXISTS filters out members who already have cancer claims in the 24-month lookback window. A member with breast cancer diagnosed in 2022 who is still receiving treatment in 2024 would have C50.x claims in both years. Without NOT EXISTS, this member would appear as a "new diagnosis" in 2024 — inflating the new-diagnosis count and distorting time-to-treatment metrics. The 24-month window is long enough to capture most cancer treatment courses while avoiding false new-diagnosis flags for members in long-term remission.*

Q5. The time-to-treatment benchmark is 60 days from diagnosis to first treatment. Which members are flagged by the query even if days_to_treatment IS NULL?

A. Members who were diagnosed in the last 60 days

B. Members with no treatment recorded in the data — meaning either treatment has not started, treatment was received outside the plan's network (out-of-network claims may not appear), or the treatment codes were not captured in the current query

C. Members with more than one cancer diagnosis type

D. Members who transferred to a different health plan after diagnosis

Answer: B. *first_treatment_date IS NULL means the query found no qualifying treatment procedure codes (chemotherapy J-codes, radiation codes, or cancer surgery codes) after the diagnosis date. This can mean: (1) treatment has not yet started (member is in the pre-treatment workup phase), (2) treatment is being delivered out-of-network and the claims are not in the warehouse, (3) the member is receiving oral oncolytics only (captured in pharmacy but not included in the first_treatments CTE), or (4) the treatment codes used do not match the query's procedure code range. These cases require clinical review to distinguish true delays from data gaps.*

Q6. Biosimilar substitution in the oncology setting is analytically similar to generic drug substitution in the pharmacy setting. What is the key analytical challenge unique to biosimilars?

A. Biosimilars are not covered by any insurance plans

B. Biosimilars do not share the same NDC prefix as the reference biologic, requiring a separate biosimilar reference table (ref_biosimilar_crosswalk) to identify substitution opportunities — unlike generic drugs which share the same GPI as their brand equivalent

C. Biosimilars are always more expensive than the reference biologic

D. Biosimilar substitution requires CMS approval for each individual member

Answer: B. *For small-molecule drugs, generics and brands share the same GPI code — making substitution identification straightforward (join on gpi_14_drug). Biosimilars are large, complex biological molecules that do not share a GPI code with the reference product. Bevacizumab (Avastin) and its biosimilar bevacizumab-awwb (Mvasi) have different GPIs and different J-codes. Identifying biosimilar substitution opportunities requires a dedicated crosswalk table mapping reference biologic J-codes to approved biosimilar J-codes. This is a key data infrastructure requirement for oncology cost management programs.*

Q7. Explain the oncology patient identification methodology including the 2+ visits rule, the ICD-10 cancer code range, and the classification CASE WHEN logic for cancer type.

(Short answer)

Sample Answer:

Identification methodology: Collect all paid claims with primary_diag BETWEEN 'C00' AND 'C96.9' (ICD-10-CM malignant neoplasms chapter) for the measurement year. Group by member_id and COUNT(DISTINCT service_date). HAVING COUNT(DISTINCT service_date) >= 2 retains members with cancer as the primary diagnosis on at least two different service dates. This 2-visit rule reduces false positives from rule-out coding. ICD-10 range: C00–C96.9 covers all malignant neoplasms in ICD-10-CM: C00–C14 = lip/oral cavity/pharynx, C15–C26 = digestive organs, C30–C39 = respiratory/thorax, C40–C41 = bone, C43–C44 = skin, C50 = breast, C51–C58 = female genitalia, C60–C63 = male genitalia (C61 = prostate), C64–C68 = urinary, C69–C72 = eye/brain/CNS, C73–C75 = thyroid/endocrine, C76–C80 = ill-defined, C81–C96 = hematologic (lymphoma, leukemia, myeloma). Cancer type classification CASE WHEN: WHEN primary_diag LIKE 'C50%' THEN 'Breast' / WHEN LIKE 'C34%' THEN 'Lung' / WHEN BETWEEN 'C18' AND 'C20.9' THEN 'Colorectal' / WHEN BETWEEN 'C81' AND 'C96.9' THEN 'Hematologic' / WHEN = 'C61' THEN 'Prostate' / ELSE 'Other Oncology'. Note: use MIN(primary_diag) in the GROUP BY query to get a single cancer type per member when grouping — the MIN of C-codes within a cancer group is deterministic for classification.

Q8. Describe how UNION ALL is used to combine medical and pharmacy claims for the oncology cost decomposition and explain what happens to cost_per_member when a high-cost member appears in both data sources.

(Short answer)

Sample Answer:

UNION ALL structure: the oncology_claims CTE pulls from two tables with different schemas but common fields mapped to the same column aliases. Medical claims table: SELECT member_id, cancer_type, service_year, care_site (classified from procedure code / TOB / POS / revenue code), allowed_amount (plan's contractual cost), drug_cost (J-code claims only, others = 0). Pharmacy claims table: SELECT member_id, cancer_type, service_year, 'Oral Oncolytic (Pharmacy)' AS care_site, plan_paid_amount AS allowed_amount (pharmacy uses plan_paid, not allowed_amount field), plan_paid_amount AS drug_cost (all pharmacy cost is drug cost). After UNION ALL, every oncology claim — medical and pharmacy — is in one table with consistent column structure. The final GROUP BY aggregates by cancer_type, care_site, and service_year. cost_per_member = SUM(allowed_amount) / COUNT(DISTINCT member_id). If a breast cancer member has $45,000 in IV drug J-code medical claims AND $22,000 in oral oncolytic pharmacy claims, both contribute to the breast cancer cost total. COUNT(DISTINCT member_id) counts her once regardless of how many rows she generates. So cost_per_member correctly reflects her total $67,000 annual oncology spend. This is why COUNT(DISTINCT member_id) is used instead of COUNT(member_id) — the DISTINCT prevents double-counting the member across multiple claim rows.

Q9. Write the complete SQL to flag oncology members with >60 days from diagnosis to first treatment. Explain the LEFT JOIN pattern and the NULLS FIRST sort order.

(Short answer)

Sample Answer:

See the fully annotated SQL block in Chapter 10. Key explanations: LEFT JOIN in the final query: FROM new_diagnoses nd LEFT JOIN first_treatments ft ON nd.member_id = ft.member_id. LEFT JOIN is required because some newly diagnosed members have not yet received a first treatment — they have no row in first_treatments. An INNER JOIN would silently drop these members from the output, meaning the most actionable cases (no treatment recorded) would never be seen. LEFT JOIN preserves all new diagnoses; members with no treatment appear with first_treatment_date = NULL. NULLS FIRST in ORDER BY days_to_treatment DESC NULLS FIRST: NULL values represent the cases where no treatment date was found. In standard SQL, NULLs sort last in DESC order — meaning the most urgent cases (no treatment at all) would appear at the bottom of the results, hidden from the care management team. NULLS FIRST pushes NULL rows to the top of the output, ensuring the most at-risk members (no treatment recorded) are reviewed immediately. The access_flag CASE WHEN has two FLAG conditions: days > 60 and first_treatment_date IS NULL — together they capture both delayed treatment and missing treatment.

Q10. Describe the four oncology care settings and explain which two create the most complex analytics challenges for a health plan.

(Short answer)

Sample Answer:

Four oncology care settings: (1) Physician office (place_of_service = 11): medical oncologist administers IV chemotherapy or conducts evaluation visits. Claims appear as professional CMS-1500 with J-codes for drugs. Typically the most common setting for community oncology. (2) Outpatient hospital (place_of_service = 22): same services as physician office but in a hospital-affiliated infusion center. Claims appear as UB-04 institutional outpatient. Hospital outpatient rates are typically 2–3× higher than physician office for the same J-code drug due to facility fees. (3) Inpatient hospital (TOB 11X): hospitalizations for surgery, high-dose chemotherapy, or oncologic emergencies. UB-04 institutional with DRG. (4) Specialty pharmacy (pharmacy claims): oral oncolytics dispensed from a specialty pharmacy — no medical claim involved; appears only in fact_pharmacy_claims with oncology_drug_flag = 'Y'. Two most complex: (A) Inpatient — complex DRG-based pricing, multiple revenue codes across a single stay, COB for dual-eligible members, LOS outlier risk, and readmission patterns all require separate analytical layers. (B) Specialty pharmacy for oral oncolytics — these drugs are covered under the pharmacy benefit (not medical), are not captured in J-code analysis, may be dispensed by a PBM specialty pharmacy with different data feeds, and have biosimilar substitution opportunities that require a crosswalk table. Plans that analyze only the medical benefit miss the oral oncolytic cost entirely, understating total oncology spend by 15–30% for solid tumors with available oral agents.

Key Takeaways

What every analyst must remember from this chapter.

Oncology patient identification: ICD-10 C00–C96.9 = malignant neoplasms. Require 2+ service dates with cancer as primary diagnosis (COUNT(DISTINCT service_date) >= 2) to reduce false positives from rule-out coding. This is the standard filter used by health plan oncology analytics programs.

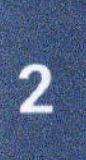

Cancer type classification: LIKE 'C50%' = Breast, 'C34%' = Lung, BETWEEN 'C18' AND 'C20.9' = Colorectal, = 'C61' = Prostate, BETWEEN 'C81' AND 'C96.9' = Hematologic. Use MIN(primary_diag) when grouping to get a deterministic cancer type per member.

3 J-codes (J9000–J9999) = IV/injected chemotherapy drugs billed on medical claims. Oral oncolytics = pharmacy claims with oncology_drug_flag = 'Y'. Complete oncology cost analysis requires UNION ALL of both sources. UNION drops legitimate dual-source rows; only UNION ALL preserves both.

4 Oncology cost decomposition uses UNION ALL to combine medical claims (allowed_amount) and pharmacy claims (plan_paid_amount). Rename to a common column. COUNT(DISTINCT member_id) in the final GROUP BY prevents double-counting members who appear in both data sources.

5 New oncology diagnosis: NOT EXISTS (SELECT 1 FROM fact_medical_claims h WHERE h.member_id = c.member_id AND h.primary_diag BETWEEN 'C00' AND 'C96.9' AND h.service_date < c.service_date AND h.service_date >= c.service_date - INTERVAL '24 months'). The 24-month lookback confirms the diagnosis is new.

6 Time-to-treatment benchmark: < 60 days from first cancer diagnosis to first treatment (J-code, radiation, or cancer surgery). Flag > 60 days AND NULL (no treatment recorded). Use ORDER BY days_to_treatment DESC NULLS FIRST to surface the most urgent cases — no treatment records — at the top of the output.

7 LEFT JOIN in time-to-treatment final query is mandatory. An INNER JOIN drops members with no treatment date (first_treatment_date IS NULL), which are the most actionable cases for care management. Always use LEFT JOIN when a missing row is itself a meaningful finding.

8 Outpatient hospital oncology (POS 22) costs 2–3× more than physician office (POS 11) for the same J-code drug due to hospital facility fees. Site-of-care analysis — comparing IV drug administration cost by POS — is one of the highest-value oncology cost management analytics.

9 Biosimilar substitution requires a ref_biosimilar_crosswalk table mapping reference biologic J-codes to approved biosimilar J-codes. Unlike small-molecule generics (same GPI as brand), biosimilars have different GPIs and J-codes than the reference product. Build and maintain this crosswalk table as FDA approves new biosimilars.

PART V Clinical Domain Analytics

Rung 5 · Chapters 11–13

Part V moves from transactional data to clinical episodes. Chapter 11 covers Behavioral Health — the MHPAEA regulatory foundation, FUH/FUM quality measures, OUD treatment gap, and psychiatric readmission. Chapter 12 covers Maternal & Neonatal — delivery identification, NTSV C-section benchmarking, mother-newborn linkage, NICU analysis, and postpartum depression screening. Chapter 13 covers Post-Acute Care — SNF LOS benchmarking, PAC-stratified readmission, end-of-life care intensity, and home health agency profiling. Every SQL block carries phase-by-phase inline comments. Every chapter ends with a unit test and key takeaways.

Part V · Clinical Domain Analytics

Chapter 11: Behavioral Health Analytics

Behavioral health conditions affect one in five Americans and produce a cost uplift — BH members cost 2.5–3.5× more in total PMPM than non-BH members, not primarily from BH services, but from the indirect medical cost caused by untreated or undertreated conditions. Understanding BH analytics requires clinical coding knowledge, regulatory expertise (MHPAEA), and SQL patterns specific to a population that shares claims infrastructure with medical but follows different code conventions.

11.1 Behavioral Health Data Landscape

Behavioral health claims are identified by specific ICD-10 diagnosis ranges, therapy CPT codes, and HCPCS H-codes for community mental health services. The analyst must know these code families before writing any BH query.

Code type	Range / values	Clinical meaning	SQL filter
ICD-10 BH diagnoses	F01–F99	Mental, behavioral & neurodevelopmental disorders	WHERE primary_diag BETWEEN 'F01' AND 'F99'
Psychiatric inpatient TOB	110, 113, 114	Inpatient psychiatric facility claims	WHERE type_of_bill IN ('110','113','114')
Individual therapy CPT	90791, 90832–90838	Psychiatric evaluation and psychotherapy	WHERE procedure_code IN ('90791','90832','90834','90837')
Group therapy CPT	90853	Group psychotherapy	WHERE procedure_code = '90853'
Crisis services CPT	90839, 90840	Psychiatric crisis intervention	WHERE procedure_code IN ('90839','90840')
HCPCS H-codes	H0001–H9999	Community mental health, SUD services	WHERE procedure_code LIKE 'H%'
MOUD drugs (pharmacy)	NDC for buprenorphine, naltrexone	Medications for opioid use disorder	JOIN ref_moud_drugs ON ndc_code

Code type	Range / values	Clinical meaning	SQL filter
OUD diagnosis	F11.x	Opioid-related disorders	WHERE primary_diag LIKE 'F11%'

> **42 CFR Part 2:** Substance use disorder records are subject to stricter confidentiality requirements under 42 CFR Part 2 than other medical records. Unlike HIPAA, Part 2 requires explicit patient consent for disclosure even to other treating providers. Analytics teams handling SUD data must ensure their data use agreements and access controls comply — this affects who can see query results and how they can be used.

11.2 Mental Health Parity — The Regulatory Foundation

The Mental Health Parity and Addiction Equity Act (MHPAEA) requires health plans to cover mental health and substance use disorder services at parity with medical/surgical services. Parity applies to both quantitative treatment limits (visit limits, day limits) and non-quantitative treatment limits (prior authorization requirements, medical necessity criteria). Failure to maintain parity is a compliance violation with significant regulatory exposure.

Parity type	What must be equal	Common violation pattern	SQL detection approach
Quantitative Treatment Limits (QTL)	Annual visit limits, day limits, episode limits must be no more restrictive for MH/SUD than for medical/surgical	Plan allows 30 therapy visits/year but 60 physical therapy visits/year	Compare visit limits from ref_benefit_design by benefit_type
Non-Quantitative Treatment Limits (NQTL)	PA requirements, fail-first/step therapy, out-of-network coverage	PA required for outpatient therapy but not for comparable medical services	Calculate PA requirement rate and denial rate by benefit_type = MH_SUD vs MEDICAL
Cost-sharing	Copays, deductibles, coinsurance must be equal	Higher copay for psychiatry than for primary care	Compare cost_share_pct from ref_benefit_design
Out-of-network access	OON coverage must be equal to medical/surgical OON coverage	No OON MH coverage but OON surgical coverage exists	Join claims to network_status flag; compare OON rates by benefit type

11.3 Behavioral Health Code Families

The behavioral health CPT code landscape has add-on codes (90833, 90836, 90838) that can only be billed alongside a primary E&M or psychotherapy code. Counting these add-on codes as standalone visits overstates utilization. Always identify the primary service and treat add-on codes as modifiers of that service, not independent encounters.

> **FUH measure window:** The Follow-Up After Hospitalization for Mental Illness (FUH) measure credits a follow-up visit on day 1 through day 7 after discharge — not including the discharge day itself. The 7-day window uses service_date, not claim_date. Claims adjudicated after the window still count if the service_date falls within it. Always filter on service_date for HEDIS measure calculations.

11.4 Behavioral Health Scenarios

Scenario 11.1 · Population Health / Financial

BH Prevalence and Cost Burden Analysis

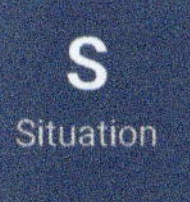

The CMO wants to quantify the total cost impact of behavioral health conditions — both the direct BH service cost and the indirect medical cost uplift. This analysis will inform the plan's care management investment strategy for the coming year.

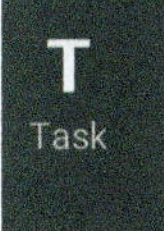

Identify BH members (2+ claims with F01–F99 primary diagnosis on different dates). Calculate total PMPM and BH-specific PMPM for BH members vs. non-BH members. Quantify the cost multiplier. Output: executive summary table for CMO presentation.

ANSI SQL — Scenario 11.1: BH Prevalence and Cost Burden

```
-- ════════════════════════════════════════════════════════════
-- SCENARIO 11.1: Behavioral Health Cost Burden Analysis
-- Goal: Compare total PMPM for BH members vs. non-BH members
-- to quantify the indirect medical cost uplift from BH conditions.
-- ════════════════════════════════════════════════════════════

-- STEP 1: Identify BH members
-- Use 2+ claims on different dates to reduce false positives
-- from rule-out coding (single claim may represent a screening)
WITH bh_members AS (
  SELECT DISTINCT member_id
  FROM  fact_medical_claims
  WHERE primary_diag BETWEEN 'F01' AND 'F99'  -- ICD-10 BH chapter
   AND claim_status = 'PAID'
   AND EXTRACT(YEAR FROM service_date) = EXTRACT(YEAR FROM CURRENT_DATE)
  GROUP BY member_id
  HAVING COUNT(DISTINCT service_date) >= 2  -- 2+ dates = confirmed BH
),

-- STEP 2: Tag all members as BH or non-BH and sum their total costs
-- LEFT JOIN preserves all members; NULL from bh_members = non-BH
all_costs AS (
  SELECT
    c.member_id,
    CASE WHEN bh.member_id IS NOT NULL
       THEN 'BH Member' ELSE 'Non-BH Member' END AS cohort,
    SUM(c.allowed_amount)                    AS total_allowed,
    -- Isolate BH-specific costs (F-code claims only)
    SUM(CASE WHEN c.primary_diag BETWEEN 'F01' AND 'F99'
         THEN c.allowed_amount ELSE 0 END)     AS bh_allowed
  FROM  fact_medical_claims c
  LEFT JOIN bh_members bh ON c.member_id = bh.member_id
  WHERE c.claim_status = 'PAID'
   AND EXTRACT(YEAR FROM c.service_date) = EXTRACT(YEAR FROM CURRENT_DATE)
  GROUP BY c.member_id,
       CASE WHEN bh.member_id IS NOT NULL THEN 'BH Member'
          ELSE 'Non-BH Member' END
),

-- STEP 3: Pull member months by cohort for the PMPM denominator
-- Member months must come from enrollment, not claims
cohort_mm AS (
  SELECT
```

```sql
        CASE WHEN bh.member_id IS NOT NULL
            THEN 'BH Member' ELSE 'Non-BH Member' END AS cohort,
        SUM(mm.member_months) AS total_mm
    FROM  fact_member_months mm
    LEFT JOIN bh_members bh ON mm.member_id = bh.member_id
    WHERE EXTRACT(YEAR FROM mm.month_start) = EXTRACT(YEAR FROM CURRENT_DATE)
    GROUP BY CASE WHEN bh.member_id IS NOT NULL
               THEN 'BH Member' ELSE 'Non-BH Member' END
)

-- STEP 4: Calculate PMPM for each cohort and derive the cost multiplier
SELECT
    ac.cohort,
    COUNT(DISTINCT ac.member_id)            AS member_count,
    cmm.total_mm                            AS member_months,
    ROUND(SUM(ac.total_allowed)
        / NULLIF(cmm.total_mm, 0), 2)       AS total_pmpm,
    ROUND(SUM(ac.bh_allowed)
        / NULLIF(cmm.total_mm, 0), 2)       AS bh_pmpm,
    -- Cost multiplier: how much more do BH members cost than non-BH?
    ROUND(SUM(ac.total_allowed) / NULLIF(cmm.total_mm, 0)
        / NULLIF(MIN(CASE WHEN ac.cohort = 'Non-BH Member'
            THEN SUM(ac.total_allowed)/NULLIF(cmm.total_mm,0) END
            ) OVER (), 0), 2)               AS cost_multiplier_vs_nonbh
FROM  all_costs ac
JOIN  cohort_mm cmm ON ac.cohort = cmm.cohort
GROUP BY ac.cohort, cmm.total_mm
ORDER BY total_pmpm DESC;
```

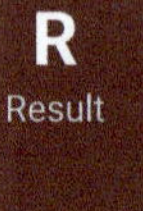

R Result

Typical finding: BH member total PMPM = $650–$900 vs. non-BH = $220–$320 — a 2.5–3.5× multiplier. The bh_pmpm column typically represents only $120–$180 of the total, meaning 75–85% of the BH cost burden is indirect medical spend driven by comorbidities, avoidable admissions, and ED utilization in untreated BH members. Present to CMO: investing in BH care management reduces the larger indirect cost, not just the BH service cost.

Scenario 11.2 · Quality / HEDIS

Follow-Up After Hospitalization for Mental Illness (FUH/FUM)

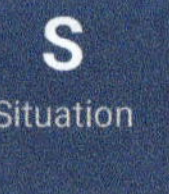

S Situation

The Stars team needs the FUH-7 and FUH-30 measure rates by attributed PCP. FUH is a HEDIS and Star Ratings measure — improving it counts in both quality submissions. The team needs a gap list to drive outreach to psychiatrists and PCPs for members who had a psychiatric discharge but no follow-up.

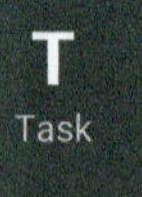

T Task

Identify all qualifying psychiatric discharges in the measurement year. For each discharge, check for a qualifying follow-up visit within 7 days (FUH-7) and 30 days (FUH-30). Flag members who met neither. Output: gap list by attributed PCP with discharge facility and diagnosis group.

ANSI SQL — Scenario 11.2: FUH Measure — Follow-Up After Psychiatric Discharge

```sql
-- ============================================================
-- SCENARIO 11.2: FUH Measure Calculation
-- FUH-7: follow-up visit within 7 days of psychiatric discharge
-- FUH-30: follow-up visit within 30 days
-- NCQA: follow-up on day 1 through 7 — discharge day (day 0) does NOT count
-- ============================================================
```

```sql
-- STEP 1: Identify qualifying psychiatric discharges (denominator)
-- TOB 110/113/114 = inpatient psychiatric facility
-- F20-F99 = psychotic, mood, anxiety, and substance use disorders
-- Exclude non-qualifying discharge statuses per NCQA specification
WITH psych_discharges AS (
  SELECT
    c.member_id,
    c.claim_id,
    c.billing_npi          AS discharging_facility,
    c.discharge_date,
    c.primary_diag,
    c.discharge_status_code
  FROM  fact_medical_claims c
  WHERE c.type_of_bill   IN ('110','113','114')  -- psych inpatient
   AND c.primary_diag  BETWEEN 'F20' AND 'F99'  -- qualifying BH dx
   AND c.claim_status   = 'PAID'
   AND EXTRACT(YEAR FROM c.discharge_date) = EXTRACT(YEAR FROM CURRENT_DATE)
   -- Exclude: transfers (02), AMA (07), deceased (20), hospice (65/66)
   AND c.discharge_status_code NOT IN ('02','04','07','20','65','66')
),

-- STEP 2: Find qualifying follow-up visits after each discharge
-- NCQA qualifying: outpatient BH visit, telehealth, intensive outpatient
-- service_date must be >= discharge_date + 1 (day after discharge)
followup_visits AS (
  SELECT
    c.member_id,
    c.service_date         AS followup_date,
    c.rendering_npi        AS followup_provider
  FROM  fact_medical_claims c
  WHERE c.procedure_code IN (  -- NCQA qualifying follow-up codes
        '90791','90792',                  -- psychiatric evaluation
        '90832','90833','90834','90836',  -- individual psychotherapy
        '90837','90838',                  -- individual therapy (60 min)
        '90839','90840',                  -- crisis intervention
        '90845','90847','90853',          -- analysis, family, group therapy
        '99213','99214','99215'           -- E&M with BH dx (primary care)
    )
   AND c.claim_status = 'PAID'
),

-- STEP 3: Join each discharge to the earliest follow-up within each window
-- LEFT JOIN: discharges with no follow-up return NULL → gap members
discharge_followup AS (
  SELECT
    pd.member_id,
    pd.claim_id,
    pd.discharge_date,
    pd.primary_diag,
    -- Earliest follow-up in each window (NULL = no follow-up)
    MIN(CASE WHEN fv.followup_date BETWEEN pd.discharge_date + 1
                        AND pd.discharge_date + 7
        THEN fv.followup_date END) AS fuh7_date,
    MIN(CASE WHEN fv.followup_date BETWEEN pd.discharge_date + 1
                        AND pd.discharge_date + 30
        THEN fv.followup_date END) AS fuh30_date
  FROM  psych_discharges pd
  LEFT JOIN followup_visits fv
      ON pd.member_id  = fv.member_id
```

```
    AND fv.followup_date > pd.discharge_date -- day 1+, not discharge day
  GROUP BY pd.member_id, pd.claim_id, pd.discharge_date, pd.primary_diag
)

-- STEP 4: Calculate rates and produce gap list
SELECT
  m.attributed_pcp_npi,
  COUNT(*)                    AS total_discharges,
  SUM(CASE WHEN df.fuh7_date  IS NOT NULL THEN 1 ELSE 0 END) AS fuh7_met,
  SUM(CASE WHEN df.fuh30_date IS NOT NULL THEN 1 ELSE 0 END) AS fuh30_met,
  ROUND(100.0 * SUM(CASE WHEN df.fuh7_date IS NOT NULL
    THEN 1 ELSE 0 END) / COUNT(*), 1)        AS fuh7_rate_pct,
  ROUND(100.0 * SUM(CASE WHEN df.fuh30_date IS NOT NULL
    THEN 1 ELSE 0 END) / COUNT(*), 1)        AS fuh30_rate_pct
FROM  discharge_followup df
JOIN  dim_members m ON df.member_id = m.member_id
GROUP BY m.attributed_pcp_npi
ORDER BY fuh7_rate_pct ASC;
```

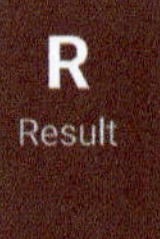

FUH-7 national average is approximately 40–45%; top-performing plans reach 60%+. PCPs with fuh7_rate_pct below 30% should receive a gap list with the specific members and discharge dates — the PCP may not know their patient was hospitalized. The discharging facility NPI enables direct outreach to psychiatric discharge planners to implement a standard follow-up scheduling protocol.

Scenario 11.3 · Clinical / Care Management

OUD Treatment Gap and ED Utilization

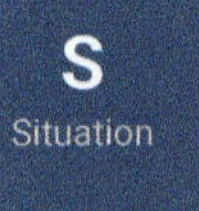

The clinical pharmacy and BH teams need to identify members with opioid use disorder (OUD) who are NOT receiving medications for OUD (MOUD — buprenorphine, naltrexone, methadone). Untreated OUD members have dramatically higher ED utilization and are at high risk of overdose.

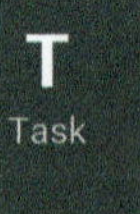

Identify members with OUD diagnosis (F11.x, 2+ dates). Flag those with no MOUD fills or MOUD medical claims in the past 12 months. Calculate their ED utilization rate. Output: treatment gap list ranked by ED visits descending for care management prioritization.

ANSI SQL — Scenario 11.3: OUD Treatment Gap and ED Utilization

```
-- ══════════════════════════════════════════════════════════════
-- SCENARIO 11.3: OUD Treatment Gap Detection
-- Goal: Identify OUD members not receiving MOUD treatment
-- and quantify their ED utilization for care management targeting.
-- ══════════════════════════════════════════════════════════════

-- STEP 1: Identify confirmed OUD members
-- F11.x = opioid-related disorders; require 2+ months to reduce
-- false positives from acute detox or single screening encounters
WITH oud_members AS (
  SELECT member_id
  FROM  fact_medical_claims
  WHERE primary_diag LIKE 'F11%' -- opioid use disorder ICD-10 range
   AND claim_status = 'PAID'
   AND service_date >= CURRENT_DATE - INTERVAL '12' MONTH
  GROUP BY member_id
  -- Require 2+ distinct calendar months with OUD diagnosis
  HAVING COUNT(DISTINCT
```

```
    EXTRACT(YEAR FROM service_date)*100
    + EXTRACT(MONTH FROM service_date)) >= 2
),

-- STEP 2: Identify members currently receiving MOUD
-- MOUD includes: buprenorphine (pharmacy), naltrexone (pharmacy + injectable)
-- and methadone maintenance (medical H0020 procedure code)
moud_treatment AS (
  -- Pharmacy: buprenorphine/naltrexone fills
  SELECT DISTINCT p.member_id
  FROM  fact_pharmacy_claims p
  JOIN  ref_moud_drugs m ON p.ndc_code = m.ndc_code
  WHERE p.claim_status    = 'PAID'
    AND p.dispensing_date >= CURRENT_DATE - INTERVAL '12' MONTH
  UNION
  -- Medical: methadone maintenance (H0020) or injectable naltrexone (J2315)
  SELECT DISTINCT member_id
  FROM  fact_medical_claims
  WHERE procedure_code IN ('H0020', 'J2315')
    AND claim_status = 'PAID'
    AND service_date >= CURRENT_DATE - INTERVAL '12' MONTH
),

-- STEP 3: Count ED visits for OUD members in the past 12 months
-- ED identified by place_of_service = 23 OR revenue code 045x
oud_ed_visits AS (
  SELECT
    c.member_id,
    COUNT(DISTINCT c.claim_id) AS ed_visit_count
  FROM  fact_medical_claims c
  JOIN  oud_members om ON c.member_id = om.member_id
  WHERE (c.place_of_service = '23'  -- ED place of service
     OR c.revenue_code BETWEEN '0450' AND '0459')
    AND c.claim_status = 'PAID'
    AND c.service_date >= CURRENT_DATE - INTERVAL '12' MONTH
  GROUP BY c.member_id
)

-- STEP 4: Produce treatment gap list — OUD members with no MOUD
-- LEFT JOIN to moud_treatment; NULL = no MOUD = treatment gap
SELECT
  om.member_id,
  m.member_name,
  m.attributed_pcp_npi,
  m.phone_number,
  COALESCE(ev.ed_visit_count, 0)  AS ed_visits_12m,
  CASE WHEN mt.member_id IS NOT NULL
     THEN 'Receiving MOUD'
     ELSE 'TREATMENT GAP — no MOUD'
  END                AS moud_status
FROM  oud_members om
JOIN  dim_members m ON om.member_id = m.member_id
LEFT JOIN moud_treatment mt ON om.member_id = mt.member_id
LEFT JOIN oud_ed_visits  ev ON om.member_id = ev.member_id
-- Focus outreach on treatment gaps only
WHERE mt.member_id IS NULL
ORDER BY ed_visits_12m DESC;
```

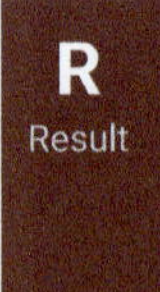
R
Result

OUD members without MOUD typically show 4–8 ED visits per year vs. 0.8–1.2 for OUD members receiving MOUD. The highest-priority members are those with 3+ ED visits in the past 12 months and no MOUD — they are in a crisis cycle that MOUD initiation can interrupt. Route to the BH care management team with the member's PCP NPI for warm handoff outreach. This report directly supports the HEDIS IET (Initiation and Engagement of SUD Treatment) measure.

Chapter 11 Review

Unit Test & Key Takeaways

Answer each question before reading the explanation. Answers immediately follow each question.

Q1. Which ICD-10 code range covers behavioral health diagnoses used in HEDIS measures like FUH?

A. F01–F99: Mental, Behavioral and Neurodevelopmental Disorders
B. G00–G99: Diseases of the Nervous System
C. R00–R99: Symptoms and Signs Not Elsewhere Classified
D. Z00–Z99: Factors Influencing Health Status

Answer: A. *F01–F99 is the ICD-10-CM chapter for all mental and behavioral health disorders. G-codes cover neurological diseases (e.g., epilepsy, Parkinson's). R-codes are unspecified symptoms. Z-codes are status/encounter codes. FUH requires F20–F99 as the primary diagnosis on the inpatient claim.*

Q2. Under MHPAEA, which statement correctly describes quantitative treatment limit (QTL) parity?

A. MH/SUD services must be covered at 100% with no cost-sharing
B. Annual visit limits and day limits for MH/SUD cannot be more restrictive than comparable medical/surgical limits
C. All MH/SUD prior authorizations must be approved within 72 hours
D. MH/SUD benefits must cover every FDA-approved treatment modality

Answer: B. *Quantitative treatment limits include visit limits, day limits, and episode limits. MHPAEA requires that these limits for MH/SUD benefits cannot be more restrictive than the predominant limits applied to substantially all medical/surgical benefits. Equal restriction — not elimination — is the standard.*

Q3. The FUH-7 measure credits a follow-up visit on which days relative to discharge?

A. Day 0 through Day 7 (including discharge day)
B. Day 1 through Day 7 (day after discharge through 7 days post-discharge)
C. Day 7 only (exactly 7 days post-discharge)
D. Day 1 through Day 14 (two weeks post-discharge)

Answer: B. *NCQA FUH specifies follow-up must occur on day 1 through day 7 after discharge. The discharge day itself (day 0) does not count. This is a common SQL error — using >= discharge_date instead of > discharge_date includes the discharge day and overstates the rate.*

Q4. Why does the OUD member identification query require 2+ claims on different service dates?

A. CMS requires 2 claims for all diagnosis-based cohort definitions
B. A single F11.x claim may represent an acute detox encounter or rule-out coding — two dates confirm a persistent condition
C. Two claims are required for HIPAA compliance in SUD analytics
D. The first claim establishes diagnosis; the second establishes active treatment

Answer: B. *Single-date diagnosis coding can represent a screening, a rule-out, or an acute crisis that resolved. Two distinct service dates indicate a persistent condition requiring ongoing management. The same 2-date criterion is used for oncology (C-codes), OUD (F11), and other high-sensitivity populations.*

Q5. In the BH cost burden query, why is the cost multiplier calculated against Non-BH members rather than the overall population average?

A. NCQA requires peer comparison against non-clinical members for all cost analyses
B. Comparing against the overall average includes BH members in the baseline, diluting the true differential — the non-BH group provides a clean counterfactual
C. Non-BH members are always the larger population, making the denominator more statistically stable
D. The overall average would include pharmacy costs which are tracked separately

Answer: B. *If BH members are included in the baseline (overall average), the comparison is circular — the high cost of BH members inflates the average, making the multiplier appear smaller than the true effect. Using non-BH members as the counterfactual provides the cleanest measure of how much BH conditions increase costs above the baseline healthy population.*

Q6. Explain how to detect a potential MHPAEA Non-Quantitative Treatment Limit (NQTL) parity violation using SQL on prior authorization data. Include the specific metrics you would calculate and the threshold that would trigger a compliance review.

(Short answer)

> **Sample Answer:**
> NQTL parity requires that PA requirements, fail-first protocols, and medical necessity criteria be no more restrictive for MH/SUD than for medical/surgical services. SQL detection methodology: (1) Classify each PA request as MH_SUD or MEDICAL_SURGICAL using primary_diag BETWEEN 'F01' AND 'F99' and BH procedure codes (90791, 90832–90838, H-codes). (2) Calculate PA approval rate, denial rate, and average decision hours separately for each benefit type. (3) Calculate PA requirement rate (what % of service claims required PA at all) by benefit type. (4) Compare: if MH/SUD PA denial rate > MEDICAL denial rate by more than 5 percentage points, or if MH/SUD requires PA for service types that medical does not, flag as potential NQTL violation. Threshold for compliance review: denial rate differential > 5pp, or PA requirement rate differential > 20pp, triggers a comparative analysis report for the compliance team.

Q7. A behavioral health analyst is asked to calculate the "indirect cost" of behavioral health conditions — the additional medical spending attributable to having a BH diagnosis, separate from the BH services themselves. Describe the methodology.

(Short answer)

> **Sample Answer:**
> Methodology: (1) Identify BH members using 2+ F01–F99 claims on different service dates. (2) Calculate total_pmpm and bh_specific_pmpm for BH members. (3) Calculate total_pmpm for non-BH members as the counterfactual baseline. (4) Indirect cost per BH member = (total_pmpm_bh_members - bh_specific_pmpm_bh_members) - total_pmpm_nonbh_members. This isolates the medical cost uplift from BH conditions: high IP admissions (especially psychiatric + medical comorbidity), ED utilization for suicidal ideation and overdose, and costly comorbidity management (e.g., diabetes poorly controlled in depressed members). The indirect cost typically exceeds the direct BH service cost by 3–4×, making untreated BH conditions a significant financial risk for the plan.

Q8. Describe the 42 CFR Part 2 compliance requirements that apply to SUD analytics and explain how they differ from standard HIPAA PHI rules.

(Short answer)

> **Sample Answer:**
> 42 CFR Part 2 governs records maintained by federally assisted SUD treatment programs (methadone clinics, buprenorphine prescribers under waiver, certified SUD treatment programs). Key differences from HIPAA: (1) Disclosure requires explicit patient consent — unlike HIPAA, which permits TPO (treatment, payment, operations) disclosure without consent. (2) Even other treating providers cannot receive SUD records without consent. (3) Re-disclosure is prohibited without a new consent. (4) Law enforcement cannot access records without a court order meeting specific criteria. For analytics teams: SUD claims data (F11–F16 diagnoses, MOUD pharmacy claims, H0020 methadone codes) should be accessed only by personnel with data use agreements that include Part 2 compliance requirements. Query results showing individual member SUD status should not be exported to platforms that allow broad access. Population-level aggregate reports (de-identified) are generally permissible.

Key Takeaways

What every analyst must remember from this chapter.

1

Behavioral health claims are identified by ICD-10 F01–F99 diagnoses, therapy CPT codes (90791, 90832–90838, 90847, 90853), and HCPCS H-codes. Psychiatric inpatient claims use TOB 110/113/114. Know these code families before writing any BH query.

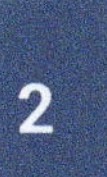

BH members typically cost 2.5–3.5× more in total PMPM than non-BH members. Only 15–25% of that cost is direct BH service spend — the majority is indirect medical cost uplift from untreated or undertreated conditions. Care management investment reduces both.

3 MHPAEA requires parity in both quantitative treatment limits (visit limits, day limits) and non-quantitative treatment limits (PA requirements, medical necessity criteria). SQL detection: compare PA denial rates and PA requirement rates between MH_SUD and MEDICAL_SURGICAL benefit types.

4 FUH-7 credits a follow-up visit on day 1 through day 7 after psychiatric discharge. Day 0 (discharge day) does not count. Always filter: service_date > discharge_date AND service_date <= discharge_date + 7. Filtering on >= discharge_date overstates the rate.

5 MOUD (buprenorphine, naltrexone, methadone) is the FDA-approved first-line treatment for OUD. OUD members without MOUD have 4–8× higher ED utilization. The OUD treatment gap report (OUD members with no MOUD fills) is the highest-ROI BH care management intervention.

6 Psychiatric add-on CPT codes (90833, 90836, 90838) can only be billed alongside a primary service. Counting them as standalone visits overstates utilization. Always identify the primary service code and treat add-on codes as modifiers.

7 Use 2+ claims on different service dates to identify BH members — the same 2-date criterion used for oncology. A single F-code claim may represent a rule-out, screening, or acute crisis. Two dates confirm a persistent condition.

8 42 CFR Part 2 imposes stricter confidentiality requirements on SUD records than HIPAA. SUD data requires explicit patient consent for disclosure — even to treating providers. Analytics teams must ensure data use agreements and access controls comply before querying MOUD fills, F11–F16 diagnoses, or methadone claims.

Chapter 12: Maternal & Neonatal Analytics

Pregnancy and childbirth represent the most common reason for hospital admission in the United States — approximately 3.6 million deliveries annually. For a health plan, maternal care is a high-cost, high-complexity domain where data quality failures have direct clinical consequences. Correctly identifying the delivery event, classifying the delivery type, linking the mother's claims to the newborn's claims, and measuring quality metrics like NTSV C-section rate and postpartum depression screening requires a combination of DRG knowledge, ICD-10 obstetric coding, and specialized SQL join patterns.

12.1 Maternal Care Data Architecture

Maternal analytics requires identifying and linking three related but distinct episodes: the prenatal care period (outpatient visits during pregnancy), the delivery hospitalization (inpatient stay), and the postpartum period (follow-up care after delivery). Each has different claim types, code systems, and timing requirements.

Episode	Claim type	Primary identifiers	Date anchor	SQL pattern
Prenatal care	Professional (CMS-1500)	CPT 59425/59426 (prenatal visits), Z34.x (prenatal encounter dx)	First prenatal visit date (estimated from delivery - 280 days)	COUNT(DISTINCT service_date) for visit count; avoid CPT 59400 (global package)
Delivery hospitalization	Institutional (UB-04)	DRG 765–782, ICD-10 O60–O84, type_of_bill 11x	discharge_date = delivery date proxy	WHERE primary_drg BETWEEN '765' AND '782'
Newborn stay	Institutional (UB-04)	DRG 790–795, Z38.x (liveborn infant), type_of_bill 11x	admit_date = birth date	JOIN to mother via delivery_facility + date proximity (± 1 day)
Postpartum visit	Professional	CPT 59430 (postpartum visit), Z39.x (postpartum care encounter)	delivery_date + 21 to 56 days (HEDIS PCR window)	service_date BETWEEN discharge_date + 21 AND discharge_date + 56

Global OB billing trap: CPT 59400 (Routine obstetric care including antepartum care, vaginal delivery and postpartum care) bundles all prenatal visits, delivery, and postpartum care into a single claim line with the delivery date. This means individual prenatal visit dates are not captured in claims. For prenatal visit timeliness analysis, use Z34.x diagnosis codes on office visit claims rather than obstetric global codes. If only 59400 claims exist, timeliness analysis from claims alone is not possible — EHR data is required.

12.2 Delivery Identification and Classification

The delivery event is the anchor for the entire maternal analytics episode. Correctly identifying the delivery date, delivery type (vaginal vs. C-section), and gestational characteristics (singleton vs. multiple gestation, term vs. preterm, vertex vs. malpresentation) is prerequisite for every downstream maternal quality measure.

ANSI SQL — 12.2: Delivery Identification and Classification

```
-- ════════════════════════════════════════════════════════════
-- Delivery identification: find all delivery hospitalizations
-- and classify by delivery type and gestational characteristics.
-- DRG 765-768 = C-section; DRG 769-782 = vaginal delivery
-- ICD-10 O60-O84 = delivery diagnoses (backup when DRG unavailable)
-- ════════════════════════════════════════════════════════════
SELECT DISTINCT
  member_id,
  admit_date      AS delivery_admit,
  discharge_date    AS delivery_discharge,
  primary_drg,
  -- Delivery type: use DRG as primary source, ICD-10 as fallback
  CASE
    WHEN primary_drg BETWEEN '765' AND '768'  THEN 'C-Section'
    WHEN primary_drg BETWEEN '769' AND '782'  THEN 'Vaginal Delivery'
    WHEN primary_diag LIKE 'O82%'            THEN 'C-Section' -- ICD fallback
    WHEN primary_diag BETWEEN 'O80' AND 'O84' THEN 'Vaginal Delivery'
    ELSE 'Unknown Delivery Type'
  END             AS delivery_type,
  -- Multiple gestation: affects NTSV eligibility (must be singleton)
  CASE
    WHEN primary_diag LIKE 'O30%'  THEN 'Multiple Gestation'
    ELSE                    'Singleton'
  END             AS gestation_type,
  -- Gestational age term/preterm: Z3A codes = gestational age in weeks
  CASE
    WHEN secondary_diag_1 LIKE 'Z3A.3%'
     OR secondary_diag_1 LIKE 'Z3A.4%' THEN 'Term (37+ weeks)'
    ELSE 'Preterm (<37 weeks)'
  END             AS gestational_term
FROM  fact_medical_claims
WHERE (primary_drg BETWEEN '765' AND '782'    -- delivery DRGs
  OR primary_diag BETWEEN 'O60' AND 'O84')  -- delivery diagnoses
 AND type_of_bill LIKE '11%'                -- inpatient only
 AND claim_status = 'PAID'
ORDER BY member_id, delivery_admit;
```

12.3 Linking Mother and Newborn Records

One of the most technically challenging aspects of maternal analytics is linking the mother's claims to the newborn's claims. The two members have different member_ids — the infant is enrolled separately, often retroactively after birth. The linkage strategy uses shared delivery facility (billing_npi) and temporal proximity (delivery date ± 1 day), because the mother's discharge_date and the infant's admit_date may differ by one day if delivery occurs near midnight.

ANSI SQL — 12.3: Mother-Newborn Record Linkage

```
-- ════════════════════════════════════════════════════════════
```

```
-- Mother-newborn linkage: join on delivery facility + date proximity
-- Mother: DRG 765-782 (delivery) at facility X on date Y
-- Infant: DRG 790-795 or Z38.x (liveborn) at same facility
-- 1-day tolerance: delivery may occur the day before discharge
-- ═══════════════════════════════════════════════════════════════
WITH mothers AS (
   -- Identify all delivery hospitalizations for the mother
   SELECT member_id,
          billing_npi    AS delivery_facility,
          discharge_date AS delivery_date    -- proxy for delivery date
   FROM  fact_medical_claims
   WHERE primary_drg BETWEEN '765' AND '782'
    AND claim_status = 'PAID'
),
newborns AS (
   -- Identify newborn admissions
   -- DRG 790-795 = newborn-specific DRGs; Z38.x = liveborn infant codes
   SELECT member_id    AS infant_id,
          billing_npi  AS birth_facility,
          admit_date   AS birth_date
   FROM  fact_medical_claims
   WHERE (primary_drg BETWEEN '790' AND '795'
          OR primary_diag LIKE 'Z38%')        -- liveborn infant diagnosis
    AND claim_status = 'PAID'
)
SELECT
   m.member_id    AS maternal_member_id,
   n.infant_id    AS infant_member_id,
   m.delivery_date,
   n.birth_date
FROM  mothers m
JOIN  newborns n
  ON m.delivery_facility = n.birth_facility  -- same hospital
  -- 1-day tolerance: handles midnight delivery date boundary
  AND ABS(DATEDIFF('day', m.delivery_date, n.birth_date)) <= 1
ORDER BY m.delivery_date;
```

Why the 1-day tolerance: The mother's discharge_date is used as a proxy for delivery date. If delivery occurs at 11 PM, the infant's birth_date is recorded as that day, but the mother's discharge_date may be the following day. Without a 1-day tolerance, these mother-infant pairs fail to join and the link is lost. A tolerance greater than 1 day risks false matches between mothers and infants from different deliveries at the same facility.

12.4 Maternal & Neonatal Scenarios

Scenario 12.1 · Quality / Network

NTSV C-Section Rate by Hospital

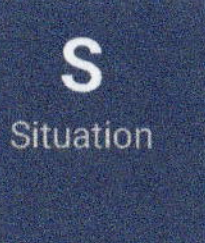

The VP of Quality needs a NTSV C-section rate by hospital for the annual network quality report. NTSV (Nulliparous, Term, Singleton, Vertex) is the gold standard denominator for measuring avoidable C-sections — it isolates first-time mothers with term, head-down, singleton pregnancies where clinical indication for C-section should be rare. The Leapfrog benchmark is ≤23.9%.

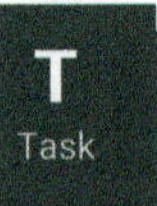

Calculate C-section rate with NTSV stratification by hospital NPI for the current year. For each hospital, report overall C-section rate and NTSV C-section rate. Flag hospitals exceeding 23.9% NTSV threshold with minimum 30 NTSV deliveries for statistical stability.

ANSI SQL — Scenario 12.1: NTSV C-Section Rate by Hospital

```
-- ══════════════════════════════════════════════════════════════
-- NTSV C-Section Rate: gold standard avoidable C-section metric
-- NTSV = Nulliparous (first delivery) + Term (≥37 wks) +
-- Singleton + Vertex (head-down presentation)
-- Leapfrog benchmark: NTSV C-section rate ≤ 23.9%
-- ══════════════════════════════════════════════════════════════

-- STEP 1: Classify all deliveries by type and NTSV eligibility
WITH all_deliveries AS (
  SELECT
    c.member_id,
    c.billing_npi        AS hospital_npi,
    c.discharge_date,
    -- C-section flag: DRG 765-768
    CASE WHEN c.primary_drg BETWEEN '765' AND '768'
      THEN 'C-Section' ELSE 'Vaginal' END AS delivery_type,
    -- Term: Z3A codes 37-42 weeks in secondary diagnoses
    CASE WHEN c.secondary_diag_1 LIKE 'Z3A.3%'
       OR c.secondary_diag_1 LIKE 'Z3A.4%'
      THEN 1 ELSE 0 END  AS is_term,
    -- Singleton: O30.x = multiple gestation; absence = singleton
    CASE WHEN c.secondary_diag_1 LIKE 'O30%'
       OR c.primary_diag   LIKE 'O30%'
      THEN 1 ELSE 0 END  AS is_multiple_gestation,
    -- Malpresentation: O32.x = fetal malpresentation (non-vertex)
    CASE WHEN c.secondary_diag_1 LIKE 'O32%'
      THEN 1 ELSE 0 END  AS is_malpresentation
  FROM  fact_medical_claims c
  WHERE (c.primary_drg BETWEEN '765' AND '782'
    OR c.primary_diag BETWEEN 'O60' AND 'O84')
   AND c.type_of_bill LIKE '11%'
   AND c.claim_status = 'PAID'
   AND EXTRACT(YEAR FROM c.discharge_date) = EXTRACT(YEAR FROM CURRENT_DATE)
),

-- STEP 2: Identify nulliparous members (first delivery in plan history)
-- Proxy: no prior delivery claim in the past 3 years
nulliparous AS (
  SELECT DISTINCT ad.member_id
  FROM  all_deliveries ad
  WHERE NOT EXISTS (
    SELECT 1 FROM fact_medical_claims prior_del
    WHERE prior_del.member_id  = ad.member_id
     AND (prior_del.primary_drg BETWEEN '765' AND '782'
       OR prior_del.primary_diag BETWEEN 'O60' AND 'O84')
     AND prior_del.claim_status = 'PAID'
     -- Prior delivery = any delivery before current year
     AND EXTRACT(YEAR FROM prior_del.discharge_date)
       < EXTRACT(YEAR FROM CURRENT_DATE)
  )
),

-- STEP 3: Flag NTSV eligibility: must meet ALL four criteria
```

```sql
ntsv_flagged AS (
  SELECT
    ad.*,
    CASE WHEN n.member_id IS NOT NULL  -- nulliparous
         AND ad.is_term = 1            -- term ≥37 weeks
         AND ad.is_multiple_gestation = 0  -- singleton
         AND ad.is_malpresentation = 0    -- vertex presentation
        THEN 1 ELSE 0 END AS ntsv_flag
  FROM  all_deliveries ad
  LEFT JOIN nulliparous n ON ad.member_id = n.member_id
)

-- STEP 4: Calculate overall and NTSV C-section rates by hospital
SELECT
  nf.hospital_npi,
  p.hospital_name,
  COUNT(*)                          AS total_deliveries,
  SUM(CASE WHEN nf.delivery_type = 'C-Section' THEN 1 ELSE 0 END)
                                AS total_csections,
  ROUND(100.0 * SUM(CASE WHEN delivery_type='C-Section' THEN 1 ELSE 0 END)
    / COUNT(*), 1)                   AS overall_csection_pct,
  SUM(nf.ntsv_flag)                   AS ntsv_deliveries,
  SUM(CASE WHEN nf.ntsv_flag=1 AND nf.delivery_type='C-Section'
        THEN 1 ELSE 0 END)              AS ntsv_csections,
  ROUND(100.0 * SUM(CASE WHEN nf.ntsv_flag=1 AND nf.delivery_type='C-Section'
    THEN 1 ELSE 0 END) / NULLIF(SUM(nf.ntsv_flag), 0), 1)
                                AS ntsv_csection_pct,
  -- Flag hospitals exceeding Leapfrog benchmark with sufficient volume
  CASE WHEN ROUND(100.0 * SUM(CASE WHEN nf.ntsv_flag=1
         AND nf.delivery_type='C-Section' THEN 1 ELSE 0 END)
         / NULLIF(SUM(nf.ntsv_flag),0), 1) > 23.9
       AND SUM(nf.ntsv_flag) >= 30
      THEN 'FLAG — above Leapfrog benchmark'
      ELSE 'Within benchmark' END          AS quality_flag
FROM  ntsv_flagged nf
JOIN  dim_providers p ON nf.hospital_npi = p.npi
GROUP BY nf.hospital_npi, p.hospital_name
HAVING COUNT(*) >= 10
ORDER BY ntsv_csection_pct DESC NULLS LAST;
```

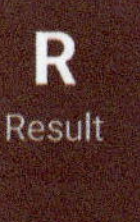

Hospitals flagged above 23.9% NTSV C-section rate with 30+ NTSV deliveries are candidates for the preferred network quality review. Present to VP Quality: each percentage point of NTSV C-section rate above benchmark represents approximately $3,500–$4,500 in excess delivery cost (C-section premium over vaginal). A hospital at 35% NTSV rate vs. 24% benchmark on 200 NTSV deliveries = $3,500 × (35-24)% × 200 = estimated $770,000 in excess annual cost.

Scenario 12.2 · Quality / Maternal Health

Postpartum Depression Screening Rate

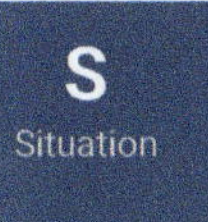

The quality team is building a maternal health quality dashboard. Postpartum depression (PPD) affects 10–15% of mothers and is the most common complication of childbirth — yet screening rates are below 50% in most health plans. The team needs the PPD screening rate by OB practice.

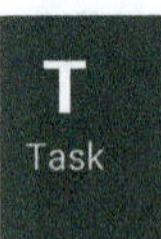

For all members with a delivery hospitalization in the current year, identify those who had a PPD screening or documented PPD diagnosis within 180 days of delivery. Rate = screened or diagnosed ÷ total deliveries. Output by OB NPI with gap count.

ANSI SQL — Scenario 12.2: Postpartum Depression Screening Rate

```
-- ════════════════════════════════════════════════════════════════
-- Postpartum Depression Screening Rate
-- Screening window: delivery date through 180 days post-delivery
-- Qualifying evidence: screening CPT codes OR F32/F33/F53.0 diagnosis
-- ════════════════════════════════════════════════════════════════

-- STEP 1: Build the denominator — all deliveries this year
-- Use discharge_date as the delivery date anchor
WITH delivery_denom AS (
  SELECT
    c.member_id,
    c.discharge_date                AS delivery_date,
    -- 180-day screening window starts on delivery date
    c.discharge_date + INTERVAL '180' DAY  AS screening_end,
    c.billing_npi                   AS delivering_ob_npi
  FROM  fact_medical_claims c
  WHERE (c.primary_drg BETWEEN '765' AND '782'
    OR c.primary_diag BETWEEN 'O60' AND 'O84')
   AND c.type_of_bill LIKE '11%'
   AND c.claim_status = 'PAID'
   AND EXTRACT(YEAR FROM c.discharge_date) = EXTRACT(YEAR FROM CURRENT_DATE)
),

-- STEP 2: Find PPD screening or diagnosis within the 180-day window
-- Screening CPTs: G0444 (annual depression screen), 96127 (brief BH assessment)
-- 96160/96161 (health risk assessment), or a documented F-code depression dx
-- F53.0 = postpartum depression (the specific ICD-10 code for PPD)
depression_screening AS (
  SELECT DISTINCT c.member_id
  FROM  fact_medical_claims c
  JOIN  delivery_denom dd ON c.member_id = dd.member_id
  WHERE (
    -- Validated screening instruments billed with these CPTs
    c.procedure_code IN ('G0444','96127','96160','96161')
    -- Or documented depression diagnosis in the postpartum period
    OR c.primary_diag LIKE 'F32%'  -- major depressive disorder
    OR c.primary_diag LIKE 'F33%'  -- recurrent depression
    OR c.primary_diag  = 'F53.0'  -- postpartum depression (specific)
  )
   AND c.claim_status = 'PAID'
   -- Must occur within 180 days of delivery
   AND c.service_date BETWEEN dd.delivery_date AND dd.screening_end
)

-- STEP 3: Calculate rate by delivering OB practice
SELECT
  dd.delivering_ob_npi,
  p.provider_full_name,
  p.specialty_group,
  COUNT(DISTINCT dd.member_id)          AS total_deliveries,
  COUNT(DISTINCT ds.member_id)          AS screened_or_diagnosed,
  COUNT(DISTINCT dd.member_id)
   - COUNT(DISTINCT ds.member_id)       AS screening_gaps,
```

```
    ROUND(100.0 * COUNT(DISTINCT ds.member_id)
      / NULLIF(COUNT(DISTINCT dd.member_id),0), 1) AS screening_rate_pct
FROM delivery_denom dd
LEFT JOIN depression_screening ds ON dd.member_id = ds.member_id
JOIN dim_providers p ON dd.delivering_ob_npi = p.npi
GROUP BY dd.delivering_ob_npi, p.provider_full_name, p.specialty_group
HAVING COUNT(DISTINCT dd.member_id) >= 10
ORDER BY screening_rate_pct ASC;
```

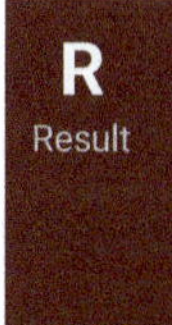

OB practices with screening_rate_pct below 40% should receive an education package on the ACOG-recommended Edinburgh Postnatal Depression Scale and the billing codes (G0444, 96127) that reimburse for its administration. Plans can increase screening rates dramatically through provider education — PPD screening is a billable service that OB practices are often not capturing. The F53.0 diagnosis flag identifies members who were diagnosed with PPD — these members need immediate routing to BH services.

Chapter 12 Review

Unit Test & Key Takeaways

Answer each question before reading the explanation.

Q1. When estimating the first day of pregnancy from a delivery date, the standard analytical assumption is:

A. Subtract 9 calendar months from the delivery date
B. Subtract 270 days (9 × 30) from the delivery date
C. Subtract 280 days (40 weeks) from the delivery date — standard gestational age
D. Use the first prenatal visit date as the pregnancy start date

Answer: C. *Standard gestational age = 280 days = 40 weeks measured from the last menstrual period (LMP). Using delivery_date - 280 days estimates the first day of the measurement period for prenatal care adequacy. This is the HEDIS PPC (Prenatal and Postpartum Care) standard. 270 days is incorrect; 9 calendar months is imprecise.*

Q2. NTSV C-section rate is the preferred quality metric for avoidable C-sections because:

A. NTSV is the only C-section metric approved by CMS for public reporting
B. NTSV isolates first-time mothers with term, singleton, head-down pregnancies where clinical indication for C-section should be rare — producing a clean measure of avoidable C-sections
C. NTSV excludes high-risk pregnancies which would otherwise inflate the C-section rate
D. NTSV is required by NCQA for all maternal HEDIS measures

Answer: B. *NTSV (Nulliparous, Term, Singleton, Vertex) isolates the lowest-risk delivery population. In this group, clinical indication for C-section (e.g., malpresentation, multiple gestation, prior C-section) has been controlled for. Variation in NTSV C-section rates across hospitals reflects practice pattern differences rather than patient acuity differences. The Leapfrog Group uses 23.9% as the benchmark.*

Q3. In the mother-newborn linkage query, why is ABS(delivery_date - birth_date) <= 1 used instead of an exact date match?

A. ANSI SQL cannot compare dates directly without the ABS() function
B. Newborns are always admitted the day after delivery
C. The mother's discharge_date is used as a delivery date proxy — if delivery occurs near midnight, the mother's discharge_date may be one day after the infant's birth_date
D. Hospitals always bill mother and infant with a 1-day offset

Answer: C. *The mother's discharge_date is used as a proxy for the delivery date, but delivery may occur at 11 PM on one day while the mother is discharged the next morning. The infant's birth_date reflects the actual delivery date. Without a 1-day tolerance, these pairs fail to join and the mother-infant linkage is lost.*

Q4. ICD-10 code F53.0 specifically identifies:

A. General major depressive disorder
B. Postpartum depression (Puerperal Depression) — the specific perinatal mood disorder code
C. Bipolar disorder with postpartum onset
D. Anxiety disorder during pregnancy

Answer: B. *F53.0 = Postpartum Depression (also called Puerperal Depression or Peripartum Depression). F32.x codes represent major depressive disorder in general and do not specify the postpartum timing. Using only F32/F33 for PPD identification misses cases that were correctly coded as F53.0 and double-counts general depression. Both F32.x/F33.x AND F53.0 should be included in PPD screening/diagnosis identification.*

Q5. CPT 59400 (global obstetric care) creates which analytical challenge?

A. It bundles inpatient and outpatient costs making cost-sharing calculation impossible

B. It bundles all prenatal visits, delivery, and postpartum care into one claim on the delivery date — making individual prenatal visit timeliness analysis impossible from claims alone

C. It is not a valid HEDIS code and must be excluded from all quality measure calculations

D. It creates a duplicate claim when combined with the hospital delivery DRG

Answer: B. *CPT 59400 is the global OB package — one code, one claim, one date (the delivery date). All prenatal visit details are rolled into this single code. If the OB practice bills globally, the analyst cannot determine when the first prenatal visit occurred or count individual visits from claims. Solution: use Z34.x (prenatal encounter) diagnosis codes on office visit claims, or rely on EHR data for timeliness analysis.*

Q6. Describe the complete SQL methodology for calculating the HEDIS Prenatal and Postpartum Care (PPC) measure, including how to handle the global OB billing problem.

(Short answer)

Sample Answer:

PPC has two rates: Timeliness of Prenatal Care (first visit in first trimester) and Postpartum Care (visit 21–56 days after delivery). Methodology: (1) Denominator: all members with a delivery claim (DRG 765–782 or O60–O84 on inpatient) who were enrolled at delivery and meet NCQA CE criteria. (2) For Timeliness: identify first prenatal visit before delivery_date - 182 days (end of first trimester). Global OB billing problem: CPT 59400 bundles all prenatal visits into one claim on the delivery date — it cannot be used for first visit timing. Solution A: use Z34.x diagnosis codes on office visit claims (99213–99215) as prenatal visit proxies. Solution B: use EHR-supplement data where available. If only 59400 data exists, timeliness cannot be measured from claims. (3) For Postpartum: find CPT 59430 or Z39.x claims between delivery_date + 21 and delivery_date + 56. (4) Report rates separately for prenatal timeliness and postpartum visit.

Q7. A plan's maternal analytics team identifies 47 hospital deliveries where the mother's claims show a vaginal delivery DRG but the newborn's claims show a NICU admission (DRG 790–792). Describe the clinical and financial implications and explain what SQL analysis should follow.

(Short answer)

Sample Answer:

Clinical implication: vaginal delivery + NICU admission indicates a term or near-term infant who required intensive care after a vaginal birth — common causes include meconium aspiration, respiratory distress syndrome, infection, or birth trauma. This is NOT unusual. Financial implication: NICU admissions are among the highest-cost neonatal events — average $4,000–$8,000/day with average LOS of 7–14 days for term infants. These cases significantly inflate the cost per delivery for the affected hospital. SQL follow-up: (1) Link mothers to infants using the mother-newborn linkage query. (2) Stratify NICU admissions by gestational age group (Z3A codes on infant claim or P07.x prematurity codes). (3) Calculate NICU rate by hospital: NICU admissions ÷ total live births. (4) Flag hospitals with NICU rate > 2 standard deviations above plan average for case management review. Hospitals with unexpectedly high NICU rates may have care quality issues or data anomalies warranting investigation.

Q8. Explain how to identify maternal severe morbidity (MSM) from claims data using the CDC indicator list, and describe two limitations of the claims-based approach.

(Short answer)

Sample Answer:

CDC MSM methodology: (1) Build delivery_hospitalizations CTE: all inpatient claims with delivery DRG or O60–O84 primary diagnosis. (2) Join to ref_msm_indicators which contains the CDC's 21 indicator conditions as ICD-10-CM codes (e.g., eclampsia O15.x, sepsis A41.x, blood transfusion 30230N0, hysterectomy 0UT90ZZ) and ICD-10-PCS procedure codes. (3) Flag any delivery claim where secondary diagnoses or procedure codes match a CDC indicator. (4) Rate = deliveries with ≥1 indicator ÷ total deliveries × 10,000. Limitations: (1) Claims-based MSM underestimates true MSM because not all indicators are coded — clinical documentation of transfusions, for example, is inconsistent across hospitals. The indicator requiring a blood transfusion procedure code will be missed if the hospital bills a revenue code instead of a procedure code. (2) Secondary diagnosis coding completeness varies by hospital — a hospital that codes all secondary diagnoses will appear to have higher MSM rates than one that codes only primary and 3 secondaries, creating spurious variation. Both limitations mean claims-based MSM should be used for trend analysis within the same hospital over time, not for absolute comparisons across hospitals.

Key Takeaways

What every analyst must remember from this chapter.

1. Maternal analytics anchors on the delivery hospitalization (DRG 765–782, ICD-10 O60–O84). Use discharge_date as the delivery date proxy. The 280-day gestation estimate (delivery_date - 280 days) is the standard for first prenatal visit calculations.

2. NTSV (Nulliparous, Term, Singleton, Vertex) C-section rate is the gold standard measure of avoidable C-sections. The Leapfrog benchmark is ≤23.9%. NTSV controls for patient acuity — variation above the benchmark reflects practice patterns, not patient complexity.

3. Mother-newborn linkage uses billing_npi (delivery facility) + date proximity (ABS(delivery_date - birth_date) ≤ 1 day). The 1-day tolerance is required because delivery may occur near midnight, causing the mother's discharge_date to differ by 1 day from the infant's birth_date.

4. CPT 59400 (global obstetric package) bundles all prenatal visits, delivery, and postpartum care into one claim on the delivery date. Individual prenatal visit timeliness cannot be measured from 59400-billed claims alone. Use Z34.x diagnosis codes on office visit claims as prenatal proxies.

5. NICU admission rate stratified by gestational age group (extremely preterm, very preterm, moderate-late preterm, term) reveals the cost cliff: term infants 20–50/1,000; extremely preterm infants 850+/1,000. Gestational age is captured via Z3A.xx secondary diagnosis codes or P07.x prematurity codes.

6. ICD-10 F53.0 is the specific code for postpartum depression — distinct from F32.x (general major depression). PPD screening is identified by CPT G0444, 96127, 96160, or 96161. The 180-day postpartum window is the standard for screening rate calculation.

7. Maternal severe morbidity (MSM) uses the CDC's 21 indicator conditions as secondary diagnoses or ICD-10-PCS procedure codes on delivery claims. Claims-based MSM underestimates true MSM due to variable coding completeness — use it for within-hospital trend analysis, not cross-hospital ranking.

8. Global OB billing is the single biggest source of maternal analytics data quality failures. Always confirm with the clinical data team whether OBs in your network bill globally (59400) or component-coded before building prenatal visit count or timeliness reports.

Chapter 13: Post-Acute Care & Transitions of Care

Post-acute care is the bridge between the hospital and the community. How well a patient transitions from an acute inpatient stay to the appropriate post-acute setting — and how efficiently that post-acute care is managed — determines both the clinical outcome and the total episode cost. For health plans and value-based care programs, post-acute care analytics identifies SNF LOS outliers, measures PAC-stratified readmission rates, evaluates home health agency quality, and flags members receiving aggressive end-of-life care who may benefit from hospice enrollment.

13.1 The Post-Acute Care Continuum

Post-acute care encompasses five distinct care settings, each with its own billing structure, quality metrics, and analytical patterns. The primary identifier for each setting is the Type of Bill (TOB) code on the institutional claim.

PAC Setting	TOB code	DRG range	Primary quality metrics	Cost driver
Skilled Nursing Facility (SNF)	21X	None (daily billing)	LOS vs. DRG benchmark, functional improvement rate, 30-day readmission	Daily rate × LOS — excess LOS is the primary lever
Home Health Agency (HHA)	32X, 33X	None (episode billing)	First visit within 24h of discharge, 30-day readmission, hospitalizations per episode	Visit count per episode — therapy-heavy agencies may be over-utilizing
Inpatient Rehabilitation Facility (IRF)	11X with DRG 945-946	945, 946	Functional Independence Measure (FIM) score improvement, LOS	Higher cost than SNF — appropriate use criteria are key
Long-Term Acute Care Hospital (LTACH)	11X with DRG 207, 208	207, 208	Ventilator weaning success, discharge to community rate	Highest per-diem cost — appropriate for vent-dependent patients only
Hospice	81X, 82X	None (daily benefit billing)	Hospice enrollment in last 6 months, aggressive EOL care rate	Total per-diem cost vs. avoidance of high-cost acute care

Discharge status codes: UB-04 discharge status codes are the primary stratifier for PAC analytics: 01=home self-care, 02=transfer to another hospital, 03=SNF, 06=home health, 20=expired, 51=hospice home, 61=hospice facility, 62=IRF. These codes drive both the PAC episode construction and the 30-day readmission denominator exclusions. Always verify your data model's discharge status code values — some systems normalize these to text.

13.2 PAC Episode Construction

Unlike acute care where an inpatient stay has clear admit and discharge dates, post-acute care episodes require grouping multiple claims across different settings. The standard approach anchors the episode on the acute discharge date and includes all PAC claims within 90 days that are not a readmission to the same hospital.

ANSI SQL — 13.2: PAC Episode Construction

```
-- ============================================================================
-- PAC Episode Construction: anchor on acute hospital discharge
-- Include all PAC service claims within 90 days of discharge
-- Exclude: readmission to same hospital (not PAC — it's a readmission)
-- PAC setting identified by TOB: SNF=21X, HHA=32X/33X, Hospice=81X/82X
-- ============================================================================

-- STEP 1: Identify index acute discharges (the anchor event)
WITH acute_discharges AS (
  SELECT
    member_id,
    claim_id          AS index_claim_id,
    billing_npi       AS discharging_hospital,
    discharge_date        AS index_discharge_date,
    primary_drg,
    discharge_status_code
  FROM  fact_medical_claims
  WHERE type_of_bill LIKE '11%'  -- inpatient acute
   AND claim_status = 'PAID'
   -- Exclude: expired (20) and transfers (02) — not true discharges
   AND discharge_status_code NOT IN ('20','02')
   AND EXTRACT(YEAR FROM discharge_date) = EXTRACT(YEAR FROM CURRENT_DATE)
),

-- STEP 2: Find all PAC claims within 90 days of each acute discharge
-- Classify by PAC setting using TOB codes
pac_claims AS (
  SELECT
    ad.member_id,
    ad.index_claim_id,
    ad.index_discharge_date,
    c.claim_id          AS pac_claim_id,
    c.billing_npi       AS pac_provider,
    c.service_date        AS pac_service_date,
    c.allowed_amount,
    -- Classify PAC setting by TOB
    CASE
      WHEN c.type_of_bill LIKE '21%' THEN 'SNF'
      WHEN c.type_of_bill IN ('32X','33X') THEN 'Home Health'
      WHEN c.type_of_bill LIKE '11%'
       AND c.primary_drg IN ('945','946') THEN 'IRF'
      WHEN c.type_of_bill IN ('81X','82X') THEN 'Hospice'
      ELSE 'Other PAC'
    END AS pac_setting
  FROM  acute_discharges ad
  JOIN  fact_medical_claims c
   ON c.member_id   = ad.member_id
   AND c.service_date BETWEEN ad.index_discharge_date
```

```
              AND ad.index_discharge_date + INTERVAL '90' DAY
      -- Exclude readmission to the SAME hospital (not PAC)
      AND c.billing_npi <> ad.discharging_hospital
      AND c.claim_status = 'PAID'
    WHERE c.type_of_bill LIKE '21%'          -- SNF
       OR c.type_of_bill IN ('32X','33X')  -- HHA
       OR c.type_of_bill IN ('81X','82X')  -- Hospice
       OR (c.type_of_bill LIKE '11%'
           AND c.primary_drg IN ('945','946'))  -- IRF
)

-- STEP 3: Summarize PAC episode cost and setting by index discharge
SELECT
    ad.member_id,
    ad.index_discharge_date,
    ad.primary_drg,
    ad.discharge_status_code,
    MAX(pc.pac_setting)                      AS primary_pac_setting,
    COUNT(DISTINCT pc.pac_claim_id)          AS pac_claim_count,
    ROUND(SUM(pc.allowed_amount), 0)         AS total_pac_cost,
    DATEDIFF('day', ad.index_discharge_date,
         MAX(pc.pac_service_date))           AS pac_episode_days
FROM  acute_discharges ad
LEFT JOIN pac_claims pc ON ad.index_claim_id = pc.index_claim_id
GROUP BY ad.member_id, ad.index_discharge_date,
       ad.primary_drg, ad.discharge_status_code
ORDER BY total_pac_cost DESC NULLS LAST;
```

13.3 Post-Acute Care Scenarios

Scenario 13.1 · Utilization Management / Network

SNF Length of Stay Benchmarking

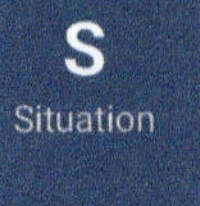

The network team is building a preferred SNF network. They need to identify which SNFs have outlier length of stay for the plan's highest-volume DRGs. SNF excess LOS is a $300–$600/day cost driver — identifying outlier facilities is a direct financial management action.

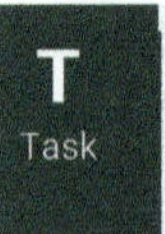

For each SNF-DRG combination with minimum 10 admissions, compare actual average SNF LOS to the DRG benchmark LOS. Calculate excess cost per facility. Flag SNFs where actual LOS exceeds benchmark by more than 20% with minimum volume.

ANSI SQL — Scenario 13.1: SNF LOS Benchmarking with Excess Cost

```
-- ══════════════════════════════════════════════════════════════════════
-- SNF LOS Benchmarking: actual LOS vs. DRG-expected benchmark
-- Links each SNF stay to the preceding inpatient DRG
-- Excess cost = (actual_los - benchmark_los) × daily_rate
-- ══════════════════════════════════════════════════════════════════════

-- STEP 1: Identify all SNF stays this year
-- TOB 21X = skilled nursing facility institutional claims
WITH snf_stays AS (
    SELECT
        c.member_id,
```

```
        c.billing_npi            AS snf_npi,
        c.admit_date             AS snf_admit,
        c.discharge_date         AS snf_discharge,
        -- LOS = days in SNF; same-day = 0 (valid for assessment-only)
        DATEDIFF('day', c.admit_date, c.discharge_date) AS snf_los,
        c.allowed_amount         AS snf_cost
    FROM  fact_medical_claims c
    WHERE c.type_of_bill LIKE '21%'  -- SNF TOB
     AND c.claim_status = 'PAID'
     AND EXTRACT(YEAR FROM c.admit_date) = EXTRACT(YEAR FROM CURRENT_DATE)
),

-- STEP 2: Link each SNF admission to the preceding inpatient DRG
-- Join to inpatient claim where hospital discharged to SNF (status 03)
-- within 3 days before SNF admission
snf_with_drg AS (
    SELECT
        s.member_id,
        s.snf_npi,
        s.snf_admit,
        s.snf_discharge,
        s.snf_los,
        s.snf_cost,
        h.primary_drg            AS preceding_drg,
        h.billing_npi            AS sending_hospital_npi
    FROM  snf_stays s
    JOIN  fact_medical_claims h
      ON h.member_id    = s.member_id
     AND h.type_of_bill LIKE '11%'            -- preceding inpatient
     AND h.claim_status = 'PAID'
     AND h.discharge_status_code = '03'       -- discharged to SNF
     -- SNF admission must start within 3 days of hospital discharge
     AND DATEDIFF('day', h.discharge_date, s.snf_admit) BETWEEN 0 AND 3
),

-- STEP 3: Join to DRG benchmark LOS table
-- ref_drg_snf_benchmarks contains expected SNF LOS by DRG
snf_benchmarked AS (
    SELECT
        sd.*,
        b.benchmark_snf_los,
        b.avg_daily_snf_rate,
        -- Excess LOS = actual - benchmark (negative = more efficient than benchmark)
        sd.snf_los - b.benchmark_snf_los AS excess_los,
        -- Excess cost = excess days × daily rate
        ROUND((sd.snf_los - b.benchmark_snf_los) * b.avg_daily_snf_rate, 0)
          AS excess_cost_estimate
    FROM  snf_with_drg sd
    JOIN  ref_drg_snf_benchmarks b ON sd.preceding_drg = b.drg_code
)

-- STEP 4: Summarize by SNF facility and DRG, flag outliers
SELECT
    sb.snf_npi,
    p.facility_name,
    p.county,
    sb.preceding_drg,
    d.drg_description,
    COUNT(*)                     AS admissions,
```

```
    ROUND(AVG(sb.snf_los), 1)          AS actual_avg_los,
    MAX(sb.benchmark_snf_los)          AS benchmark_los,
    ROUND(AVG(sb.excess_los), 1)       AS avg_excess_los,
    ROUND(SUM(sb.excess_cost_estimate),0) AS total_excess_cost,
    CASE WHEN AVG(sb.snf_los)
            > MAX(sb.benchmark_snf_los) * 1.20
        AND COUNT(*) >= 10
       THEN 'FLAG — outlier LOS' ELSE 'Within range' END AS los_flag
FROM  snf_benchmarked sb
JOIN  dim_providers p ON sb.snf_npi = p.npi
JOIN  ref_drg d      ON sb.preceding_drg = d.drg_code
GROUP BY sb.snf_npi, p.facility_name, p.county, sb.preceding_drg, d.drg_description
HAVING COUNT(*) >= 10
ORDER BY total_excess_cost DESC;
```

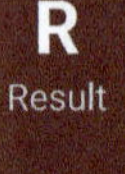

R Result

Sort by total_excess_cost to find the highest-impact SNF-DRG combinations. A SNF with +5 excess LOS days on 50 joint replacement admissions at $450/day = $112,500 in estimated excess spend annually. Present to the network team: these facilities are candidates for preferred network exclusion or performance-based contracts. The total_excess_cost column directly translates to the financial case for preferred SNF program investment.

Scenario 13.2 · Clinical / Hospice

End-of-Life Care Intensity Analysis

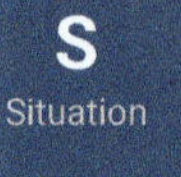

S Situation

The palliative care team wants to identify decedents who received aggressive end-of-life care — ICU in last 30 days, ED visits in last 30 days, chemotherapy in last 30 days — and flag those with no hospice enrollment. This population is a clinical quality concern and a care management intervention opportunity.

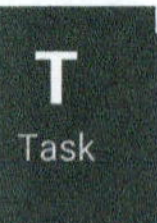

T Task

Identify all members who died in the current year (discharge_status_code = 20). For each decedent, calculate indicators of aggressive EOL care in the last 30 days of life. Flag those with 2+ aggressive care indicators and no hospice enrollment.

ANSI SQL — Scenario 13.2: End-of-Life Care Intensity

```
-- ═══════════════════════════════════════════════════════════════
-- End-of-Life Care Intensity: identify decedents receiving
-- aggressive care in last 30 days with no hospice enrollment.
-- Aggressive EOL indicators: ICU, ED, chemo, multiple IP admissions.
-- discharge_status_code = 20 is the claims-based death identifier.
-- ═══════════════════════════════════════════════════════════════

-- STEP 1: Identify all decedents this year
-- discharge_status_code 20 = expired; discharge_date = date of death
WITH decedents AS (
    SELECT
        member_id,
        MAX(discharge_date) AS death_date  -- most recent expiration
    FROM  fact_medical_claims
    WHERE discharge_status_code = '20'  -- expired
      AND claim_status = 'PAID'
      AND EXTRACT(YEAR FROM discharge_date) = EXTRACT(YEAR FROM CURRENT_DATE)
    GROUP BY member_id
),

-- STEP 2: Check for hospice enrollment in last 30 days of life
```

```
-- Hospice TOB 81X = hospice home care; 82X = hospice inpatient
hospice_last30 AS (
  SELECT DISTINCT c.member_id
  FROM  fact_medical_claims c
  JOIN  decedents d ON c.member_id = d.member_id
  WHERE c.type_of_bill IN ('81X','82X')  -- hospice claims
   AND c.claim_status = 'PAID'
   AND c.service_date BETWEEN d.death_date - INTERVAL '30' DAY
                 AND d.death_date
),

-- STEP 3: Calculate aggressive EOL care indicators for last 30 days
-- Each indicator is a CASE WHEN aggregation within the 30-day window
eol_care_flags AS (
  SELECT
    d.member_id,
    d.death_date,
    -- Hospice flag: was member on hospice in last 30 days?
    CASE WHEN h.member_id IS NOT NULL THEN 1 ELSE 0 END AS hospice_flag,
    -- ICU admission: revenue code 0200 = ICU
    MAX(CASE WHEN c.revenue_code BETWEEN '0200' AND '0219'
          AND c.service_date >= d.death_date - INTERVAL '30' DAY
         THEN 1 ELSE 0 END)    AS icu_last30,
    -- Emergency department visit
    MAX(CASE WHEN (c.place_of_service = '23'
            OR c.revenue_code BETWEEN '0450' AND '0459')
          AND c.service_date >= d.death_date - INTERVAL '30' DAY
         THEN 1 ELSE 0 END)    AS ed_last30,
    -- Chemotherapy administration: J9000-J9999
    MAX(CASE WHEN c.procedure_code BETWEEN 'J9000' AND 'J9999'
          AND c.service_date >= d.death_date - INTERVAL '30' DAY
         THEN 1 ELSE 0 END)    AS chemo_last30,
    -- Multiple inpatient admissions (2+)
    SUM(CASE WHEN c.type_of_bill LIKE '11%'
          AND c.service_date >= d.death_date - INTERVAL '30' DAY
         THEN 1 ELSE 0 END)    AS ip_admits_last30
  FROM  decedents d
  LEFT JOIN hospice_last30 h ON d.member_id = h.member_id
  JOIN  fact_medical_claims c ON d.member_id = c.member_id
    AND c.claim_status = 'PAID'
  GROUP BY d.member_id, d.death_date,
       CASE WHEN h.member_id IS NOT NULL THEN 1 ELSE 0 END
)

-- STEP 4: Calculate aggressive EOL score and flag high-intensity cases
SELECT
  ecf.member_id,
  m.member_name,
  m.attributed_pcp_npi,
  ecf.death_date,
  ecf.hospice_flag,
  ecf.icu_last30,
  ecf.ed_last30,
  ecf.chemo_last30,
  ecf.ip_admits_last30,
  -- Aggregate indicator score: 0-4+ (each indicator = 1 point)
  ecf.icu_last30 + ecf.ed_last30 + ecf.chemo_last30
  + CASE WHEN ecf.ip_admits_last30 >= 2 THEN 1 ELSE 0 END AS eol_intensity_score,
  CASE WHEN ecf.hospice_flag = 0
```

```
        AND (ecf.icu_last30 + ecf.ed_last30 + ecf.chemo_last30
           + CASE WHEN ecf.ip_admits_last30 >= 2 THEN 1 ELSE 0 END) >= 2
       THEN 'HIGH INTENSITY — no hospice'
       WHEN ecf.hospice_flag = 1 THEN 'Hospice enrolled'
       ELSE 'Low intensity'
    END AS eol_flag
FROM  eol_care_flags ecf
JOIN  dim_members m ON ecf.member_id = m.member_id
ORDER BY eol_intensity_score DESC, ecf.hospice_flag;
```

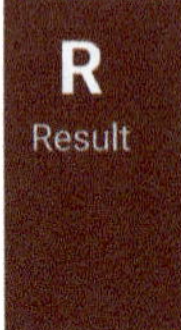

Members flagged HIGH INTENSITY — no hospice with eol_intensity_score ≥ 3 represent the highest clinical and financial concern. The average cost of aggressive EOL care in the last 30 days exceeds $30,000. Earlier hospice enrollment for appropriate members reduces cost by 30–50% while significantly improving quality of life. Present to the palliative care team: PCPs whose patients have high EOL intensity scores without hospice enrollment may benefit from palliative care training or navigation services.

Chapter 13 Review

Unit Test & Key Takeaways

Answer each question before reading the explanation.

Q1. Which discharge status code on an inpatient claim indicates discharge to a skilled nursing facility?

A. 01 — Discharged to home or self-care
B. 02 — Transfer to another short-term hospital
C. 03 — Discharged to skilled nursing facility
D. 06 — Discharged to home with home health services

Answer: C. *UB-04 Patient Discharge Status Code 03 = Discharged/transferred to a skilled nursing facility (SNF). This is the primary field used to identify SNF transitions in PAC episode construction and to stratify 30-day readmission rates by discharge destination. Code 06 = home health; 62 = IRF; 51/61 = hospice.*

Q2. In the PAC episode construction query, the condition c.billing_npi <> ad.discharging_hospital is included to:

A. Prevent the same provider from appearing in both acute and PAC sections
B. Exclude readmissions to the same hospital — a return to the index hospital within 90 days is a readmission, not post-acute care
C. Filter out duplicate billing from the same facility
D. Satisfy a HIPAA requirement that PAC and acute claims be kept separate

Answer: B. *If the member returns to the same hospital that discharged them within 90 days, that is a readmission — not a post-acute care transition. Including those claims in the PAC episode would double-count them as both a readmission and a PAC encounter. The billing_npi comparison correctly separates these two events.*

Q3. What does discharge status code 20 indicate on an inpatient claim?

A. The patient was transferred to a long-term care facility
B. The patient expired — this is the claims-based death identifier; discharge_date = date of death
C. The patient left against medical advice
D. The patient was discharged to hospice home care

Answer: B. *UB-04 discharge status code 20 = expired. When code 20 appears, the discharge_date is the date of death. This is used to identify decedents for EOL care analysis, to build the 30-day readmission denominator (expired patients cannot be readmitted and must be excluded), and to calculate mortality rates. Code 51/61 = hospice; code 07 = AMA.*

Q4. Home health episodes are grouped using FLOOR(days_since_episode_start / 60). Why 60 days?

A. 60 days is the NCQA-specified home health quality measurement window
B. 60 days aligns with the Medicare Home Health Prospective Payment System episode unit — each HHA billing episode is 60 days
C. 60 days ensures readmissions up to 2 months after home health are captured
D. ANSI SQL FLOOR functions are most accurate with multiples of 60

Answer: B. *Medicare HH PPS pays HHAs in 60-day episode units. Using 60 days as the grouping window aligns the analytical episode with the payment episode, enabling meaningful cost-per-episode comparisons across HHAs. This is also the period used in CMS's Home Health Quality Reporting Program (HHQRP) for readmission rate calculation.*

Q5. When identifying decedents from claims data, which limitation must analysts acknowledge?

A. Claims cannot identify deaths from non-healthcare causes

B. Claims-based decedent identification (discharge_status_code = 20) only captures members who die in a hospital or SNF — deaths at home, in hospice, or outside a facility-based setting may not appear

C. Death records cannot be used in PMPM calculations

D. Discharge status code 20 includes transfers to long-term care as well as deaths

Answer: B. *discharge_status_code = 20 only appears on inpatient facility claims. Members who die at home (with or without hospice), in outpatient settings, or outside the healthcare system entirely will not have a code-20 claim. Claims-based death detection underestimates true mortality, particularly for populations that avoid hospitalization at end of life. For complete mortality analysis, link to state vital records or the SSA death master file.*

Q6. Describe the complete methodology for building a preferred SNF network using LOS benchmarking data, including how to handle the DRG linkage challenge and what to do when DRG data is unavailable for a PAC claim.

(Short answer)

> **Sample Answer:**
> Preferred SNF network methodology: (1) Collect all SNF claims (TOB 21X) for the prior 12–24 months. (2) Link each SNF admission to the preceding inpatient claim: join on member_id where inpatient discharge_status_code = 03 (to SNF) and the SNF admission is within 3 days of discharge. (3) Extract the preceding_drg from the inpatient claim — this is the clinical context for expected SNF LOS. (4) Join to ref_drg_snf_benchmarks to get the expected LOS for that DRG. (5) Calculate excess LOS = actual_snf_los - benchmark_snf_los. (6) Calculate excess cost = excess_los × avg_daily_snf_rate. DRG linkage challenge: some SNF admissions have no preceding inpatient claim within 3 days (direct SNF admissions from the community). For these: (a) use the member's most recent inpatient DRG in the past 30 days as a proxy, (b) group them into a "community admission" category, or (c) exclude them from DRG-benchmarked analysis. When DRG is unavailable: benchmark against overall average SNF LOS by facility without DRG stratification, with appropriate caveats about case mix differences. Preferred network criteria: SNFs with ≥30 admissions where actual LOS is within benchmark ± 15%, and 30-day readmission rate below plan average.

Q7. Explain why a 90-day PAC episode window is used rather than 30 days, and describe a scenario where using 30 days would materially undercount PAC costs.

(Short answer)

> **Sample Answer:**
> A 90-day PAC window captures the full post-acute episode for most DRG categories. The rationale: (1) SNF stays for major joint replacement (DRG 470) average 17–25 days; home health following SNF can add another 30–45 days; the total episode extends well beyond 30 days. (2) Long-term acute care (LTACH) stays for ventilator-dependent patients average 25–35 days, often transitioning to SNF afterward — capturing the full cascade requires 90 days. (3) IRF episodes average 12–16 days but may be preceded by SNF evaluation. Scenario where 30 days undercount: a patient discharged after stroke (DRG 061) goes to SNF for 21 days, then to home health for 30 days, then to outpatient therapy for 2 months. A 30-day window captures the SNF only; a 90-day window captures SNF + home health, tripling the measured PAC cost. For value-based care episode payment models (bundled payment for joint replacement, CJR), the 90-day window is the contractual standard — using 30 days would systematically understate episode cost and distort provider performance comparisons.

Q8. A palliative care program director asks: "What is our hospice utilization rate for members who died, and how does it compare to the national benchmark?" Describe the SQL approach and identify at least two data quality caveats.

(Short answer)

> **Sample Answer:**
> SQL approach: (1) Identify decedents: members with discharge_status_code = 20 in the measurement year (MAX(discharge_date) per member where code = 20). (2) Identify hospice enrollment: LEFT JOIN to hospice claims (TOB 81X/82X) for each decedent; presence of any hospice claim = hospice enrolled. (3) Hospice utilization rate = COUNT(decedents with hospice) / COUNT(total decedents). (4) For quality: also calculate "hospice in last 6 months" and "hospice LOS" (days between first hospice claim and death_date). National benchmark: approximately 50% of Medicare decedents enroll in hospice; for commercial and younger populations, rates are typically 20–35%. Data quality caveats: (1) Claims-based death detection misses deaths outside hospital settings — members who die at home without calling 911 or receiving acute care may not have a code-20 claim. This systematically overestimates the hospice rate (the denominator is

smaller than true deaths). Link to state vital records or SSA death master file for complete mortality. (2) Hospice election in another plan year is invisible — a member who enrolled in hospice in December and died in January of the next year will appear as non-hospice in the prior year's data. Cross-year lookback for hospice enrollment is required for members who died early in the year.

Key Takeaways

What every analyst must remember from this chapter.

1. Post-acute care settings are identified by Type of Bill (TOB) codes: SNF = 21X, Home Health = 32X/33X, Hospice = 81X/82X, IRF = 11X with DRG 945–946. Discharge status codes drive PAC stratification: 03=SNF, 06=HHA, 51/61=hospice, 62=IRF, 01=home self-care, 20=expired.

2. PAC episode construction anchors on the acute discharge date and includes all PAC claims within 90 days. Exclude readmissions to the same hospital (billing_npi = discharging_hospital) — these are readmissions, not PAC transitions.

3. SNF LOS benchmarking requires linking each SNF admission to the preceding inpatient DRG. The join condition: discharge_status_code = 03 AND SNF admit within 3 days of hospital discharge. Excess cost = (actual_los - benchmark_los) × daily_rate.

4. Discharge status code 03 = SNF; 06 = home health; 20 = expired (claims-based death). Code 20 on inpatient claim makes discharge_date = date of death. Exclude code 02 (transfer) and 20 (expired) from readmission index admission denominators.

5. Home health 60-day episode grouping aligns with the Medicare HH PPS payment episode. First HHA visit within 24 hours of hospital discharge is the strongest predictor of preventing readmission — agencies below 80% on-time first visit have higher readmission rates.

6. Aggressive EOL care indicators: ICU in last 30 days, ED visit in last 30 days, chemotherapy in last 30 days, 2+ inpatient admissions in last 30 days. Members with 2+ indicators and no hospice enrollment are the highest clinical priority for palliative care program outreach.

7. Claims-based decedent identification (discharge_status_code = 20) only captures facility deaths. Deaths at home, in hospice only settings, or outside the healthcare system are invisible. For complete mortality analysis, link to state vital records or the SSA death master file.

8. PAC readmission rates stratified by discharge destination reveal which transitions carry the highest readmission risk. SNF-to-hospital readmissions average 20–25%; home-to-hospital readmissions average 12–15%. The difference reflects patient acuity at discharge and PAC quality — both are addressable.

Heading into Part VI: Part VI enters the financial, provider, and network analytics domain — the analytical layer that determines how the plan contracts, prices, and evaluates its provider ecosystem. Financial Analytics, Actuarial Pricing, Provider Scorecards, Network Contracting, Revenue Cycle, and Value-Based Care each build on the clinical episode knowledge from Part V. Every SQL block continues to carry phase-by-phase inline comments, and every chapter ends with unit tests and key takeaways.

Part VI — Financial, Provider & Network Analytics

Chapters 14–19

Cost Trend · Actuarial Pricing · Provider Scorecards · Network Contracting · RCM · Value-Based Care

Part VI moves from clinical episodes into the financial and operational engine of a health plan. These six chapters cover medical economics, actuarial pricing, provider network performance, fee schedule benchmarking, revenue cycle management, and value-based care analytics. Every chapter contains conceptual explanation, fully annotated SQL with plain-English inline comments, a 10-question unit test (6 MC + 4 SA), and key takeaways.

Chapter 14: Financial Analytics & Medical Economics

Cost trend · MLR · IBNR completion factors · Budget variance decomposition

14.1 Medical Cost Trend

Medical cost trend is the annualized rate of change in PMPM. It has two multiplicative components: utilization trend (services per member per month) and unit cost trend (price per service). Total trend = (1 + util_trend) × (1 + cost_trend) - 1. Decomposing them routes accountability correctly — utilization to care management, unit cost to contracting.

> **Key Formula** Annualized trend over N years: POWER(current_pmpm / prior_pmpm, 1.0/N) - 1. For 2 years: POWER(end/start, 0.5) - 1. The geometric average, not arithmetic, is correct — it accounts for compounding.

14.2 Medical Loss Ratio (MLR)

MLR = Total Claims Cost / Premium Revenue. The ACA mandates minimum MLR of 80% for small group/individual plans and 85% for large group plans. Plans below the floor must issue premium rebates. Stop-loss reinsurance comes in two forms: specific (per-member threshold, e.g., $250K/year) and aggregate (plan-wide, e.g., 120% of expected total claims). Both require weekly SQL monitoring.

14.3 IBNR Lag Triangle & Completion Factors

IBNR (Incurred But Not Reported) completion factors convert incomplete recent-month data into an estimated final PMPM. A lag triangle cross-tabs service months against elapsed months — each cell shows cumulative

PMPM received by that elapsed point divided by the eventual final PMPM. The reciprocal of each factor is the multiplier applied to current incomplete data.

ANSI SQL — 14.3: IBNR Lag Triangle & Completion Factors (Fully Annotated)

```
-- PURPOSE: Build a claims-lag triangle showing what % of final PMPM has
-- been received at 1, 2, 3, 6, and 12 months after each service month.
-- completion_factor_at_1m = 0.42 means: at 1 month maturity we have
-- received only 42% of the final PMPM. IBNR multiplier = 1/0.42 = 2.38.

-- STEP 1: Sum paid claims by service month AND paid month.
-- paid_month = the month the claim was processed (lags behind service_date).
WITH monthly_paid AS (
  SELECT
    DATE_TRUNC('month', c.service_date) AS svc_month,
    DATE_TRUNC('month', c.paid_date)    AS paid_month,
    SUM(c.allowed_amount)               AS paid_in_month
  FROM  fact_medical_claims c
  WHERE c.claim_status = 'PAID'
   AND c.line_of_business = 'COMMERCIAL'
   AND c.service_date >= CURRENT_DATE - INTERVAL '36' MONTH
  GROUP BY 1, 2
),

-- STEP 2: Compute cumulative paid using a running window SUM.
-- lag_months = how many months elapsed between service and payment.
lagged AS (
  SELECT
    svc_month,
    DATEDIFF('month', svc_month, paid_month)  AS lag_months,
    SUM(paid_in_month) OVER (
      PARTITION BY svc_month        -- one running total per service month
      ORDER BY paid_month          -- accumulate in chronological order
      ROWS BETWEEN UNBOUNDED PRECEDING AND CURRENT ROW
    )                             AS cumulative_paid
  FROM  monthly_paid
),

-- STEP 3: Convert cumulative paid to PMPM by joining to member months.
lagged_pmpm AS (
  SELECT l.svc_month, l.lag_months,
     ROUND(l.cumulative_paid / NULLIF(mm.total_mm, 0), 2) AS cumulative_pmpm
  FROM  lagged l
  JOIN (
    SELECT DATE_TRUNC('month', month_start) AS svc_month,
       SUM(member_months)           AS total_mm
    FROM  fact_member_months
    WHERE line_of_business = 'COMMERCIAL'
    GROUP BY 1
  ) mm ON l.svc_month = mm.svc_month
),

-- STEP 4: Pivot cumulative PMPM at each key lag point into one row per service month.
-- MAX(CASE WHEN lag = X THEN pmpm END) is the standard SQL pivot pattern.
-- HAVING MAX(lag_months) >= 12 keeps only fully matured months for calibration.
completion_factors AS (
  SELECT svc_month,
     MAX(CASE WHEN lag_months =  1 THEN cumulative_pmpm END) AS pmpm_at_1m,
     MAX(CASE WHEN lag_months =  2 THEN cumulative_pmpm END) AS pmpm_at_2m,
     MAX(CASE WHEN lag_months =  3 THEN cumulative_pmpm END) AS pmpm_at_3m,
     MAX(CASE WHEN lag_months =  6 THEN cumulative_pmpm END) AS pmpm_at_6m,
     MAX(CASE WHEN lag_months >= 12 THEN cumulative_pmpm END) AS final_pmpm
```

```
    FROM  lagged_pmpm
    GROUP BY svc_month
    HAVING MAX(lag_months) >= 12
)
-- STEP 5: Average completion factors across all matured months.
-- These averages become multipliers applied to current incomplete months.
-- e.g., if avg_completion_at_1m = 0.42, multiply 1-month-old PMPM by 1/0.42.
SELECT
    ROUND(AVG(pmpm_at_1m / NULLIF(final_pmpm,0)), 3) AS avg_completion_at_1m,
    ROUND(AVG(pmpm_at_2m / NULLIF(final_pmpm,0)), 3) AS avg_completion_at_2m,
    ROUND(AVG(pmpm_at_3m / NULLIF(final_pmpm,0)), 3) AS avg_completion_at_3m,
    ROUND(AVG(pmpm_at_6m / NULLIF(final_pmpm,0)), 3) AS avg_completion_at_6m
FROM  completion_factors;
```

14.4 Budget Variance Decomposition

Budget variance = Actual PMPM - Budget PMPM. Three decomposition layers: (1) Enrollment mix — did the population's risk profile change? (2) Utilization — more services per member? (3) Unit cost — higher price per service? Each layer routes to a different owner: mix to Actuarial, utilization to CMO, unit cost to VP Network.

ANSI SQL — 14.4: Three-Layer Budget Variance Decomposition (Fully Annotated)

```
-- PURPOSE: Decompose total PMPM variance into utilization and unit cost
-- components, side-by-side for current and prior year.
-- util_variance_pmpm = prior unit cost × utilization change
-- cost_variance_pmpm = prior utilization × unit cost change

-- STEP 1: Build current-year metrics by service category.
WITH actuals AS (
    SELECT p.service_category,
        ROUND(SUM(c.allowed_amount)/NULLIF(SUM(mm.member_months),0),2) AS actual_pmpm,
        -- Claims per 1,000 member months = utilization rate
        ROUND(1000.0*COUNT(DISTINCT c.claim_id)
          /NULLIF(SUM(mm.member_months),0),1)                AS util_per_1k,
        -- Average allowed per claim = unit cost
        ROUND(SUM(c.allowed_amount)/NULLIF(COUNT(DISTINCT c.claim_id),0),0) AS unit_cost
    FROM  fact_medical_claims c
    JOIN  ref_procedure_codes p  ON c.procedure_code = p.procedure_code
    JOIN  fact_member_months  mm
      ON c.member_id = mm.member_id
     AND mm.membership_year = EXTRACT(YEAR FROM CURRENT_DATE)
    WHERE c.claim_status = 'PAID'
     AND EXTRACT(YEAR FROM c.service_date) = EXTRACT(YEAR FROM CURRENT_DATE)
    GROUP BY p.service_category
),

-- STEP 2: Same query for prior year (used as the baseline for comparison).
prior_yr AS (
    SELECT p.service_category,
        ROUND(SUM(c.allowed_amount)/NULLIF(SUM(mm.member_months),0),2) AS prior_pmpm,
        ROUND(1000.0*COUNT(DISTINCT c.claim_id)
          /NULLIF(SUM(mm.member_months),0),1)                AS prior_util,
        ROUND(SUM(c.allowed_amount)/NULLIF(COUNT(DISTINCT c.claim_id),0),0) AS prior_unit_cost
    FROM  fact_medical_claims c
    JOIN  ref_procedure_codes p  ON c.procedure_code = p.procedure_code
    JOIN  fact_member_months  mm
      ON c.member_id = mm.member_id
     AND mm.membership_year = EXTRACT(YEAR FROM CURRENT_DATE) - 1
    WHERE c.claim_status = 'PAID'
     AND EXTRACT(YEAR FROM c.service_date) = EXTRACT(YEAR FROM CURRENT_DATE) - 1
    GROUP BY p.service_category
```

```
)
-- STEP 3: Join years, compute variance and decompose into components.
-- util_variance = change in volume × prior price (isolates volume effect)
-- cost_variance = prior volume × change in price (isolates price effect)
SELECT a.service_category,
   a.actual_pmpm, py.prior_pmpm,
   ROUND(a.actual_pmpm - py.prior_pmpm, 2)                AS pmpm_variance,
   -- How much of variance is from utilization change (price held constant)?
   ROUND((a.util_per_1k - py.prior_util)/1000.0 * py.prior_unit_cost, 2) AS util_variance_pmpm,
   -- How much is from unit cost change (volume held constant)?
   ROUND(py.prior_util/1000.0 * (a.unit_cost - py.prior_unit_cost), 2)  AS cost_variance_pmpm,
   a.util_per_1k, py.prior_util,
   a.unit_cost,  py.prior_unit_cost
FROM  actuals a
JOIN  prior_yr py ON a.service_category = py.service_category
ORDER BY ABS(a.actual_pmpm - py.prior_pmpm) DESC; -- largest variances first
```

Chapter 14 Review

Unit Test · Key Takeaways

Answer each question before reading the explanation.

Q1. The ACA MLR floor for large group commercial plans is:

A. 75%
B. 80%
C. 85%
D. 90%

Answer: C. *85% for large group (50+ employees); 80% for small group/individual. Plans below the floor must rebate the difference to members. MLR = Total Claims / Premium Revenue. An MLR above 100% means the plan paid more in claims than it collected — an underwriting loss.*

Q2. The correct annualized 2-year trend formula in SQL is:

A. (current_pmpm - prior_pmpm) / prior_pmpm / 2
B. POWER(current_pmpm / NULLIF(prior_pmpm,0), 0.5) − 1
C. AVG(current_pmpm, prior_pmpm) / prior_pmpm − 1
D. SQRT(current_pmpm − prior_pmpm)

Answer: B. *POWER(end/start, 1.0/years) − 1 is the geometric compound annual growth formula. For 2 years: POWER(end/start, 0.5) − 1. Arithmetic averaging underestimates trend when growth compounds. NULLIF prevents divide-by-zero if any category had zero PMPM in the base year.*

Q3. Blended medical cost trend with utilization up 4% and unit cost up 6% equals:

A. 10.0%
B. 10.24%
C. 10.12%
D. 8.0%

Answer: B. *(1 + 0.04) × (1 + 0.06) − 1 = 1.04 × 1.06 − 1 = 1.1024 − 1 = 10.24%. Trend components multiply, they do not add. Rate filings that use additive trend systematically underprice, creating adverse MLR outcomes in future years.*

Q4. IBNR completion factor at 1-month maturity of 0.42 means the IBNR multiplier is:

A. 0.42
B. 0.58
C. 2.38
D. 1.42

Answer: C. *IBNR multiplier = 1 / completion_factor = 1 / 0.42 = 2.38. Multiply the current 1-month PMPM by 2.38 to estimate the fully-developed PMPM. Typical completion rates at 1 month: pharmacy ≈90%, professional ≈60%, outpatient ≈50%, inpatient ≈35–42%.*

Q5. Specific stop-loss reinsurance differs from aggregate stop-loss in that:

A. Specific applies to inpatient only; aggregate applies to all service lines

B. Specific triggers when a single member's annual claims exceed a threshold (e.g., $250K); aggregate triggers when the plan's total claims exceed a % of expected (e.g., 120%)

C. Specific is purchased by members; aggregate is purchased by the plan

D. Specific covers pharmacy; aggregate covers medical

Answer: B. *Both are reinsurance products purchased by the plan from an external carrier. Specific stop-loss protects against catastrophic individual members. Aggregate stop-loss protects against a bad year for the entire book. Both require SQL monitoring: weekly for specific (members approaching threshold), monthly for aggregate (plan-wide exposure).*

Q6. Budget variance decomposition formula util_variance_pmpm = (actual_util - prior_util)/1000 × prior_unit_cost holds unit cost constant to:

A. Remove the effect of enrollment changes from the variance

B. Isolate the pure volume effect — shows how much PMPM would have changed from utilization alone if price had stayed the same, routing the problem to care management

C. Calculate the weighted average of utilization and cost changes

D. Normalize the variance to a per-member basis

Answer: B. *By holding unit cost at the prior year level, the formula isolates exactly what the utilization change contributed to PMPM variance. Similarly, cost_variance_pmpm holds utilization at the prior year level and isolates the price effect. Together they decompose the total variance into two actionable components with clear organizational owners.*

Q7. Explain how the IBNR lag triangle is built and how completion factors are applied to produce an estimated final PMPM for an incomplete month.

(Short answer)

> **Sample Answer:**
> Building the triangle: For each historical service month, track cumulative paid claims at 1, 2, 3, 6, and 12 months elapsed. Each cell = cumulative_paid_at_lag / total_member_months_for_service_month = cumulative PMPM. At 12+ months, the month is considered fully developed. Completion factor at lag X = AVG(cumulative_pmpm_at_X / final_pmpm) across all matured service months. SQL: MAX(CASE WHEN lag_months = X THEN cumulative_pmpm END) pivot pattern; HAVING MAX(lag_months) >= 12 limits to matured months only. Application: if October PMPM at 1-month maturity = $285 and avg_completion_at_1m = 0.42, estimated final October PMPM = $285 / 0.42 = $678. This replaces the raw $285 in executive dashboards. Always label estimated months as IBNR-adjusted in every report — never present them as final.

Q8. Write the SQL to identify members approaching the specific stop-loss threshold and explain the operational response at each alert tier.

(Short answer)

> **Sample Answer:**
> SELECT m.member_id, m.member_name, m.plan_id, ROUND(SUM(c.allowed_amount),0) AS ytd_allowed, sl.specific_threshold, ROUND(sl.specific_threshold - SUM(c.allowed_amount),0) AS remaining_to_threshold, CASE WHEN SUM(c.allowed_amount) >= sl.specific_threshold THEN 'THRESHOLD MET — submit to reinsurer' WHEN SUM(c.allowed_amount) >= sl.specific_threshold * 0.80 THEN 'ALERT — within 20% of threshold' ELSE 'Monitor' END AS stop_loss_status FROM fact_medical_claims c JOIN dim_members m ON c.member_id = m.member_id JOIN ref_stop_loss_contracts sl ON m.plan_id = sl.plan_id WHERE c.claim_status IN ('PAID','PROCESSED','APPROVED') AND EXTRACT(YEAR FROM c.service_date) = EXTRACT(YEAR FROM CURRENT_DATE) GROUP BY m.member_id, m.member_name, m.plan_id, sl.specific_threshold HAVING SUM(c.allowed_amount) >= sl.specific_threshold * 0.70 ORDER BY ytd_allowed DESC. Operational response: THRESHOLD MET = immediately submit a specific stop-loss claim to the reinsurer within the contract's submission window (typically 90 days of threshold breach) — missing the deadline forfeits recovery. ALERT (within 20%) = flag the member's case manager; the next inpatient admission will likely breach the threshold. Monitor = watch weekly. Run every Monday morning as the first financial analytics task.

Q9. Explain the three-layer budget variance decomposition. Assign each layer an organizational owner and write the SQL formula for each component.

(Short answer)

> **Sample Answer:**
> Three layers: (1) Enrollment mix variance — did the membership become sicker (higher RAF) or healthier? Owner: Actuarial/Underwriting. If the plan enrolled more high-risk members than assumed, PMPM will exceed budget even with perfect care management. SQL: not directly computable from claims alone — requires comparing current avg RAF to budget assumption. (2) Utilization variance — more services per member? Owner: CMO and Care Management. SQL formula: util_variance_pmpm = (actual_util_per_1k - budget_util_per_1k) / 1000.0 × budget_unit_cost. This holds price constant and isolates the volume effect. (3) Unit cost variance — higher price per service? Owner: VP Network and Contracting. SQL formula:

cost_variance_pmpm = budget_util_per_1k / 1000.0 × (actual_unit_cost - budget_unit_cost). This holds volume constant and isolates the price effect. Check: util_variance_pmpm + cost_variance_pmpm should ≈ total_pmpm_variance (small cross-term from simultaneous changes). Present all three components in the monthly financial package — the combined table routes each variance row to the correct accountable team automatically.

Q10. A plan's inpatient PMPM shows a +$22 favorable variance vs. budget in October. The IBNR completion factor for inpatient at 1 month is 0.38. Before reporting this as a success, what must the analyst do?

(Short answer)

Sample Answer:

The analyst must apply the IBNR multiplier before interpreting the October result. October inpatient is only 38% complete at 1-month maturity. The estimated final inpatient PMPM = observed PMPM × (1/0.38) = observed × 2.63. If the budget was $280 inpatient PMPM and the observed is $258, the "favorable" variance of $22 actually suggests the final PMPM will be approximately $258/0.38 = $679 — far above both the budget and the prior year. Steps: (1) Apply the completion factor: estimated_final = observed_pmpm / avg_completion_at_1m. (2) Compare estimated_final to budget — the true variance may be unfavorable. (3) Label the month in the dashboard as "IBNR-adjusted estimate — subject to revision." (4) Add the IBNR flag CASE WHEN: CASE WHEN svc_month >= DATE_TRUNC('month', CURRENT_DATE) - INTERVAL '3 months' THEN 'IBNR-adjusted' ELSE 'Final' END. Never present IBNR-impacted months as final performance results — premature favorable reporting leads to incorrect operational decisions and surprises at financial close.

Key Takeaways

What every analyst must remember from this chapter.

1. MLR = Claims / Premium Revenue. ACA floors: 85% large group, 80% small group/individual. Monitor weekly. MLR trending above floor for 3+ months = pricing or adverse selection issue requiring actuarial escalation.

2. Medical cost trend is multiplicative: blended = (1 + util_trend) × (1 + unit_cost_trend) - 1. Annualized over N years: POWER(end/start, 1.0/N) - 1. Never use simple arithmetic averaging for trend factors in rate filings.

3. IBNR lag triangle: cross-tab service_month × lag_months using MAX(CASE WHEN lag_months = X THEN cumulative_pmpm END). HAVING MAX(lag_months) >= 12 for matured months only. Completion factor = AVG(cumulative_pmpm_at_X / final_pmpm). Multiplier = 1 / completion_factor.

4. Typical IBNR completion at 1 month: Pharmacy ≈90%, Professional ≈60%, Outpatient ≈50%, Inpatient ≈35–42%. Calculate plan-specific factors from your own lag triangle — never borrow from a different plan or LOB.

5. Budget variance decomposition: util_variance_pmpm = (actual_util - budget_util)/1000 × budget_unit_cost. cost_variance_pmpm = budget_util/1000 × (actual_unit_cost - budget_unit_cost). Route each component to its owner: utilization → CMO, unit cost → VP Network.

6. Specific stop-loss = per-member threshold (e.g., $250K/year). Alert at 80% of threshold. Submit to reinsurer immediately when threshold is met — missing the submission window forfeits recovery. Run monitoring every Monday.

7. Aggregate stop-loss triggers when total plan claims exceed a % of expected (e.g., 120%). Monitor monthly: SUM(allowed_amount) for the year vs. (expected_pmpm × total_member_months × aggregate_attachment_pct).

8. Never present IBNR-affected months as final results. Label every recent month: CASE WHEN svc_month >= CURRENT_DATE - INTERVAL '3 months' THEN 'IBNR-adjusted estimate' ELSE 'Final' END AS data_maturity.

Chapter 15: Actuarial Pricing & Rate Filing Analytics

Rate filing process · Trend factors · Credibility weighting · Large claim pooling

15.1 The Rate Filing Data Chain

Health plans file premium rates with state insurance departments annually. The analyst's role in the rate filing: supply base-period allowed PMPM, apply IBNR completion, identify large claim pooling excess, provide credibility-weighted adjustments, and calculate annualized trend factors. The actuary then adds expense loading and margin.

> **Why allowed_amount, not paid_amount** Paid PMPM varies by benefit design — a high-deductible plan has lower paid PMPM than a rich-benefit plan for identical services. Allowed PMPM represents the true cost of services regardless of member cost-sharing. Premium must cover allowed cost.

15.2 Trend Factors by Service Category

ANSI SQL — 15.2: Multi-Year Service Category Trend (Fully Annotated)

```
-- PURPOSE: Calculate annualized PMPM, utilization, and unit cost trend
-- by service category for rate filing trend selection.
-- Two years of data used for the 2-year geometric trend.

-- STEP 1: Annual metrics for current year and base year.
WITH annual_metrics AS (
  SELECT
    EXTRACT(YEAR FROM c.service_date)                    AS yr,
    p.service_category,
    -- PMPM from enrollment denominator (never from claims)
    ROUND(SUM(c.allowed_amount)/NULLIF(SUM(mm.member_months),0),2)  AS pmpm,
    ROUND(1000.0*COUNT(DISTINCT c.claim_id)
      /NULLIF(SUM(mm.member_months),0),1)                AS util_per_1k,
    ROUND(SUM(c.allowed_amount)/NULLIF(COUNT(DISTINCT c.claim_id),0),0) AS unit_cost
  FROM  fact_medical_claims c
  JOIN  ref_procedure_codes  p  ON c.procedure_code = p.procedure_code
  JOIN  fact_member_months   mm
    ON c.member_id = mm.member_id
   AND mm.membership_year = EXTRACT(YEAR FROM c.service_date)
  WHERE c.claim_status = 'PAID'
   AND c.line_of_business = 'COMMERCIAL'
   AND EXTRACT(YEAR FROM c.service_date) IN (:base_year, :current_year)
  GROUP BY 1, 2
)
-- STEP 2: Self-join to compare current year to base year.
-- POWER(end/start, 1.0/2) = geometric annual trend over 2 years.
SELECT
  a2.service_category,
  a2.pmpm    AS pmpm_current,
  a1.pmpm    AS pmpm_base,
  -- Annualized 2-year PMPM trend (geometric compound rate)
  ROUND(POWER(a2.pmpm / NULLIF(a1.pmpm,0), 0.5) - 1, 4)          AS pmpm_trend_2yr,
  -- Utilization component of trend
  ROUND(POWER(a2.util_per_1k/NULLIF(a1.util_per_1k,0), 0.5) - 1, 4) AS util_trend,
  -- Unit cost component of trend
  ROUND(POWER(a2.unit_cost/NULLIF(a1.unit_cost,0), 0.5) - 1, 4)     AS cost_trend
FROM  annual_metrics a2          -- current (most recent) year
```

```sql
JOIN annual_metrics a1            -- base year (2 years prior)
  ON a2.service_category = a1.service_category
 AND a2.yr = :current_year AND a1.yr = :base_year
ORDER BY a2.service_category;
```

15.3 Credibility Theory

Credibility blends a plan's own experience with an industry benchmark. Z = MIN(1, √(member_months / 1082)). The 1,082 threshold is derived from classical credibility theory at 90% confidence, 5% precision. Credibility-weighted PMPM = Z × plan_pmpm + (1−Z) × benchmark_pmpm. A plan with 272 MM has Z = 0.50 — half own experience, half benchmark.

15.4 Large Claim Pooling

Claims above a pooling threshold (commonly $50K–$250K per member per year) are removed from base period experience and replaced with a uniform pooling charge per MM. This prevents one catastrophic case from distorting the entire rate. The total rate base PMPM is unchanged — pooling redistributes, it does not eliminate, catastrophic cost.

ANSI SQL — 15.4: Large Claim Pooling Adjustment (Fully Annotated)

```sql
-- PURPOSE: Identify members exceeding the large claim pooling threshold,
-- remove the excess from base period experience, and calculate the
-- uniform pooling charge PMPM that replaces it.
-- Total rate base PMPM is unchanged -- pooling only redistributes cost.

-- STEP 1: Sum each member's annual allowed amount for the base period.
WITH member_ytd AS (
   SELECT c.member_id, m.plan_id,
          SUM(c.allowed_amount) AS ytd_allowed
   FROM  fact_medical_claims c
   JOIN  dim_members m ON c.member_id = m.member_id
   WHERE c.claim_status = 'PAID'
     AND c.line_of_business = 'COMMERCIAL'
     AND EXTRACT(YEAR FROM c.service_date) = :base_year
   GROUP BY c.member_id, m.plan_id
),

-- STEP 2: Flag members above threshold; calculate excess and capped amounts.
-- Excess = amount ABOVE the threshold (removed from experience).
-- Capped = amount that STAYS in experience (floored at threshold).
pooled AS (
   SELECT member_id, plan_id, ytd_allowed,
          -- Amount removed from experience (the pooled excess)
          GREATEST(0, ytd_allowed - :pooling_threshold) AS pooled_excess,
          -- Amount kept in experience (no more than the threshold per member)
          LEAST(ytd_allowed, :pooling_threshold)     AS capped_allowed
   FROM  member_ytd
)
-- STEP 3: Calculate pooling charge PMPM.
-- Pooling charge = total excess / total member months.
-- This spreads the catastrophic cost uniformly across all members.
SELECT
   p.plan_id,
   COUNT(DISTINCT CASE WHEN pooled_excess > 0 THEN member_id END) AS large_claim_members,
   SUM(ytd_allowed)                         AS total_experience,
   SUM(pooled_excess)                        AS total_pooled_excess,
   SUM(ytd_allowed) - SUM(pooled_excess)              AS pooled_experience,
   mm.total_mm,
   -- Base PMPM after removing large claim excess
```

```
  ROUND((SUM(ytd_allowed)-SUM(pooled_excess))/NULLIF(mm.total_mm,0),2) AS base_pmpm_pooled,
  -- Uniform pooling charge added back across all members
  ROUND(SUM(pooled_excess)/NULLIF(mm.total_mm,0),2)          AS pooling_charge_pmpm,
  -- Final rate base = pooled experience + pooling charge (= original total)
  ROUND(SUM(ytd_allowed)/NULLIF(mm.total_mm,0),2)            AS rate_base_pmpm
FROM  pooled p
JOIN (
  SELECT plan_id, SUM(member_months) AS total_mm
  FROM  fact_member_months
  WHERE membership_year = :base_year AND line_of_business = 'COMMERCIAL'
  GROUP BY plan_id
) mm ON p.plan_id = mm.plan_id
GROUP BY p.plan_id, mm.total_mm;
```

Chapter 15 Review

Unit Test · Key Takeaways

Answer each question before reading the explanation.

Q1. Allowed_amount is the correct base for rate filing (not paid_amount) because:

A. Allowed is required by CMS for all commercial rate filings

B. Paid varies with benefit design — a high-deductible plan has lower paid even for identical services. Allowed represents the contractual cost of services, which is what the premium must cover regardless of how cost-sharing is structured.

C. Paid_amount always understates the true cost by exactly the deductible amount

D. Paid_amount includes pharmacy costs; allowed_amount does not

Answer: B. *If a plan changes from a $500 to a $2,000 deductible, paid_amount drops but allowed_amount is unchanged — the cost of services did not change, only who pays the first dollars. Using paid as the rate base would produce an artificially low premium, leaving the plan underpriced for its actual medical cost exposure.*

Q2. A plan with 272 member months has a credibility weight of:

A. 0.25

B. 0.50

C. 0.75

D. 1.00

Answer: B. *Z = MIN(1, √(272/1082)) = MIN(1, √0.251) = MIN(1, 0.501) ≈ 0.50. At 1,082+ MM, Z = 1.0 (full credibility). The 1,082 threshold comes from classical credibility theory: $(1.645/0.05)^2$ = 1,082, representing 90% confidence that the observed mean is within ±5% of the true mean.*

Q3. Large claim pooling does NOT change the total rate base PMPM because:

A. The pooling charge is paid by the reinsurer, not the plan

B. Pooling only redistributes cost: it removes the excess above the threshold from experience and re-introduces it as a uniform pooling charge per MM. The sum (pooled_experience_pmpm + pooling_charge_pmpm) equals the original total PMPM.

C. Only claims below the threshold are used for pricing; above-threshold claims are excluded entirely

D. The pooling charge is recovered from the member via increased deductibles

Answer: B. *Example: $3M total experience, $50K threshold, one $1.2M member. Excess = $1.15M. Pooled experience = $1.85M. Over 6,000 MM: pooled_experience_pmpm = $308, pooling_charge = $192, total = $500 PMPM — same as $3M/6,000 = $500 without pooling. The stabilization benefit: the $308 component is much more predictable year-over-year than the original $500 driven by one catastrophic case.*

Q4. Credibility-weighted PMPM formula is:

A. Z × benchmark_pmpm + (1−Z) × plan_pmpm

B. Z × plan_pmpm + (1−Z) × benchmark_pmpm — Z portion from own experience; (1−Z) from benchmark

C. (plan_pmpm + benchmark_pmpm) / 2

D. plan_pmpm × (1 + Z × trend_factor)

Answer: B. *Z is the weight given to the plan's own experience; (1−Z) is the weight given to the external benchmark. A plan with Z ... nd plan_pmpm = $440, benchmark = $425: credibility_weighted = 0.50 × $440 + 0.50 × $425 = $432.50. This prevents ... being priced entirely on statistically unreliable own-experience data.*

Q5. The rate filing data chain analyst role includes all of the following EXCEPT:

A. Supplying base period allowed PMPM by service category
B. Applying IBNR completion factors to the most recent months
C. Setting the administrative expense load and risk margin
D. Calculating large claim pooling excess and uniform pooling charge

Answer: C. *Expense loading (administrative costs as % of premium) and risk margin (profit) are actuarial determinations certified by the appointed actuary. The analyst owns the data layers — experience, IBNR, pooling, trend calculation. The actuary owns judgment calls — which trend point to select, what expense load to apply, what risk margin is appropriate for the market.*

Q6. For rate filing purposes, the full credibility threshold of 1,082 member months represents:

A. The minimum enrollment required to offer a product in most states
B. The number of observations needed for 90% confidence that the observed PMPM is within ±5% of the true PMPM — derived from classical credibility theory: $(z_{0.05}/r)^2 = (1.645/0.05)^2 = 1{,}082$
C. The average enrollment of a small employer group in the US
D. CMS's minimum denominator for risk adjustment credibility

Answer: B. *Classical credibility full credibility threshold for a PMPM metric: $n_{full} = (z_\alpha/r)^2$ where $z_\alpha = 1.645$ (90% confidence) and $r = 0.05$ (5% precision). Plans below this threshold blend own experience with a benchmark using $Z = \sqrt{n/n_{full}}$. Below 270 MM ($Z < 0.50$), plans should lean heavily on the external benchmark.*

Q7. Walk through the complete rate filing data chain. Identify the analyst's SQL deliverable at each step.

(Short answer)

> **Sample Answer:**
> Step 1 — Base period allowed PMPM: SELECT p.service_category, ROUND(SUM(c.allowed_amount)/NULLIF(SUM(mm.member_months),0),2) AS allowed_pmpm FROM fact_medical_claims c JOIN ref_procedure_codes p ON ... JOIN fact_member_months mm ON ... WHERE c.claim_status='PAID' AND EXTRACT(YEAR FROM c.service_date) = :base_year GROUP BY p.service_category. Analyst deliverable: allowed PMPM table by service category for base period. Step 2 — IBNR adjustment: apply completion factors to the most recent 12 months of the base period to ensure fully developed data. Deliverable: completion factor table from lag triangle, and adjusted PMPM for recent months. Step 3 — Large claim pooling: run the pooling query to identify members above threshold, calculate total_pooled_excess and pooling_charge_pmpm. Deliverable: pooling summary table with rate_base_pmpm. Step 4 — Credibility: provide total_mm so actuary can compute Z. Deliverable: member months by plan_id and base year. Step 5 — Trend calculation: run multi-year service category trend query, provide util_trend and cost_trend by category. Deliverable: trend factor table for actuary selection. The actuary then applies expense load and margin — the analyst does not set these. Every SQL query must be versioned, documented, and stored with the filing submission for regulatory audit.

Q8. A plan has 650 member months, plan PMPM of $440, and a benchmark PMPM of $425. Calculate the credibility-weighted PMPM and write the SQL.

(Short answer)

> **Sample Answer:**
> Z = MIN(1, SQRT(650/1082)) = MIN(1, SQRT(0.601)) = MIN(1, 0.775) = 0.775. Credibility-weighted PMPM = 0.775 × $440 + 0.225 × $425 = $341.00 + $95.63 = $436.63. SQL: SELECT :plan_pmpm AS plan_pmpm, :benchmark_pmpm AS benchmark_pmpm, ROUND(LEAST(1.0, SQRT(:member_months/1082.0)),3) AS credibility_z, ROUND(LEAST(1.0, SQRT(:member_months/1082.0)) * :plan_pmpm + (1 - LEAST(1.0, SQRT(:member_months/1082.0))) * :benchmark_pmpm, 2) AS credibility_weighted_pmpm. Interpretation: at Z=0.775, the plan has about 77.5% statistical reliability — meaning 22.5% of the rate base comes from the external benchmark. The $436.63 is the correct rate base, not the raw $440. A plan that uses its own $440 without credibility blending overstates its rate reliability and may face adverse regulatory review.

Q9. Explain what happens to the rate base if large claim pooling is NOT applied. Give a numerical example.

(Short answer)

> **Sample Answer:**
> Without pooling: a 500-member group with one $1.2M catastrophic member has total_experience = $1.2M + (499 × ~$3,600/yr) = $1.2M + $1.796M = $2.996M. Over 6,000 MM, rate_base_pmpm = $499.33. This rate priced next year's premium — but there is no statistical basis to expect another $1.2M member next year. With $50K pooling threshold: excess = $1.15M; capped = $50K. pooled_experience = $1.846M; pooled_experience_pmpm = $307.67. pooling_charge_pmpm = $1.15M/6,000 = $191.67. Rate base PMPM = $307.67 + $191.67 = $499.33 — identical total, but now the $307.67 component is statistically stable (driven by the normal 499-member population), while the $191.67 pooling charge represents the expected average cost of catastrophic cases spread uniformly. In a year with no catastrophic members, the experience PMPM drops to ≈$307 — which the pooling charge already priced. The mechanism stabilizes rates without changing the expected cost.

Q10. Describe the difference between trend selection (analyst role) and trend application (actuary role). Why can the analyst not simply pick the lowest trend factor?

(Short answer)

> **Sample Answer:**
> Trend selection is an actuarial judgment requiring certification by the appointed actuary. The analyst's role is data preparation: run the multi-year lag triangle, calculate geometric trends at 1-year, 2-year, and 3-year intervals for each service category, and present the data with clear labels. The actuary then selects which trend point to apply, considering: external benchmarks (industry trend surveys from Milliman, Segal), credibility of the plan's own data (small plans have high-variance trends), COVID/pandemic distortions in recent years (depressed utilization 2020–2021, elevated 2022+), and regulatory guidance from the state insurance department on acceptable trend ranges. Why the analyst cannot pick the lowest trend: premium rates must be actuarially sound — they must cover expected claims with a reasonable confidence margin. A rate filing that uses an artificially low trend will produce a premium that is insufficient to cover actual claims, leading to adverse MLR, financial losses, and potential regulatory action. State actuaries review rate filings and flag trend selections that are outliers from benchmarks. If the selected trend is unjustifiably low, the state can reject the filing or require a rebate. The analyst's integrity obligation is to present accurate, complete trend data — not to optimize for the lowest premium.

Key Takeaways

What every analyst must remember from this chapter.

1. Rate filing analyst deliverables (in order): base period allowed PMPM by service category → IBNR-adjusted recent months → large claim pooling summary → member months for credibility → trend factor table. The actuary adds expense load and margin.

2. Always use allowed_amount (not paid_amount) for rate filing base. Paid varies with benefit design; allowed represents the contractual cost of services regardless of member cost-sharing structure.

3. Credibility: Z = MIN(1, SQRT(n/1082)). Full credibility at 1,082 MM. Credibility-weighted PMPM = Z × plan_pmpm + (1−Z) × benchmark_pmpm. Below 270 MM (Z < 0.50), lean heavily on the external benchmark.

4. Large claim pooling: GREATEST(0, ytd_allowed − threshold) = pooled_excess. Pooling charge PMPM = total_pooled_excess / total_MM. Rate base PMPM = pooled_experience_pmpm + pooling_charge_pmpm = original total PMPM (unchanged).

5. Trend components are multiplicative: blended = (1 + util_trend) × (1 + cost_trend) − 1. Annualized N-year trend = POWER(end/start, 1.0/N) − 1. Calculate separately for each service category — inpatient trend differs significantly from professional or pharmacy trend.

6. Base period IBNR adjustment: before using the most recent 12 months as the rate base, apply completion factors to fully develop each month. An undeveloped month underestimates the rate base, leading to underpricing.

7. Trend selection is actuarial judgment (appointed actuary certifies). Trend calculation is analyst SQL. The analyst presents options; the actuary decides. Never advocate for a specific trend selection — present the data neutrally.

8. State insurance regulators review all commercial rate filings. Trend selections that are outliers below industry benchmarks trigger additional justification requests. Maintain complete documentation of every SQL query used in the filing for regulatory audit response.

Chapter 16: Provider Analytics & Network Performance

Provider scorecards · Risk-adjusted cost · Referral leakage · OIG compliance · Network adequacy

16.1 Provider Scorecard Framework

A provider scorecard evaluates each in-network provider on cost efficiency and clinical quality simultaneously. Cost dimension: risk-adjusted PMPM vs. peer average. Quality dimension: HEDIS gap closure rate for attributed panel. Both are required for top-tier designation — cheap but low-quality or expensive but high-quality providers cannot earn Tier 1.

ANSI SQL — 16.1: Provider Risk-Adjusted Scorecard (Fully Annotated)

```
-- PURPOSE: Calculate a composite provider scorecard combining risk-adjusted
-- cost PMPM vs. peer average AND HEDIS gap closure rate.
-- Risk adjustment prevents penalizing providers who manage sicker panels.

-- STEP 1: Pull attributed panel with RAF scores.
WITH attributed_panel AS (
  SELECT a.attributed_pcp_npi, a.member_id,
      COALESCE(r.total_raf_score, 1.0) AS raf_score  -- default 1.0 if no HCCs
  FROM  dim_pcp_attribution a
  LEFT JOIN raf_scores r ON a.member_id = r.member_id
  WHERE a.attribution_year = EXTRACT(YEAR FROM CURRENT_DATE)
),

-- STEP 2: Calculate actual and risk-adjusted PMPM per PCP.
-- Risk-adjusted PMPM = actual_pmpm / avg_panel_raf.
-- This credits providers for managing appropriately expensive sick panels.
pcp_cost AS (
  SELECT ap.attributed_pcp_npi,
      COUNT(DISTINCT ap.member_id)                AS panel_size,
      ROUND(AVG(ap.raf_score),3)                AS avg_panel_raf,
      ROUND(SUM(c.allowed_amount)/NULLIF(SUM(mm.member_months),0),2) AS actual_pmpm,
      -- Divide actual PMPM by panel average RAF to remove sickness effect
      ROUND(SUM(c.allowed_amount)/NULLIF(SUM(mm.member_months),0)
        / NULLIF(AVG(ap.raf_score),0), 2)          AS ra_pmpm
  FROM  attributed_panel ap
  JOIN  fact_medical_claims c  ON ap.member_id = c.member_id
  JOIN  fact_member_months  mm ON ap.member_id = mm.member_id
              AND mm.membership_year = EXTRACT(YEAR FROM CURRENT_DATE)
  WHERE c.claim_status = 'PAID'
   AND EXTRACT(YEAR FROM c.service_date) = EXTRACT(YEAR FROM CURRENT_DATE)
  GROUP BY ap.attributed_pcp_npi
),

-- STEP 3: HEDIS gap closure rate per PCP.
-- Gap closure rate = members with all HEDIS gaps closed / total attributed.
pcp_quality AS (
  SELECT ap.attributed_pcp_npi,
      COUNT(DISTINCT ap.member_id)                AS total_attributed,
      -- Members with zero open gaps across all HEDIS measures
      COUNT(DISTINCT CASE WHEN hg.open_gap_count = 0
              THEN ap.member_id END)           AS fully_closed,
      ROUND(100.0 * COUNT(DISTINCT CASE WHEN hg.open_gap_count = 0
              THEN ap.member_id END)
        / NULLIF(COUNT(DISTINCT ap.member_id),0), 1)        AS gap_closure_pct
```

```sql
    FROM  attributed_panel ap
    LEFT JOIN (
      SELECT member_id, COUNT(*) AS open_gap_count
      FROM  fact_hedis_gaps
      WHERE measurement_year = EXTRACT(YEAR FROM CURRENT_DATE)
        AND gap_status = 'OPEN'
      GROUP BY member_id
    ) hg ON ap.member_id = hg.member_id
    GROUP BY ap.attributed_pcp_npi
),

-- STEP 4: Plan-wide peer average RA PMPM for benchmarking.
peer_avg AS (SELECT ROUND(AVG(ra_pmpm),2) AS avg_ra_pmpm FROM pcp_cost)

-- STEP 5: Final scorecard with composite tier assignment.
SELECT
    pc.attributed_pcp_npi,
    p.provider_full_name, p.specialty_group, p.county,
    pc.panel_size,
    pc.avg_panel_raf,
    pc.actual_pmpm, pc.ra_pmpm,
    pa.avg_ra_pmpm             AS peer_avg_ra_pmpm,
    ROUND(pc.ra_pmpm - pa.avg_ra_pmpm, 2) AS ra_pmpm_vs_peer,  -- positive = above peer
    pq.gap_closure_pct,
    -- Tier 1: at/below peer cost AND high quality. Tier 3: neither.
    CASE
      WHEN pc.ra_pmpm <= pa.avg_ra_pmpm AND pq.gap_closure_pct >= 70
      THEN 'TIER 1 — High Value'
      WHEN pc.ra_pmpm <= pa.avg_ra_pmpm * 1.10 AND pq.gap_closure_pct >= 50
      THEN 'TIER 2 — Average Value'
      ELSE 'TIER 3 — Below Benchmark'
    END AS performance_tier
FROM  pcp_cost pc
JOIN  pcp_quality pq ON pc.attributed_pcp_npi = pq.attributed_pcp_npi
JOIN  dim_providers p ON pc.attributed_pcp_npi = p.npi
CROSS JOIN peer_avg pa
WHERE pc.panel_size >= 30   -- minimum panel for statistical validity
ORDER BY pc.ra_pmpm ASC;
```

16.2 Referral Leakage

Referral leakage = specialist claims where the rendering provider is out-of-network, for members attributed to in-network PCPs. High-leakage specialties: orthopedics, oncology, behavioral health, advanced imaging. SQL: identify specialist (non-primary-care) claims, JOIN to dim_providers for network_status, GROUP BY PCP × specialty × network_status.

16.3 OIG Exclusion Monitoring

Health plans that pay claims from OIG-excluded providers face False Claims Act liability. Load the OIG exclusion list monthly from exclusions.oig.hhs.gov and JOIN it to claims. Exclusion check must run at credentialing, re-credentialing, and weekly via automated SQL. Escalate any match to Compliance immediately.

ANSI SQL — 16.3: OIG Exclusion Compliance Check (Fully Annotated)

```sql
-- PURPOSE: Identify any paid claims where the rendering or billing provider
-- appears on the OIG exclusion list on the date of service.
-- Any match = potential False Claims Act violation — escalate to Compliance.

SELECT
    c.rendering_npi, c.billing_tin,
```

```
    p.provider_full_name, p.specialty_group,
    COUNT(DISTINCT c.claim_id)           AS claim_count,
    ROUND(SUM(c.allowed_amount),0)       AS total_allowed,
    MIN(c.service_date)                  AS first_excluded_claim,
    oig.exclusion_date,
    oig.exclusion_type,
    oig.reinstatement_date
FROM  fact_medical_claims c
JOIN  dim_providers p ON c.rendering_npi = p.npi
-- Join on NPI or TIN (excluded entities may appear in either field)
JOIN  ref_oig_exclusions oig
  ON (c.rendering_npi = oig.npi OR c.billing_tin = oig.tin)
 -- Service date must fall within the exclusion period
 AND oig.exclusion_date <= c.service_date
 AND (oig.reinstatement_date IS NULL        -- still excluded today
      OR oig.reinstatement_date > c.service_date) -- not yet reinstated at claim date
WHERE c.claim_status IN ('PAID','PROCESSED','APPROVED')
 AND EXTRACT(YEAR FROM c.service_date) = EXTRACT(YEAR FROM CURRENT_DATE)
GROUP BY c.rendering_npi, c.billing_tin, p.provider_full_name,
      p.specialty_group, oig.exclusion_date, oig.exclusion_type, oig.reinstatement_date
ORDER BY total_allowed DESC;

-- Compliance response for any results:
-- 1. Immediately notify the Compliance Officer.
-- 2. Stop all future payments to the excluded provider.
-- 3. Request refund of all payments during the exclusion period.
-- 4. Report under OIG self-disclosure protocol if required.
-- 5. Investigate how the provider passed credentialing -- fix the gap.
```

Chapter 16 Review

Unit Test · Key Takeaways

Answer each question before reading the explanation.

Q1. Risk-adjusted PMPM = actual_pmpm / avg_panel_raf because:

A. RAF scores are required denominators for all provider payment calculations

B. A PCP with a sicker (higher RAF) panel will always have higher actual PMPM even with perfect efficiency. Dividing by panel average RAF removes the sickness effect — only cost above what the RAF predicts is attributable to provider behavior.

C. CMS mandates risk-adjusted PMPM for all provider scorecards

D. Average panel RAF is always close to 1.0 so the division has minimal effect

Answer: B. *Example: PCP A panel avg RAF 0.8, actual PMPM $280 → ra_pmpm $350. PCP B panel avg RAF 1.8, actual PMPM $630 → ra_pmpm $350. Both are equally efficient. Without risk adjustment, PCP B appears 2.25× more expensive — creating a perverse incentive to avoid high-need patients, harming health equity.*

Q2. The minimum panel size of 30 in the HAVING clause of the provider scorecard serves to:

A. Meet CMS network adequacy requirements for primary care panels

B. Ensure statistical validity — a PCP with 5 attributed members has too small a sample for their PMPM or gap closure rate to distinguish performance from random noise. Label sub-threshold providers as "insufficient data" rather than assigning a tier.

C. Limit the output to the top 30 providers by panel size

D. Exclude providers who are new to the network and lack history

Answer: B. *A PCP with 5 attributed members and one complex member showing $1,400 PMPM is statistically indistinguishable from a high-cost provider — it is random sample variation. Most plans use 30 members as a minimum for reporting and 50+ for performance-based payment decisions. Never assign a performance tier below the minimum volume threshold.*

Q3. OIG exclusion monitoring must run at which frequency:

A. Annually at the time of provider re-credentialing only

B. Monthly OIG list download; weekly SQL JOIN of the updated list to current claims. Also at initial credentialing and re-credentialing. Any gap in monitoring creates liability exposure.

C. Quarterly, aligned with the financial close cycle

D. Only when a provider complaint is received

Answer: B. *OIG exclusions can be added at any time. A provider who was in good standing when credentialed may be excluded 6 months later. Weekly monitoring catches the exclusion before significant claims are paid under the excluded provider's NPI. The cost of the monitoring SQL is trivial compared to the potential False Claims Act exposure.*

Q4. Referral leakage is analytically significant because:

A. Out-of-network specialist claims are automatically denied by the plan

B. Plans pay higher out-of-network rates for the same service, reducing financial efficiency and care coordination. High-leakage PCPs may not have a relationship with in-network specialists or may be routing patients based on personal preference rather than network participation.

C. Referral leakage triggers a HEDIS measure exclusion for affected members

D. Out-of-network claims do not appear in fact_medical_claims

Answer: B. *Leakage identification SQL: JOIN specialist (non-primary-care CPT codes) claims to dim_providers on rendering_npi, filter WHERE network_status = 'OUT_OF_NETWORK'. GROUP BY attributed_pcp_npi, specialty_group. Sort by total_allowed DESC. High-leakage specialties: orthopedics, oncology, behavioral health, advanced imaging. Engage high-leakage PCPs through provider relations with an in-network specialist directory.*

Q5. Network adequacy analysis checks whether:

A. Every member has been seen by an in-network provider in the past 12 months

B. Sufficient in-network providers of each specialty exist within required distance/time standards for each county or service area — meeting CMS and state regulatory minimums

C. The plan's network includes at least one provider in every ZIP code

D. All in-network providers have current NCQA PCMH recognition

Answer: B. *Network adequacy SQL: GROUP BY county_fips × specialty_group, COUNT(DISTINCT in-network NPI where accepting_new_patients = Y), compare to ref_adequacy_standards minimum_required. Flag counties below the minimum as ADEQUACY DEFICIENCY. Run quarterly and before regulatory filings. Inadequate networks trigger enrollment caps and access-to-care penalties from CMS or state departments of insurance.*

Q6. A provider scorecard Tier 1 designation requires:

A. Quality score alone — the top quartile of HEDIS gap closure rates

B. Both at-or-below-peer risk-adjusted cost AND above-quality-threshold gap closure rate. Two-dimensional requirement prevents gaming by being cheap through under-treatment OR high quality at far above peer cost.

C. More than 100 attributed members AND positive patient experience scores

D. Zero OIG flags AND no malpractice history in the past 3 years

Answer: B. *The two-dimensional Tier 1 criterion (ra_pmpm <= peer_avg AND gap_closure_pct >= 70%) ensures that savings come from genuine efficiency, not from withholding necessary care. A provider who is below-peer cost because they skip expensive-but-necessary referrals would have a low quality score and fail the Tier 1 threshold.*

Q7. Describe the risk-adjusted PMPM calculation and explain why skipping risk adjustment systematically penalizes providers who serve high-need populations.

(Short answer)

Sample Answer:

Risk-adjusted PMPM: (1) Pull all members attributed to each PCP from dim_pcp_attribution. (2) LEFT JOIN to raf_scores; COALESCE to 1.0 for members without an RAF score (no HCCs documented). (3) Calculate avg_panel_raf = AVG(raf_score) across all attributed members. (4) actual_pmpm = SUM(c.allowed_amount) / SUM(mm.member_months). (5) ra_pmpm = actual_pmpm / avg_panel_raf. Without risk adjustment: a PCP serving Medicaid, dual-eligible, or high-chronic-disease patients will have higher actual_pmpm because their patients have more conditions and generate more claims. Without adjustment they appear to be high-cost outliers and receive Tier 3 ratings. Perverse incentive created: providers rationally stop accepting high-need patients to protect their scorecard tier. PCPs close their panels to Medicaid members; specialists stop taking complex referrals. The result: high-need populations lose access to the most capable providers, health equity deteriorates, and the plan's cost-shifting from sick to healthy panels is invisible in the data. Risk adjustment removes this incentive — only costs above what the RAF score predicts are attributable to the provider's behavior rather than their patients' conditions.

Q8. Write the SQL for network adequacy by county and specialty and describe what a plan should do when a deficiency is found.

(Short answer)

Sample Answer:
SELECT mzc.county_fips, inp.specialty_group, COUNT(DISTINCT mzc.member_id) AS members_in_county, COUNT(DISTINCT CASE WHEN inp.network_status='IN_NETWORK' AND inp.accepting_new_patients='Y' THEN inp.npi END) AS accepting_providers, ref.min_required_providers, CASE WHEN COUNT(DISTINCT CASE WHEN inp.network_status='IN_NETWORK' AND inp.accepting_new_patients='Y' THEN inp.npi END) < ref.min_required_providers THEN 'ADEQUACY DEFICIENCY' ELSE 'Meets standard' END AS adequacy_status FROM (SELECT DISTINCT member_id, county_fips FROM dim_members WHERE coverage_status='ACTIVE') mzc JOIN dim_providers inp ON inp.county_fips = mzc.county_fips JOIN ref_adequacy_standards ref ON ref.specialty_group = inp.specialty_group GROUP BY mzc.county_fips, inp.specialty_group, ref.min_required_providers ORDER BY adequacy_status DESC. When deficiency is found: (1) Identify which county and specialty has the gap. (2) Search for providers in adjacent counties who are within the CMS distance/time standard (e.g., 30 minutes or 30 miles). (3) Contact those providers for network participation – offer a temporary single-case agreement if needed. (4) If no provider within standard distance exists, file a network adequacy exception with CMS/state explaining the shortage area and alternative access plan. (5) If deficiency cannot be resolved, the plan must offer members cost-sharing waivers for out-of-network access to that specialty in the deficient county. Document everything – regulators review network adequacy reports and can issue corrective action plans.

Q9. A provider is flagged by the OIG exclusion check with $45,000 in claims paid during the exclusion period. Walk through the complete compliance response.

(Short answer)

Sample Answer:
Step 1 – Immediate notification: contact the Compliance Officer and General Counsel within 24 hours. Provide the SQL output showing claim_count, total_allowed, exclusion_date, and the provider's NPI and TIN. Step 2 – Payment halt: place an immediate hold on all future claims from this provider's rendering NPI and billing TIN. Do not issue any pending checks. Step 3 – Network action: suspend the provider from the network directory immediately. Notify the credentialing team – the provider must not be listed as in-network during the exclusion period. Step 4 – Recovery: send a refund request to the provider for the $45,000 paid during the exclusion period. If the provider does not respond within 30 days, initiate a formal recovery process under the provider contract. Step 5 – Self-disclosure: evaluate whether to self-disclose to the OIG under the Self-Disclosure Protocol (SDP). Self-disclosure is generally advisable for inadvertent violations – it typically results in lower penalties than a formal OIG investigation would. Step 6 – Root cause: determine how the excluded provider passed credentialing. Was the exclusion list not checked at the credentialing date? Was it checked against NPI but not TIN? Fix the credentialing workflow. Step 7 – Preventive controls: verify that the weekly OIG exclusion JOIN query is running correctly with current data. Add a pre-payment edit in the adjudication system to flag claims from excluded providers before they are paid.

Q10. Describe the provider scorecard tiering process end-to-end and explain what SQL a provider would receive in a Tier 3 appeal packet.

(Short answer)

Sample Answer:
Tiering process: (1) Calculate risk-adjusted PMPM vs. peer average (cost dimension) – require minimum 30-member panel. (2) Calculate HEDIS gap closure rate for attributed panel (quality dimension). (3) Apply two-dimensional tier rules. (4) Validate results – check that tier assignments are stable across the prior 3 months (single-month anomalies should not trigger tier changes). (5) Communicate to providers 60–90 days before tiers take effect – state law in most jurisdictions requires advance notice for network tiering. (6) Provide a 30-day appeal window. Appeal packet SQL (member-level detail file): SELECT attr.member_id, m.member_name, m.date_of_birth, hg.measure_id, hg.measure_description, hg.gap_status, hg.numerator_date, hg.numerator_provider FROM dim_pcp_attribution attr JOIN dim_members m ON attr.member_id = m.member_id LEFT JOIN fact_hedis_gaps hg ON attr.member_id = hg.member_id AND hg.measurement_year = EXTRACT(YEAR FROM CURRENT_DATE) WHERE attr.attributed_pcp_npi = :appeal_npi ORDER BY hg.measure_id, hg.gap_status. This lets the provider verify: (a) which members were attributed to them, (b) which HEDIS gaps are shown as open, (c) whether any numerator services occurred that should have closed the gap but were not captured in the data. Common legitimate appeal bases: attribution error (member did not actually see this PCP), numerator service occurred but claim was not processed before the measurement snapshot date, member met an exclusion criterion that was not applied.

Key Takeaways

What every analyst must remember from this chapter.

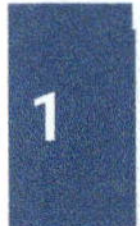
1 Risk-adjusted PMPM = actual_pmpm / avg_panel_raf. Without risk adjustment, providers serving sicker populations are systematically penalized, creating a perverse incentive to avoid high-need patients. Always use RAF-adjusted cost for provider scorecards.

2 Provider scorecard two dimensions: (1) Risk-adjusted cost vs. peer average. (2) HEDIS gap closure rate. Both required for Tier 1. A cheap but clinically poor provider, or a high-quality but far-above-peer-cost provider, cannot achieve Tier 1.

3 Minimum panel size: 30 members for scorecard reporting, 50+ for performance-based payment. Below threshold = "insufficient data" label, not a tier assignment. Never rank providers on statistically unreliable small samples.

4 OIG exclusion monitoring: load exclusion list monthly. Run weekly JOIN of claims to ref_oig_exclusions on NPI and TIN. Check at credentialing and re-credentialing. Any match = escalate to Compliance immediately within 24 hours.

5 Referral leakage = specialist claims where network_status = 'OUT_OF_NETWORK' for members attributed to in-network PCPs. Top leakage specialties: orthopedics, oncology, BH, imaging. Engage high-leakage PCPs with an in-network specialist directory.

6 Network adequacy SQL: GROUP BY county × specialty, COUNT(DISTINCT in-network NPIs accepting new patients), compare to ref_adequacy_standards minimum. ADEQUACY DEFICIENCY when count < minimum. Run quarterly. Deficiencies trigger CMS/state corrective action plans.

7 NPI types: Type 1 = individual clinician (rendering_npi). Type 2 = organization (billing_npi). A claim with a Type 2 NPI in the rendering_npi field means the individual clinician's identity was not captured — HEDIS crediting and quality attribution are impossible.

8 Provider scorecard appeals: provide member-level HEDIS gap detail (member_id, measure_id, gap_status, numerator_date) for the attributed panel. Allow 30-day appeal window. Common valid disputes: attribution error, numerator service not captured before snapshot, member exclusion criterion not applied.

Chapter 17: Network Contracting & Fee Schedule Analytics

Fee schedule compliance · Rate achievement vs. Medicare · Contract renewal risk scoring

17.1 Fee Schedule Architecture

A fee schedule is the contractual allowed amount for each procedure code at each provider. Stored as: billing_tin, procedure_code, effective_date, expiration_date, allowed_amount. The point-in-time JOIN (service_date >= effective_date AND service_date < COALESCE(expiration_date, '2099-12-31')) retrieves the rate in effect on the claim date — identical to the SCD-2 join pattern.

> **Rate Achievement** Rate achievement = plan_allowed / Medicare_rate. 1.00× = paying exactly Medicare. Most commercial plans target 130–175% of Medicare. Providers above 185% are high-priority renegotiation targets.

ANSI SQL — 17.2: Fee Schedule Compliance — Actual vs. Contracted Rate (Fully Annotated)

```
-- PURPOSE: Compare what the plan actually paid on each claim against the
-- contractual fee schedule rate. rate_variance > 0 = potential overpayment.
-- Common causes: new rates not loaded on time; outlier provisions missed.

-- Point-in-time fee schedule join: retrieve the contracted rate in effect
-- on the claim's service_date (same pattern as SCD-2 dimension join).
WITH fee_schedule_join AS (
  SELECT c.claim_id, c.rendering_npi, c.billing_tin, c.procedure_code,
      c.service_date,
      c.allowed_amount            AS actual_allowed,
      fs.allowed_amount           AS contracted_rate,
      ROUND(c.allowed_amount - fs.allowed_amount, 2)          AS rate_variance,
      ROUND(100.0*(c.allowed_amount-fs.allowed_amount)
        /NULLIF(fs.allowed_amount,0),1)                       AS variance_pct
  FROM  fact_medical_claims c
  JOIN  ref_fee_schedule fs
    ON fs.billing_tin    = c.billing_tin
   AND fs.procedure_code = c.procedure_code
   -- Retrieve rate active on the service date (SCD-2 point-in-time pattern)
   AND c.service_date  >= fs.effective_date
   AND c.service_date  <  COALESCE(fs.expiration_date, '2099-12-31')
  WHERE c.claim_status = 'PAID'
   AND EXTRACT(YEAR FROM c.service_date) = EXTRACT(YEAR FROM CURRENT_DATE)
)
SELECT billing_tin, p.provider_group_name, procedure_code, r.procedure_description,
  COUNT(*)                         AS claim_count,
  ROUND(SUM(actual_allowed),0)         AS total_actual,
  ROUND(SUM(contracted_rate),0)        AS total_contracted,
  ROUND(SUM(rate_variance),0)          AS total_overpayment,
  ROUND(100.0*SUM(rate_variance)
    /NULLIF(SUM(contracted_rate),0),1) AS overpayment_pct,
  CASE WHEN SUM(rate_variance)>5000 AND AVG(variance_pct)>5
     THEN 'FLAG — systemic overpayment' ELSE 'Within tolerance' END AS flag
FROM  fee_schedule_join
JOIN  dim_providers p ON billing_tin = p.billing_tin
JOIN  ref_procedure_codes r ON procedure_code = r.procedure_code
GROUP BY billing_tin, p.provider_group_name, procedure_code, r.procedure_description
HAVING SUM(rate_variance) > 0
ORDER BY total_overpayment DESC;
```

ANSI SQL — 17.3: Rate Achievement vs. Medicare Fee Schedule (Fully Annotated)

```sql
-- PURPOSE: Calculate how much more (or less) the plan pays relative to
-- what Medicare pays for the same service at each provider.
-- rate_achievement = plan_allowed / medicare_rate.
-- 1.50 = plan is paying 150% of what Medicare pays.
-- Used by contracting to prioritize which hospital contracts to renegotiate.

WITH claim_medicare AS (
  SELECT c.billing_npi, c.procedure_code, c.primary_drg,
      c.allowed_amount          AS plan_allowed,
      mfs.medicare_rate         AS medicare_benchmark,
      -- Rate achievement: plan rate as multiple of Medicare rate
      ROUND(c.allowed_amount / NULLIF(mfs.medicare_rate,0), 3) AS rate_achievement
  FROM  fact_medical_claims c
  JOIN  ref_medicare_fee_schedule mfs
    ON mfs.procedure_code  = c.procedure_code
   AND mfs.effective_year  = EXTRACT(YEAR FROM c.service_date)
   AND mfs.locality_code   = c.service_locality -- geographic adjustment
  WHERE c.claim_status = 'PAID'
   AND c.allowed_amount > 0
   AND EXTRACT(YEAR FROM c.service_date) = EXTRACT(YEAR FROM CURRENT_DATE)
)
SELECT cm.billing_npi, p.hospital_name, p.county,
  COUNT(*)                        AS claim_count,
  ROUND(SUM(cm.plan_allowed),0)         AS total_plan_paid,
  ROUND(SUM(cm.medicare_benchmark),0)     AS total_medicare_equiv,
  -- Weighted average rate achievement across all claims for this provider
  ROUND(SUM(cm.plan_allowed)/NULLIF(SUM(cm.medicare_benchmark),0),3) AS weighted_rate_achievement,
  -- Annualized cost of paying above 1.50× Medicare at this provider
  ROUND(SUM(CASE WHEN cm.rate_achievement > 1.50
    THEN cm.plan_allowed - cm.medicare_benchmark*1.50 ELSE 0 END),0)
                   AS excess_above_150pct_medicare
FROM  claim_medicare cm
JOIN  dim_providers p ON cm.billing_npi = p.npi
GROUP BY cm.billing_npi, p.hospital_name, p.county
HAVING COUNT(*) >= 50
ORDER BY weighted_rate_achievement DESC;
```

Chapter 17 Review

Unit Test · Key Takeaways

Answer each question before reading the explanation.

Q1. The fee schedule JOIN condition service_date >= effective_date AND service_date < COALESCE(expiration_date, '2099-12-31') is analogous to:

A. The IBNR completion factor application to incomplete months

B. The SCD-2 point-in-time join — it retrieves the contracted rate that was active on the date of service, preventing the wrong contract period from being applied to a claim

C. The member month LEFT JOIN from enrollment

D. The HAVING COUNT(*) >= 50 minimum volume filter

Answer: B. *Both SCD-2 and fee schedule joins use the same pattern: retrieve the row whose active window contains the transaction date. COALESCE(expiration_date, '2099-12-31') handles currently-active contracts with NULL expiration — without it, NULL comparisons evaluate to UNKNOWN (FALSE), silently excluding all active contracts and leaving claims without a matched rate.*

Q2. Rate achievement of 1.85× Medicare for inpatient acute services means:

A. The plan is paying 85% of what Medicare pays — a favorable, below-market contract

B. The plan is paying 185% of the Medicare fee schedule for the same DRGs. Most commercial plans target 140–175% for inpatient acute. 185% is a renegotiation priority — the excess_above_150pct_medicare field quantifies the annual cost of being above target.

C. The hospital's billed charges are 185% above Medicare allowable

D. The plan earns 85 cents of administrative margin for every Medicare dollar paid

Answer: B. *Rate achievement = plan_allowed / medicare_rate. 1.00× = paying Medicare rates. 1.85× means the plan paid $185 for every $100 Medicare pays. The excess_above_150pct_medicare field = SUM(plan_allowed - medicare_rate × 1.50) WHERE rate_achievement > 1.50 — quantifying annual savings if renegotiated to the 1.50× target.*

Q3. The most common causes of fee schedule overpayments are:

A. Provider fraud and deliberate overbilling

B. New contract rates not loaded in the fee schedule table on time (15-day gap = claims paid at wrong rate) and contract exceptions not captured in the adjudication system (outlier provisions, DRG grouper upgrades)

C. Member cost-sharing amounts not deducted before the fee schedule comparison

D. IBNR lag causing claims to be repriced after the fee schedule expired

Answer: B. *Most overpayments are systems failures. Example: new hospital contract takes effect January 1 but the fee schedule table is not updated until January 15 — all claims in those 15 days are adjudicated at the old rate. If the old rate was lower than the new contract, the plan underpays. If higher, the plan overpays. Fee schedule update verification should be part of every contract implementation process.*

Q4. Contract renewal risk is highest for providers with:

A. The most attributed members in the plan's network

B. Contracts expiring within 12 months AND high rate achievement (well above Medicare benchmark) AND high annual claim volume — the combination creates the largest financial risk if the contract lapses

C. The lowest quality scores on the provider scorecard

D. The highest OIG audit risk flags

Answer: B. *Contract renewal risk score = rate_achievement × annual_volume × (1/months_to_expiration). A hospital at 2.1× Medicare generating $22M annually with a contract expiring in 6 months is the highest risk. If the contract lapses, the hospital goes out-of-network — members face access disruption and the plan faces emergency interim agreements at disadvantageous rates.*

Q5. COALESCE(fs.expiration_date, '2099-12-31') in the fee schedule JOIN is required because:

A. NULL expiration dates cause the query to run slower without COALESCE

B. Currently-active contracts have NULL for expiration_date since they have not ended. NULL in date comparisons evaluates to UNKNOWN (treated as FALSE in JOIN conditions), which would silently exclude all active contracts from matching any claims.

C. COALESCE converts the date to a standard format for cross-database compatibility

D. NULL expiration_date indicates a terminated contract that should be excluded

Answer: B. *This is the same COALESCE pattern used in SCD-2 joins for member attributes. In both cases, NULL means "currently active with no defined end date." Setting NULL to 2099-12-31 ensures the condition c.service_date < 2099-12-31 is always TRUE for valid claim dates — making the currently-active row correctly match all recent claims.*

Q6. Percent-of-charges contracting differs from fee schedule contracting in that:

A. Percent-of-charges is used for hospitals only; fee schedule for physicians

B. In percent-of-charges, the plan pays a percentage of the provider's billed_amount — the provider controls costs by setting their charge master high. Fee schedule contracts specify a fixed rate per CPT or DRG, independent of charges.

C. Percent-of-charges contracts always result in lower plan costs than fee schedules

D. Percent-of-charges is only permitted for Medicare Advantage contracts

Answer: B. *Percent-of-charges (POC) is the least transparent payment model: a hospital charging $50,000 for a DRG at 60% of charges = $30,000. The same hospital raising charges to $70,000 at 60% = $42,000 — a $12,000 increase with no change in services. Fee schedules are fixed regardless of charges. Most sophisticated plans negotiate conversion from POC to fee-schedule at renewal — POC protects the hospital's billing flexibility at the plan's expense.*

Q7. Explain the fee schedule point-in-time JOIN. When does a claim date fall between two fee schedule periods, and what should the analyst do?

(Short answer)

Sample Answer:

The fee schedule is a history table: the same billing_tin + procedure_code has multiple rows over time, one per contract period. JOIN condition: c.service_date >= fs.effective_date AND c.service_date < COALESCE(fs.expiration_date, '2099-12-31'). This retrieves the row whose active window contains the claim date. When a claim date falls in a gap between two periods: if the prior contract expired November 30 and the new one took effect February 1, December and January claims match no fee schedule row. These claims should appear in a no-match audit: SELECT c.claim_id, c.billing_tin, c.procedure_code, c.service_date, c.allowed_amount FROM fact_medical_claims c LEFT JOIN ref_fee_schedule fs ON fs.billing_tin=c.billing_tin AND fs.procedure_code=c.procedure_code AND c.service_date>=fs.effective_date AND c.service_date<COALESCE(fs.expiration_date,'2099-12-31') WHERE c.claim_status='PAID' AND fs.allowed_amount IS NULL. Action: (1) Identify whether a contract existed for that period — if yes, load the missing data. (2) If no contract existed, claims were likely adjudicated at a default rate — determine whether the default was correct. (3) Escalate to Contracting to ensure no future contract gaps. Run this no-match audit weekly as part of fee schedule maintenance.

Q8. A hospital's contract expires in 90 days. Rate achievement is 2.0× Medicare. Annual claim volume is $18M. Walk through the contracting analytics package.

(Short answer)

Sample Answer:
Pre-negotiation analytics: (1) Rate achievement by DRG: SELECT primary_drg, d.drg_description, COUNT(*) AS admits, ROUND(SUM(plan_allowed)/SUM(medicare_rate),3) AS drg_rate_achievement FROM claim_medicare cm JOIN ref_drg d ON cm.primary_drg=d.drg_code WHERE billing_npi=:hospital GROUP BY primary_drg, d.drg_description ORDER BY drg_rate_achievement DESC. Which DRG families drive the 2.0× average — surgical DRGs at 2.4× vs. medical at 1.7×? (2) Volume and case mix: admissions by service line, average DRG weight (case mix index trend). If case mix is rising, hospital may argue for a rate increase — be prepared with data. (3) Network dependency: % of plan members in the hospital's county who used this hospital in the past 12 months. A hospital with 80% market share in its county is non-negotiable without creating a serious member access disruption. (4) Savings model at target rate: if current = 2.0× Medicare on $18M, savings at 1.75× target = $18M × (2.0−1.75)/2.0 = $18M × 0.125 = $2.25M annually. Present to CFO as the financial justification for investing negotiation resources. (5) In-network alternative: are there comparable hospitals within CMS distance standards at 1.50−1.65× Medicare? If yes, the plan has leverage to redirect volume. If no, accept a less favorable rate. All five analyses complete before entering the room.

Q9. Write the SQL to score contract renewal risk and build the annual renegotiation calendar.

(Short answer)

Sample Answer:
SELECT c.billing_tin, p.provider_group_name, p.county, con.contract_expiration_date, DATEDIFF('day', CURRENT_DATE, con.contract_expiration_date) AS days_to_expiration, ROUND(SUM(c.allowed_amount),0) AS annual_allowed, ROUND(SUM(c.allowed_amount)/NULLIF(SUM(mfs.medicare_rate),0),3) AS rate_achievement, ROUND(SUM(c.allowed_amount)/NULLIF(SUM(mfs.medicare_rate),0) * SUM(c.allowed_amount) / NULLIF(365.0/DATEDIFF('day',CURRENT_DATE,con.contract_expiration_date),0),0) AS renewal_risk_score, CASE WHEN DATEDIFF('day',CURRENT_DATE,con.contract_expiration_date) <= 180 AND SUM(c.allowed_amount)/NULLIF(SUM(mfs.medicare_rate),0) > 1.50 THEN 'URGENT — high cost, renews in 6 months' WHEN DATEDIFF('day',CURRENT_DATE,con.contract_expiration_date) <= 365 AND SUM(c.allowed_amount)/NULLIF(SUM(mfs.medicare_rate),0) > 1.40 THEN 'PRIORITY — begin negotiations' ELSE 'Routine — monitor' END AS renegotiation_priority FROM fact_medical_claims c JOIN ref_medicare_fee_schedule mfs ON mfs.procedure_code=c.procedure_code AND mfs.effective_year=EXTRACT(YEAR FROM c.service_date) JOIN ref_provider_contracts con ON c.billing_tin=con.billing_tin AND con.contract_type='ACTIVE' JOIN dim_providers p ON c.billing_tin=p.billing_tin WHERE c.claim_status='PAID' AND EXTRACT(YEAR FROM c.service_date)=EXTRACT(YEAR FROM CURRENT_DATE) GROUP BY c.billing_tin, p.provider_group_name, p.county, con.contract_expiration_date ORDER BY renegotiation_priority, annual_allowed DESC. Present to VP Network monthly as the contract action calendar.

Q10. Explain the excess_above_150pct_medicare field and how it is used to justify renegotiation budget to the CFO.

(Short answer)

Sample Answer:
Field definition: SUM(CASE WHEN rate_achievement > 1.50 THEN plan_allowed - medicare_rate × 1.50 ELSE 0 END) AS excess_above_150pct_medicare. This calculates, for each claim above 1.50× Medicare, the dollar amount the plan paid above the 1.50× target. Summed across all claims for a provider for the year, it represents the annual savings opportunity if that provider is renegotiated to exactly 1.50× Medicare. How it justifies the budget: if a hospital shows excess_above_150pct_medicare = $3.2M annually, the contracting team can tell the CFO: "If we renegotiate this hospital to 1.50× Medicare, we save $3.2M per year — and the negotiation will take approximately 6 months of contracting team time. The ROI is $3.2M in year 1." This builds the financial case for allocating negotiating resources to high-rate providers rather than spreading effort uniformly across all renewals. Important caveat: 1.50× Medicare is a target, not a guarantee. The actual negotiated rate depends on market conditions, hospital leverage, and competitive alternatives. The excess_above_150pct_medicare figure is the maximum potential savings, not the expected outcome. Present it as an opportunity estimate, not a committed saving.

Key Takeaways

What every analyst must remember from this chapter.

1 Fee schedule JOIN: JOIN ref_fee_schedule ON billing_tin, procedure_code, service_date >= effective_date AND service_date < COALESCE(expiration_date, '2099-12-31'). SCD-2 point-in-time pattern — retrieves the contracted rate in effect on the claim date. Run no-match audit weekly to catch claims with no fee schedule match.

2 Rate achievement = plan_allowed / medicare_benchmark. Target: 130–160% professional, 140–175% outpatient, 150–185% inpatient acute. Providers above 185% are high-priority renegotiation. Use POWER(end/start, 0.5) - 1 for 2-year annualized trend.

3 Fee schedule overpayment detection: WHERE SUM(actual_allowed - contracted_rate) > 0 GROUP BY billing_tin × procedure_code. Common causes: new rates not loaded on time, outlier provisions not captured, DRG grouper upgrade mismatch. Run weekly; route to Payment Integrity.

4 Contract renewal risk = rate_achievement × annual_volume × urgency (1/months_to_expiration). Sort descending. URGENT flag: expiring in ≤6 months AND rate_achievement > 1.50. Begin negotiations immediately for URGENT contracts.

5 excess_above_150pct_medicare = SUM(plan_allowed - medicare_rate × 1.50) WHERE rate_achievement > 1.50. This is the annual savings opportunity if renegotiated to the 1.50× target. Present to CFO as the ROI justification for contracting team investment.

6 Percent-of-charges contracts: provider sets charge master, plan pays X% of charges. Identify POC claims: ABS(allowed_amount - billed_amount × pct_of_charges) <= $1.00. Convert to fee-schedule at renewal — POC is the least transparent payment model.

7 Network adequacy deficiency response: (1) Identify deficient county × specialty. (2) Search adjacent counties within CMS distance standard. (3) Offer single-case agreements to OON providers. (4) If no solution: file adequacy exception with CMS/state. (5) Provide members with OON cost-sharing waivers for deficient specialty.

8 Contract gap audit: LEFT JOIN claims to fee_schedule; WHERE fs.allowed_amount IS NULL. These are claims with no contracted rate match — they were adjudicated at a default rate. Investigate weekly. Each gap represents either a missing fee schedule row or a legitimate period with no contract (out-of-network claim adjudicated at plan-defined default).

Chapter 18: Revenue Cycle & RCM Analytics

A/R aging · CARC denial analysis · Days in A/R · Clean claim rate · Write-off decisions

18.1 Revenue Cycle Overview

Revenue cycle management (RCM) analytics serves two audiences: (1) Providers use RCM to maximize collections and reduce denials. (2) Payers use RCM to monitor claims processing efficiency and payment accuracy. Key metrics: Days in A/R = total_AR_balance / (annual_gross_charges / 365). Clean claim rate = first-pass adjudication success rate. Denial rate = denied / total submitted.

> **Benchmarks** Days in A/R: < 30 days for physician groups, < 45 days for community hospitals, < 60 days for teaching hospitals. Clean claim rate target: > 95%. Denial rate target: < 5%. Collection rate target: > 95% of contractual allowable.

ANSI SQL — 18.1: A/R Aging Analysis by Payer and Service Line (Fully Annotated)

```
-- PURPOSE: Build the standard A/R aging report — buckets outstanding
-- balances by days since service date.
-- Standard buckets: 0-30, 31-60, 61-90, 91-120, 120+ days.
-- pct_over_120days > 15% signals bad debt risk -- collection probability
-- drops to 40-50% beyond 120 days.

WITH unpaid_claims AS (
  SELECT c.billing_tin, c.payer_id, p.service_category,
      -- Balance = billed minus any partial payments received so far
      c.billed_amount - COALESCE(c.paid_amount, 0)      AS balance_due,
      DATEDIFF('day', c.service_date, CURRENT_DATE)      AS days_outstanding
  FROM  fact_medical_claims c
  JOIN  ref_procedure_codes p ON c.procedure_code = p.procedure_code
  -- All claims NOT in a final resolved status
  WHERE c.claim_status NOT IN ('PAID','DENIED','REVERSED','WRITTEN_OFF')
   AND c.service_date >= CURRENT_DATE - INTERVAL '18' MONTH
)
SELECT payer_id, service_category,
  COUNT(*)                                   AS claim_count,
  ROUND(SUM(balance_due),0)                  AS total_balance,
  -- Age each balance into the standard 30-day buckets
  ROUND(SUM(CASE WHEN days_outstanding BETWEEN  0 AND  30 THEN balance_due ELSE 0 END),0) AS bucket_0_30,
  ROUND(SUM(CASE WHEN days_outstanding BETWEEN 31 AND  60 THEN balance_due ELSE 0 END),0) AS bucket_31_60,
  ROUND(SUM(CASE WHEN days_outstanding BETWEEN 61 AND  90 THEN balance_due ELSE 0 END),0) AS bucket_61_90,
  ROUND(SUM(CASE WHEN days_outstanding BETWEEN 91 AND 120 THEN balance_due ELSE 0 END),0) AS bucket_91_120,
  ROUND(SUM(CASE WHEN days_outstanding > 120         THEN balance_due ELSE 0 END),0) AS bucket_120_plus,
  -- % in oldest bucket: the primary bad debt risk indicator
  ROUND(100.0*SUM(CASE WHEN days_outstanding>120 THEN balance_due ELSE 0 END)
    /NULLIF(SUM(balance_due),0),1)           AS pct_over_120days
FROM  unpaid_claims
GROUP BY payer_id, service_category
ORDER BY total_balance DESC;
```

ANSI SQL — 18.2: Denial Root Cause by CARC Code (Fully Annotated)

```
-- PURPOSE: Identify the top denial reason codes (CARC codes) by provider
-- and quantify the recoverable revenue among appealable denials.
-- Each CARC code maps to a specific operational fix for the billing team.

WITH denial_detail AS (
  SELECT c.billing_tin, c.procedure_code,
      c.denial_reason_code            AS carc_code,
```

```
        r.carc_description,
        r.denial_category,        -- Authorization, Coding, Eligibility, etc.
        c.billed_amount,
        -- Flag denials that can be appealed with supporting documentation
        CASE WHEN r.appealable_flag = 'Y' THEN 1 ELSE 0 END AS appealable
    FROM  fact_medical_claims c
    JOIN  ref_carc_codes r ON c.denial_reason_code = r.carc_code
    WHERE c.claim_status IN ('DENIED','DENY','D')
      AND c.claim_frequency_code <> '8'  -- exclude void transactions
      AND EXTRACT(YEAR FROM c.service_date) = EXTRACT(YEAR FROM CURRENT_DATE)
),
-- Total submitted claims per provider (for denial rate denominator)
total_submitted AS (
    SELECT billing_tin, COUNT(*) AS total_claims
    FROM  fact_medical_claims
    WHERE claim_frequency_code <> '8'
      AND EXTRACT(YEAR FROM service_date) = EXTRACT(YEAR FROM CURRENT_DATE)
    GROUP BY billing_tin
)
SELECT dd.billing_tin, p.provider_group_name,
    dd.carc_code, dd.carc_description, dd.denial_category,
    COUNT(*)                              AS denial_count,
    ROUND(SUM(dd.billed_amount),0)                  AS denied_billed_value,
    SUM(dd.appealable)                        AS appealable_count,
    -- Recoverable revenue = appealable_count × average billed per denial
    ROUND(SUM(dd.appealable) * AVG(dd.billed_amount),0) AS recoverable_revenue,
    ROUND(100.0*SUM(dd.appealable)/COUNT(*),1)         AS appealable_pct,
    ROUND(100.0*COUNT(*)/NULLIF(ts.total_claims,0),1)  AS denial_rate_pct
FROM  denial_detail dd
JOIN  dim_providers p  ON dd.billing_tin = p.billing_tin
JOIN  total_submitted ts ON dd.billing_tin = ts.billing_tin
GROUP BY dd.billing_tin, p.provider_group_name, dd.carc_code,
       dd.carc_description, dd.denial_category, ts.total_claims
HAVING COUNT(*) >= 10
ORDER BY denied_billed_value DESC;
```

Chapter 18 Review

Unit Test · Key Takeaways

Answer each question before reading the explanation.

Q1. Days in A/R is calculated as:

A. Total claims count / claims paid per day

B. Total outstanding receivables / (annual gross charges / 365) — measures how many days of revenue are sitting uncollected. Benchmark < 30 days for physician groups, < 45 community hospitals.

C. Number of denied claims × average days to appeal resolution

D. Total billed amount / total collected amount × 365

Answer: B. *Example: $30M outstanding A/R and $450M annual gross charges → $30M / ($450M/365) = 24.4 days in A/R. A rising days-in-A/R signals slower payer payment, increased denials, or billing backlogs. SQL: SUM(balance_due) / (SUM(billed_amount) / 365.0) WHERE service_date >= CURRENT_DATE - INTERVAL '365 days'.*

Q2. CARC code 97 on a remittance advice means:

A. The claim was a duplicate of a previously paid claim

B. The service is included in the payment for another procedure already adjudicated — a bundling denial, often triggered by NCCI edits. Billing 99213 and 93000 separately when the ECG is bundled into the E&M generates CARC 97 for the ECG.

C. The claim was denied for lack of prior authorization

D. The member's eligibility was not verified at time of service

Answer: B. *CARC 97 is one of the most common codes. Fix: the billing team must understand which CPT/HCPCS combinations are bundled under NCCI edits and either submit only the primary code or document separate clinical encounters justifying both codes. A high CARC 97 rate from a provider indicates a coding education gap.*

Q3. The clean claim rate measures:

A. Percentage of claims paid within 15 business days

B. Percentage of claims passing first-pass adjudication without requiring manual review, additional information, or denial — a clean claim has no missing fields, valid eligibility, covered procedure code, and met authorization requirements

C. Percentage of claims submitted electronically vs. paper

D. Percentage of claims with zero member cost-sharing

Answer: B. *Clean claim rate = claims auto-adjudicated on first pass / total submitted. Target > 95%. Every percentage point below 95% represents administrative rework cost for both provider (rebilling, appeals) and payer (manual review queues). Common dirty claim causes: invalid member ID, missing referring NPI, procedure inconsistent with diagnosis, missing prior authorization number.*

Q4. The pct_over_120days field in the A/R aging report is a risk indicator because:

A. Claims over 120 days are excluded from financial statements per GAAP

B. Collection probability drops sharply after 90–120 days — from ~75% at 61–90 days to ~40–50% at 120+ days. Claims approaching the payer's timely filing limit (typically 12 months from service) may become permanently non-collectable.

C. HIPAA requires all claims over 120 days to be written off

D. Payers are legally prohibited from paying claims submitted after 120 days

Answer: B. *Collection probability by age band: 0–30 days ≈95%, 31–60 days ≈85%, 61–90 days ≈75%, 91–120 days ≈60%, 120+ days ≈40–50%, 180+ days ≈25%. Timely filing limits vary by payer: CMS/Medicare requires 12 months, many commercial payers require 90 days from service or date of EOB. The 120+ day bucket drives write-off decisions and bad debt reserve calculations.*

Q5. The recoverable_revenue field in the denial query is calculated as:

A. Total billed amount for all denied claims

B. appealable_count × avg_billed_amount_per_denial — the estimated revenue that can be recovered if all appealable denials are successfully appealed. This prioritizes appeal resources to the highest financial return.

C. denied_billed_value × historical appeal success rate

D. Total denied claims × average days to appeal resolution

Answer: B. *Not all denied revenue is recoverable. CARC 50 (non-covered service) is patient responsibility, not appealable. CARC 197 (prior auth required) may be appealable with retro-auth documentation. Focusing appeal resources on appealable denials × average billed amount maximizes ROI. The billing director uses recoverable_revenue sorted descending to prioritize the appeals team's weekly workload.*

Q6. A provider group's days in A/R is 68 days vs. a benchmark of 35 days. The most likely root cause to investigate first is:

A. The provider sees too many Medicare patients who pay slower

B. High denial rate from one specific payer — one payer with a 28% denial rate requiring extensive rework and resubmission can push overall days-in-A/R above 60 days even if all other payers pay within 20 days

C. The billing team is understaffed and behind on submissions

D. The provider recently switched billing software

Answer: B. *Investigation sequence: (1) Break days-in-A/R by payer — which payer has the oldest A/R? (2) For that payer, run the CARC code denial root cause query — what are the top 3 denial codes? (3) Check clean claim rate for that payer — are initial submissions being rejected at a higher rate? (4) Verify timely filing compliance for that payer — are claims approaching the timely filing window? One payer relationship with 25% denial rate and 45-day payment cycle can explain 33 extra days in A/R for a multi-payer practice.*

Q7. Write the SQL for days in A/R by payer and explain what each result tells the billing director.

(Short answer)

Sample Answer:
SELECT c.payer_id, pay.payer_name, SUM(c.billed_amount - COALESCE(c.paid_amount,0)) AS total_ar, ROUND((SELECT SUM(c2.billed_amount)/365.0 FROM fact_medical_claims c2 WHERE c2.payer_id=c.payer_id AND c2.service_date>=CURRENT_DATE-INTERVAL '365 days') ,2) AS avg_daily_charges, ROUND(SUM(c.billed_amount-COALESCE(c.paid_amount,0)) / NULLIF((SELECT SUM(c2.billed_amount)/365.0 FROM fact_medical_claims c2 WHERE c2.payer_id=c.payer_id AND c2.service_date>=CURRENT_DATE-INTERVAL '365 days'),0),1) AS days_in_ar FROM fact_medical_claims c JOIN ref_payers pay ON c.payer_id=pay.payer_id WHERE c.claim_status NOT IN ('PAID','DENIED','WRITTEN_OFF') GROUP BY c.payer_id, pay.payer_name ORDER BY days_in_ar DESC. Interpretation: A payer at 72 days is paying 72 days after service on average vs. a 30–45 day contract standard. This triggers: (1) Review the provider

contract — most commercial contracts require payment within 30 or 45 days of clean claim receipt. (2) Calculate the finance charge on delayed balances — most state prompt pay laws require interest on late commercial payments. (3) Escalate to Provider Relations — the payer may have a systematic processing issue. (4) If the payer routinely exceeds contract terms, the provider has grounds for a formal dispute and potentially early contract termination notice.

Q8. Describe the five major CARC denial categories and give one operational fix for each.

(Short answer)

Sample Answer:

Five CARC denial categories: (1) Authorization/Pre-certification (CARC 15): the service required prior authorization that was not obtained. Fix: implement real-time PA workflow integrated with the scheduling system; establish a retro-authorization process for emergent cases. (2) Eligibility (CARC 31): member cannot be identified as the insured. Fix: run 270/271 real-time eligibility verification at registration, not just at scheduling; re-verify on day of service. (3) Coding/Bundling (CARC 97): service is bundled into another already-paid service under NCCI edits. Fix: implement NCCI edit checking in the charge capture system before claim submission; educate billing team on bundling rules. (4) Non-covered service (CARC 96): service not covered by the benefit plan. Fix: verify benefit plan details at registration; if the service is covered under a different benefit category, reclassify the claim. (5) Timely filing (CARC 29): claim submitted after the payer's filing deadline. Fix: implement automated submission monitoring that flags claims approaching 80% of the filing window; escalate to billing manager for priority submission. Each CARC code routes to a specific operational team: PA workflow to utilization management, eligibility to registration/front desk, coding to HIM/coding team, non-covered to benefits team, timely filing to billing operations.

Q9. A provider group has a 22% denial rate with one commercial payer. Describe the SQL-driven investigation methodology.

(Short answer)

Sample Answer:

Step 1 — Trend the denial rate monthly: SELECT DATE_TRUNC('month',service_date) AS mo, COUNT(*) AS total, SUM(CASE WHEN claim_status IN ('DENIED','DENY') THEN 1 ELSE 0 END) AS denied, ROUND(100.0*SUM(CASE WHEN claim_status IN ('DENIED','DENY') THEN 1 ELSE 0 END)/COUNT(*),1) AS denial_rate FROM fact_medical_claims WHERE payer_id=:payer AND billing_tin=:provider GROUP BY 1 ORDER BY 1. Did the rate spike in a specific month? Was there a contract change, fee schedule update, or benefit design change at that time? Step 2 — CARC code breakdown: GROUP BY denial_reason_code, carc_description, COUNT(*), SUM(billed_amount). Top 3 codes driving the 22%? If CARC 15 = 40% of denials → PA workflow problem. If CARC 97 = 30% → coding education gap. Step 3 — Procedure code breakdown: which CPT codes have the highest denial rate? 99215 at 35% denial vs. 99213 at 8% → potential upcoding flagged by payer. Step 4 — Revenue at risk: SUM(billed_amount) WHERE claim_status = 'DENIED' AND appealable_flag = 'Y'. This is the recoverable revenue if appeals are filed. Step 5 — Denial speed: DATEDIFF('day', submission_date, denial_date). Denials < 15 days = auto-denial (code edit or eligibility check). Denials > 45 days = manual clinical review. Different causes require different responses. Present three-priority action list to billing director with estimated recovery for each action.

Q10. Describe the write-off decision process and write the SQL that produces a write-off candidate list.

(Short answer)

Sample Answer:

Write-off criteria: (a) Non-appealable CARC code (patient responsibility, non-covered service, timely filing exceeded). (b) Appeal exhausted with no successful outcome. (c) Balance below cost-to-collect threshold (typically $10–$25). Write-off candidate SQL: SELECT c.claim_id, c.billing_tin, c.member_id, m.member_name, c.service_date, c.billed_amount, c.denial_reason_code, r.carc_description, r.appealable_flag, DATEDIFF('day',c.service_date,CURRENT_DATE) AS days_since_service, CASE WHEN r.appealable_flag='N' AND DATEDIFF('day',c.service_date,CURRENT_DATE) > 365 THEN 'WRITE-OFF — non-appealable, >1 year' WHEN r.appealable_flag='Y' AND c.appeal_status='EXHAUSTED' AND DATEDIFF('day',c.denial_date,CURRENT_DATE) > 120 THEN 'WRITE-OFF — appeal exhausted' WHEN c.billed_amount < 25 AND DATEDIFF('day',c.service_date,CURRENT_DATE) > 90 THEN 'WRITE-OFF — below cost-to-collect' ELSE 'HOLD — continue follow-up' END AS recommendation FROM fact_medical_claims c JOIN dim_members m ON c.member_id=m.member_id JOIN ref_carc_codes r ON c.denial_reason_code=r.carc_code WHERE c.claim_status='DENIED' ORDER BY c.billed_amount DESC. The billing director approves the list. Approved amounts are reclassified to the bad debt expense account. The claim record remains in the database permanently for audit purposes — writing off does not delete the claim, it changes its financial classification.

Key Takeaways

What every analyst must remember from this chapter.

1. Days in A/R = total_AR_balance / (annual_gross_charges / 365). Benchmarks: < 30 days physician groups, < 45 community hospitals, < 60 teaching hospitals. Rising days-in-A/R = denial rate increase, billing backlog, or slow payer payment. Break by payer first to identify the root cause.

2. A/R aging buckets: 0–30, 31–60, 61–90, 91–120, 120+. SQL: SUM(CASE WHEN days_outstanding BETWEEN 0 AND 30 THEN balance_due ELSE 0 END) for each bucket. pct_over_120days > 15% = bad debt risk. Collection probability: ~95% at 0–30 days, ~40% at 120+ days.

3. Clean claim rate = claims passing first-pass adjudication / total submitted. Target > 95%. Common dirty claim causes: invalid member ID, missing referring NPI, procedure inconsistent with diagnosis, missing prior auth. Each point below 95% = administrative rework cost for both provider and payer.

4. CARC denial categories and fixes: 15 (auth required) → PA workflow. 31 (eligibility) → registration verification. 97 (bundling/NCCI) → coding education. 96 (non-covered) → benefits verification. 29 (timely filing) → submission monitoring. Each code routes to a specific operational team.

5. Recoverable revenue = appealable_count × avg_billed_amount. Focus appeal resources on appealable denials with highest billed amounts. Non-appealable denials (patient responsibility, non-covered) route to patient billing or write-off, not to appeals.

6. Denial investigation sequence: (1) Trend monthly rate — find the spike. (2) CARC code breakdown — top 3 codes. (3) CPT code breakdown — high-denial procedures. (4) Denial speed (days to denial) — fast = auto-edit; slow = clinical review. (5) Calculate recoverable revenue. Present three-priority action list.

7. Write-off criteria: non-appealable + > 1 year old, OR appeal exhausted + > 120 days post-denial, OR billed < $25 + > 90 days. Write-off changes the financial classification (to bad debt expense); the claim record is preserved permanently for audit.

8. Prompt pay compliance: most state laws require commercial payers to pay clean claims within 30–45 days. Track days_to_payment = DATEDIFF('day', submission_date, paid_date) by payer. Payers consistently exceeding the contractual window owe interest and may be in contract violation.

Chapter 19 :Value-Based Care & Alternative Payment Models

Shared savings · Bundled payments · PCMH performance · Risk corridors · VBC scorecard

19.1 Value-Based Care Spectrum

Value-based care (VBC) replaces or supplements fee-for-service with incentives tied to quality and cost outcomes. Spectrum from least to most risk: (1) Pay-for-reporting. (2) Pay-for-performance. (3) Shared savings. (4) Bundled payments. (5) Full capitation. Each model requires different SQL analytics for performance measurement and financial settlement.

> **Total Cost of Care** VBC analytics must include BOTH medical and pharmacy costs. A provider who reduces medical costs by shifting to expensive specialty pharmacy has not improved total population health economics. UNION ALL fact_medical_claims and fact_pharmacy_claims for the attributed population.

19.2 Shared Savings Calculation

Shared savings programs compare actual total cost of care to a risk-adjusted benchmark. If actual < benchmark AND quality gates are met, the provider earns a savings share. Benchmark = base_pmpm × trend_factor × risk_index, where risk_index = current_avg_raf / base_avg_raf.

ANSI SQL — 19.2: Shared Savings Performance Calculation (Fully Annotated)

```sql
-- PURPOSE: Calculate shared savings performance per VBC entity.
-- Compare risk-adjusted actual total cost of care to the benchmark.
-- Provider earns savings_share_pct of savings IF quality gate is met.
-- Total cost = medical + pharmacy (both channels combined).

-- STEP 1: Medical cost for attributed population.
WITH medical_cost AS (
   SELECT v.vbc_entity_id,
         SUM(c.allowed_amount)     AS medical_allowed,
         SUM(mm.member_months)     AS member_months
   FROM  dim_vbc_attribution v
   JOIN  fact_medical_claims c  ON v.member_id = c.member_id
   JOIN  fact_member_months  mm ON v.member_id = mm.member_id
                    AND mm.membership_year = :perf_year
   WHERE c.claim_status = 'PAID'
     AND EXTRACT(YEAR FROM c.service_date) = :perf_year
   GROUP BY v.vbc_entity_id
),

-- STEP 2: Pharmacy cost for same population.
-- Must include pharmacy to prevent channel-shifting gaming.
pharmacy_cost AS (
   SELECT v.vbc_entity_id,
         SUM(p.plan_paid_amount)    AS pharmacy_allowed
   FROM  dim_vbc_attribution v
   JOIN  fact_pharmacy_claims p ON v.member_id = p.member_id
   WHERE p.claim_status = 'PAID'
     AND EXTRACT(YEAR FROM p.dispensing_date) = :perf_year
   GROUP BY v.vbc_entity_id
),

-- STEP 3: Risk-adjusted benchmark.
```

```
-- risk_index = current panel avg RAF / base year panel avg RAF.
-- If panel is sicker this year, benchmark rises proportionally.
benchmark AS (
  SELECT v.vbc_entity_id,
      b.base_pmpm, b.trend_factor, b.base_avg_raf,
      ROUND(AVG(r.total_raf_score),3)       AS current_avg_raf,
      -- Risk index: adjusts benchmark for panel risk change since base year
      AVG(r.total_raf_score)/NULLIF(b.base_avg_raf,0) AS risk_index,
      -- Benchmark = base PMPM × trend × risk_index
      ROUND(b.base_pmpm * b.trend_factor
        * (AVG(r.total_raf_score)/NULLIF(b.base_avg_raf,0)),2) AS benchmark_pmpm
  FROM  dim_vbc_attribution v
  JOIN  ref_vbc_benchmarks  b ON v.vbc_entity_id = b.vbc_entity_id
  LEFT JOIN raf_scores      r ON v.member_id   = r.member_id
  GROUP BY v.vbc_entity_id, b.base_pmpm, b.trend_factor, b.base_avg_raf
),

-- STEP 4: Quality score (must meet gate to unlock savings payment).
quality AS (
  SELECT vbc_entity_id,
      ROUND(AVG(measure_score),1) AS composite_quality_score
  FROM  fact_vbc_quality_measures
  WHERE performance_year = :perf_year
  GROUP BY vbc_entity_id
)

-- STEP 5: Final calculation -- actual vs. benchmark, apply quality gate.
SELECT mc.vbc_entity_id, e.entity_name,
  mc.member_months,
  -- Total cost PMPM = (medical + pharmacy) / member months
  ROUND((mc.medical_allowed + COALESCE(pc.pharmacy_allowed,0))
    /NULLIF(mc.member_months,0),2)                AS actual_total_pmpm,
  bm.benchmark_pmpm,
  -- Savings: positive = spending below benchmark
  ROUND(bm.benchmark_pmpm
    - (mc.medical_allowed+COALESCE(pc.pharmacy_allowed,0))
    /NULLIF(mc.member_months,0),2)                AS savings_pmpm,
  -- Annualized savings in dollars
  ROUND((bm.benchmark_pmpm
    - (mc.medical_allowed+COALESCE(pc.pharmacy_allowed,0))
    /NULLIF(mc.member_months,0)) * mc.member_months,0)    AS annualized_savings,
  q.composite_quality_score,
  vc.min_quality_threshold,
  vc.savings_share_pct,
  -- Provider earns savings ONLY IF quality gate is met AND savings are positive
  CASE
    WHEN q.composite_quality_score >= vc.min_quality_threshold
     AND bm.benchmark_pmpm > (mc.medical_allowed+COALESCE(pc.pharmacy_allowed,0))
       /NULLIF(mc.member_months,0)
    THEN ROUND(vc.savings_share_pct/100.0
       * ((bm.benchmark_pmpm
       - (mc.medical_allowed+COALESCE(pc.pharmacy_allowed,0))
        /NULLIF(mc.member_months,0)) * mc.member_months),0)
    ELSE 0
  END AS provider_savings_payment
FROM  medical_cost mc
JOIN  pharmacy_cost pc  ON mc.vbc_entity_id = pc.vbc_entity_id
JOIN  benchmark bm      ON mc.vbc_entity_id = bm.vbc_entity_id
JOIN  quality q         ON mc.vbc_entity_id = q.vbc_entity_id
JOIN  ref_vbc_contracts vc ON mc.vbc_entity_id = vc.vbc_entity_id
JOIN  ref_vbc_entities  e  ON mc.vbc_entity_id = e.vbc_entity_id
ORDER BY annualized_savings DESC;
```

19.3 Bundled Payment Episode Construction

A bundled payment pays a single price for a defined episode of care (e.g., total hip replacement + 90-day post-acute care). The plan and provider share savings below the target price. The SQL must: identify the anchor event, join all costs within the episode window, and compare total episode cost to the target price.

ANSI SQL – 19.3: Bundled Payment Episode Construction (Fully Annotated)

```
-- PURPOSE: Construct bundled payment episodes anchored on a qualifying
-- procedure and accumulate all costs within the episode window.
-- Compare total episode cost to the contractual target price.
-- episode_savings < 0 = cost overrun; provider shares loss risk.

-- STEP 1: Identify anchor events (qualifying procedures in the bundle).
WITH anchor_events AS (
  SELECT c.member_id,
      c.claim_id           AS anchor_claim_id,
      c.rendering_npi        AS performing_surgeon,
      c.service_date         AS anchor_date,
      c.procedure_code         AS anchor_procedure,
      bp.bundle_type,
      bp.target_price,       -- contractual fixed price for the episode
      bp.episode_window_days   -- how many post-procedure days are included
  FROM  fact_medical_claims c
  JOIN  ref_bundle_procedures bp ON c.procedure_code = bp.procedure_code
  WHERE c.claim_status = 'PAID'
   AND EXTRACT(YEAR FROM c.service_date) = :perf_year
),

-- STEP 2: Accumulate ALL medical costs within the episode window.
-- Readmissions within the window count as episode cost (incentivizes quality).
episode_medical AS (
  SELECT ae.anchor_claim_id, ae.member_id, ae.bundle_type,
      ae.target_price, ae.performing_surgeon, ae.anchor_date,
      SUM(c.allowed_amount)              AS medical_episode_cost,
      -- Count readmissions as a quality signal
      COUNT(DISTINCT CASE WHEN c.type_of_bill LIKE '11%'
        AND c.claim_id <> ae.anchor_claim_id
        THEN c.claim_id END)             AS readmissions
  FROM  anchor_events ae
  JOIN  fact_medical_claims c
    ON c.member_id    = ae.member_id
   -- Include all claims from anchor date through end of episode window
   AND c.service_date BETWEEN ae.anchor_date
               AND ae.anchor_date + ae.episode_window_days
   AND c.claim_status = 'PAID'
  GROUP BY ae.anchor_claim_id, ae.member_id, ae.bundle_type,
       ae.target_price, ae.performing_surgeon, ae.anchor_date
),

-- STEP 3: Pharmacy costs within the episode window (oral post-op medications).
episode_pharmacy AS (
  SELECT ae.anchor_claim_id,
      SUM(p.plan_paid_amount) AS pharmacy_episode_cost
  FROM  anchor_events ae
  JOIN  fact_pharmacy_claims p
    ON p.member_id = ae.member_id
   AND p.dispensing_date BETWEEN ae.anchor_date
                AND ae.anchor_date + ae.episode_window_days
  WHERE p.claim_status = 'PAID'
```

```
    GROUP BY ae.anchor_claim_id
)
-- STEP 4: Compare total episode cost to target price.
-- episode_savings = target_price - total_cost.
-- Positive = under target (provider earns share). Negative = overrun.
SELECT em.anchor_claim_id, em.bundle_type,
    em.performing_surgeon, p.provider_full_name AS surgeon_name,
    em.anchor_date, em.target_price,
    em.medical_episode_cost,
    COALESCE(ep.pharmacy_episode_cost,0)            AS pharmacy_episode_cost,
    em.medical_episode_cost+COALESCE(ep.pharmacy_episode_cost,0) AS total_episode_cost,
    em.target_price-(em.medical_episode_cost+COALESCE(ep.pharmacy_episode_cost,0))
                                        AS episode_savings,
    em.readmissions,
    CASE WHEN em.readmissions > 0 THEN 'FLAG — readmission within episode'
        ELSE 'No readmission' END                AS quality_flag,
    CASE WHEN em.target_price-(em.medical_episode_cost+COALESCE(ep.pharmacy_episode_cost,0)) < 0
        THEN 'OVERRUN — review for outlier protection'
        ELSE 'Within target' END               AS financial_flag
FROM  episode_medical em
LEFT JOIN episode_pharmacy ep ON em.anchor_claim_id = ep.anchor_claim_id
JOIN  dim_providers p ON em.performing_surgeon = p.npi
ORDER BY episode_savings ASC; -- largest overruns (most negative) first
```

Chapter 19 Review

Unit Test · Key Takeaways

Answer each question before reading the explanation.

Q1. The shared savings benchmark must be risk-adjusted because:

A. CMS requires risk adjustment for all value-based contracts

B. If the provider's panel becomes sicker over time, actual cost rises even with perfect care management. Without risk adjustment, rising cost falsely appears as poor performance. Risk index = current_avg_raf / base_avg_raf scales the benchmark to the panel's expected cost change.

C. Risk adjustment increases the benchmark, making it easier to earn savings

D. The savings share percentage is determined by the risk index

Answer: B. *Example: panel RAF rose from 1.2 to 1.5 — 25% sicker. Without adjustment, the provider is held to an expectation calibrated for a healthier population. Risk index = 1.5/1.2 = 1.25, so benchmark rises by 25%. Only actual spending above this adjusted benchmark represents genuine care management underperformance.*

Q2. The quality gate in shared savings prevents:

A. Providers from participating in shared savings before 3 years of network membership

B. Providers from earning savings payments by reducing costs through withholding necessary care — under-treatment reduces claims costs but harms members. The quality threshold ensures savings come from genuine efficiency, not clinical under-service.

C. Providers from earning savings if their panel size falls below a minimum

D. Double-counting pharmacy costs in the total cost calculation

Answer: B. *Without a quality gate, a provider could artificially reduce costs by skipping expensive but necessary referrals, diagnostic tests, or specialist consultations. The quality gate (e.g., composite HEDIS rate ≥ 70th percentile) ensures that cost reduction comes from genuine care efficiency. The quality gate is binary — miss the threshold by 1 point and the entire savings payment = $0.*

Q3. Total cost of care in shared savings analytics includes pharmacy because:

A. CMS requires pharmacy in all VBC calculations

B. A provider who reduces medical costs by shifting patients to expensive specialty drugs appears efficient on medical-only measures while total cost increases. Including pharmacy prevents channel-substitution gaming and measures true population health economics.

C. Pharmacy costs are always larger than medical costs for VBC populations

D. Shared savings contracts automatically include pharmacy through the PBM

Answer: B. *Total cost of care = UNION ALL of fact_medical_claims (allowed_amount) and fact_pharmacy_claims (plan_paid_amount) for the attributed population. Without pharmacy, a VBC entity could earn shared savings by prescribing $80,000 specialty drugs that shift cost to the pharmacy benefit while the medical PMPM appears favorable.*

Q4. In a bundled payment, a readmission within the episode window:

A. Is excluded from the bundle and billed as a separate episode

B. Is included in total episode cost — reducing the surgeon's episode savings (or increasing the loss). This incentivizes surgeons to invest in post-discharge care coordination and follow-up to prevent complications.

C. Automatically triggers the risk corridor protection for the surgeon

D. Is covered by the plan's stop-loss reinsurance, not the bundle

Answer: B. *A patient readmitted for surgical site infection at day 30 generates $35,000 in additional claims — all within the 90-day episode window. target_price - (original_cost + $35,000_readmission) = savings reduced by $35,000. The bundle financially aligns the surgeon's interests with preventing complications, driving investment in patient education, discharge planning, and post-acute coordination.*

Q5. The risk corridor in a VBC shared savings contract protects the provider from:

A. Regulatory penalties if quality scores fall below threshold

B. Catastrophic financial loss — the corridor caps downside risk. Below a minimum savings rate (MSR), savings are not shared. Above a cap, the plan takes a larger share of excess savings. Outside the corridor on the loss side, the plan absorbs losses above the cap.

C. Network adequacy failures that reduce attributed panel size

D. Changes in benchmark calculation methodology mid-year

Answer: B. *Risk corridor mechanics: (1) Below MSR (e.g., 5% savings rate): 0% sharing — protects both parties from paying out on random variation. (2) Sharing region (5–10% savings): provider earns share_pct of savings above MSR. (3) Above cap (>10%): plan takes a larger % — protects plan from excessive payouts on statistical outliers. On the loss side: similar structure limits provider's maximum financial exposure to a defined threshold.*

Q6. The benchmark formula benchmark_pmpm = base_pmpm × trend_factor × risk_index adjusts for:

A. Inflation only — risk is held constant across VBC contract years

B. Both medical cost inflation (trend_factor) and panel composition change (risk_index) — both are required for a fair benchmark that is neutral to factors outside the provider's direct control

C. Risk only — trend is not applied so providers bear inflation risk

D. Only the difference in member months between the base and performance year

Answer: B. *Without trend: benchmark becomes easier to beat each year as actual costs rise with inflation — provider earns savings without improving efficiency. Without risk index: providers penalized for accepting sicker patients (rising RAF) or rewarded for losing sicker patients (falling RAF). Both adjustments remove factors outside provider control, making savings attributable to genuine care management behavior.*

Q7. Calculate the shared savings payment for a VBC entity with: 8,000 member months, actual total cost PMPM $420, benchmark PMPM $460, composite quality score 74%, min quality threshold 70%, savings share 40%.

(Short answer)

> **Sample Answer:**
> Step 1 — Quality gate: 74% >= 70% ✓ gate passed. Step 2 — Savings PMPM: $460 - $420 = $40/MM. Step 3 — Annualized savings: $40 × 8,000 = $320,000. Step 4 — Provider savings payment: $320,000 × 40% = $128,000. SQL equivalent: CASE WHEN q.composite_quality_score >= vc.min_quality_threshold AND bm.benchmark_pmpm > actual_total_pmpm THEN ROUND(vc.savings_share_pct/100.0 * (bm.benchmark_pmpm - actual_total_pmpm) * mc.member_months, 0) ELSE 0 END AS provider_savings_payment. If quality score were 68% (below 70% threshold): provider_savings_payment = $0 despite $320,000 in savings. The quality gate is binary — missing by any margin forfeits the entire payment. This is the most common source of VBC contract disputes and requires precise, documented quality score calculation with a clear audit trail from each HEDIS measure numerator and denominator through to the composite score.

Q8. Explain how bundled payment episode construction differs from general episode grouper analytics.

(Short answer)

> **Sample Answer:**
> Bundled payment episode: starts from a contractually defined anchor event (specific CPT code, e.g., 27447 = total knee replacement). Episode window is fixed by contract (e.g., 90 days post-procedure). All claims from anchor_date through anchor_date + 90 days for the same member are included in the episode cost. Target price is agreed upon in the contract before the performance year. The definition is administrative — set by contractual agreement, not clinical algorithm. Episode grouper analytics: uses a clinical algorithm (e.g., Optum ETG, IBM MEG, Truven) to group all related claims into clinically

coherent episodes based on diagnosis and treatment patterns. Groupers can define episodes for chronic conditions (a diabetes episode spanning years), acute events (a pneumonia episode), or surgical procedures (including pre-operative workup). Groupers use clinical rules, not fixed calendar windows, to determine episode boundaries. Key SQL difference: bundled payment uses BETWEEN anchor_date AND anchor_date + window_days as the episode boundary. Episode groupers use a pre-computed episode_id field assigned by the grouper engine to each claim. Bundled payment SQL can be written without external software. Episode grouper SQL requires a pre-processing step where the clinical algorithm assigns episode_ids to claims before the analytics queries run.

Q9. Describe the PCMH payment model. Write the SQL for a monthly PCMH performance scorecard.

(Short answer)

Sample Answer:

PCMH (Patient-Centered Medical Home): PCPs achieve NCQA PCMH recognition by meeting access, coordination, and quality standards. In return, the plan pays an enhanced care management PMPM fee on top of FFS. Key performance metrics for PCMH scorecard: (1) HEDIS gap closure rate for PCP-attributable measures. (2) Avoidable ED rate per 1,000 MM (target < 150). (3) 30-day hospital readmission rate. (4) Generic prescribing rate for attributed panel. (5) High-risk member care plan completion rate. Monthly PCMH scorecard SQL: SELECT attr.attributed_pcp_npi, p.provider_full_name, COUNT(DISTINCT attr.member_id) AS panel_size, ROUND(100.0*COUNT(DISTINCT CASE WHEN hg.gap_status='CLOSED' THEN hg.member_id END)/NULLIF(COUNT(DISTINCT hg.member_id),0),1) AS hedis_closure_rate, ROUND(1000.0*SUM(CASE WHEN ed.nyu_category IN ('Non-Emergent','Primary Care Treatable') THEN 1 ELSE 0 END)/NULLIF(SUM(mm.member_months),0),1) AS avoidable_ed_per_1k, ROUND(100.0*COUNT(DISTINCT CASE WHEN ra.readmission_flag=1 THEN ra.member_id END)/NULLIF(COUNT(DISTINCT ha.member_id),0),1) AS readmission_rate_pct FROM dim_pcp_attribution attr JOIN dim_providers p ON attr.attributed_pcp_npi=p.npi LEFT JOIN fact_hedis_gaps hg ON attr.member_id=hg.member_id AND hg.measurement_year=EXTRACT(YEAR FROM CURRENT_DATE) LEFT JOIN ed_nyu_claims ed ON attr.member_id=ed.member_id JOIN fact_member_months mm ON attr.member_id=mm.member_id AND mm.membership_year=EXTRACT(YEAR FROM CURRENT_DATE) WHERE attr.attribution_year=EXTRACT(YEAR FROM CURRENT_DATE) GROUP BY attr.attributed_pcp_npi, p.provider_full_name HAVING COUNT(DISTINCT attr.member_id)>=30 ORDER BY hedis_closure_rate DESC.

Q10. Walk through the risk corridor calculation for a VBC entity with $3.0M benchmark, $2.8M actual cost, MSR=5%, sharing rate=40%, cap=10%.

(Short answer)

Sample Answer:

Step 1 — Total savings: $3.0M - $2.8M = $200,000. Savings rate = $200K / $3.0M = 6.67%. Step 2 — Below MSR? MSR = 5% × $3.0M = $150,000. The first $150,000 of savings is NOT shared — both plan and provider retain their respective shares without a savings payment. Step 3 — Above MSR, in sharing region (5%–10%): Shareable savings = $200,000 - $150,000 = $50,000. Provider earns: $50,000 × 40% = $20,000. Step 4 — Is savings rate above the cap (10%)? 6.67% < 10% → No cap applies. Total provider savings payment = $20,000. SQL: CASE WHEN savings_rate < min_savings_rate THEN 0 WHEN savings_rate BETWEEN min_savings_rate AND cap_rate THEN (annualized_savings - benchmark_total*min_savings_rate) * sharing_pct WHEN savings_rate > cap_rate THEN (benchmark_total*(cap_rate-min_savings_rate)*sharing_pct) + (annualized_savings - benchmark_total*cap_rate)*low_sharing_pct END AS provider_savings_payment. Always present a corridor reconciliation table showing each band calculation — VBC financial settlements require full auditability, and providers will scrutinize every line.

Key Takeaways

What every analyst must remember from this chapter.

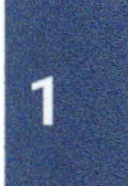

VBC spectrum: FFS (no risk) → pay-for-performance → shared savings → bundled payment → capitation (full risk). Each model needs different SQL: shared savings = total cost vs. benchmark; bundles = episode cost vs. target price; capitation = panel surplus/deficit.

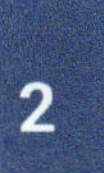

Shared savings formula: provider_savings_payment = savings_share_pct × (benchmark_pmpm - actual_pmpm) × member_months IF composite_quality_score >= min_quality_threshold. Quality gate is binary — miss by 1 point, payment = $0.

3 Benchmark = base_pmpm × trend_factor × risk_index. risk_index = current_avg_raf / base_avg_raf. Both trend and risk adjustments are required. Without trend, benchmark becomes easier to beat each year. Without risk, providers are penalized for accepting sicker patients.

4 Total cost of care = medical claims (allowed_amount) + pharmacy claims (plan_paid_amount) for the attributed population. UNION ALL both tables into one episode cost CTE. Without pharmacy, VBC entities can shift costs to the pharmacy channel and appear efficient on medical-only measures.

5 Bundled payment episode SQL: anchor_events CTE on qualifying CPT codes; JOIN all claims WHERE service_date BETWEEN anchor_date AND anchor_date + episode_window_days; sum total episode cost; episode_savings = target_price - total_cost. ORDER BY episode_savings ASC — largest overruns first.

6 Risk corridor mechanics: below MSR = 0% sharing. In sharing region (MSR to cap) = provider earns share_pct of savings above MSR. Above cap = plan takes larger % of excess savings. Present a reconciliation table for every settlement — providers will audit every calculation.

7 PCMH scorecard metrics: HEDIS gap closure rate, avoidable ED per 1,000 MM (target < 150), 30-day readmission rate, generic prescribing rate, high-risk care plan completion. Run monthly. Minimum panel size 30. Enhanced care management PMPM fee is the financial reward for PCMH recognition.

8 VBC attribution must be finalized by December 31. Attribution changes mid-year affect both the benchmark and actual cost denominators. Lock attribution at year-end for final settlement; use preliminary attribution for monthly monitoring. Attribution disputes are the #1 source of VBC contract disagreements.

Part VII — Population Health & Epidemiology

Chapters 20–26

FWA · Epidemiology · Risk Stratification · Health Equity · Prior Auth · RAPS/EDPS · Care Management

Part VII covers the population-level analytics disciplines that sit above individual episode management. Chapters 20–26 equip the analyst with SQL for fraud detection, population epidemiology, risk stratification, health equity measurement, prior authorization compliance, risk adjustment submission, and care management program ROI. Every chapter has conceptual explanation, fully annotated SQL, 6 MC + 4 SA unit tests, and key takeaways.

Chapter 20:Fraud, Waste & Abuse Detection

Upcoding · NCCI unbundling · Opioid diversion · Impossible billing

20.1 FWA Framework

Fraud = intentional misrepresentation for financial gain. Waste = overuse without fraudulent intent. Abuse = practices inconsistent with sound fiscal or medical practice. FWA analytics detects statistical outliers whose billing patterns deviate significantly from peer norms. Every flag is a hypothesis for investigation, not a conclusion.

> **OIG vs. FWA** OIG exclusion (Ch 16) = known bad actors already sanctioned. FWA detection = finding potential bad actors before sanction. Both run weekly. OIG is retrospective confirmation; FWA detection is prospective investigation.

20.2 E&M Upcoding Detection

Upcoding = billing a higher-complexity E&M code than the encounter supports. A provider whose 99215 rate far exceeds specialty peers is an upcoding candidate. The SQL compares each provider's CPT code distribution against specialty-adjusted peer benchmarks.

ANSI SQL — 20.2: E&M Upcoding Detection (Fully Annotated)

```sql
-- PURPOSE: Identify providers whose rate of billing high-complexity E&M
-- codes (99215, 99205) significantly exceeds their specialty peer benchmark.
-- Flag Z-score > 2.0 = >2 standard deviations above peer = clinical record review.
WITH em_by_provider AS (
  SELECT c.rendering_npi, p.specialty_group, c.procedure_code,
      COUNT(*) AS visit_count
  FROM  fact_medical_claims c
  JOIN  dim_providers p ON c.rendering_npi = p.npi
  WHERE c.procedure_code IN (
         '99201','99202','99203','99204','99205',
         '99211','99212','99213','99214','99215')
   AND c.claim_status = 'PAID'
   AND EXTRACT(YEAR FROM c.service_date) = EXTRACT(YEAR FROM CURRENT_DATE)
  GROUP BY c.rendering_npi, p.specialty_group, c.procedure_code
),
-- high_em_rate = visits at 99215 or 99205 / total E&M visits
provider_em_rate AS (
  SELECT rendering_npi, specialty_group,
      SUM(visit_count) AS total_em,
      SUM(CASE WHEN procedure_code IN ('99215','99205') THEN visit_count ELSE 0 END) AS high_em_count,
      ROUND(100.0*SUM(CASE WHEN procedure_code IN ('99215','99205') THEN visit_count ELSE 0 END)
```

```
        /NULLIF(SUM(visit_count),0),1) AS high_em_rate_pct
  FROM  em_by_provider
  GROUP BY rendering_npi, specialty_group
  HAVING SUM(visit_count) >= 100 -- minimum volume for statistical reliability
),
-- Specialty peer average and standard deviation for z-score denominator
peer_benchmark AS (
  SELECT specialty_group,
       ROUND(AVG(high_em_rate_pct),1)   AS peer_avg,
       ROUND(STDDEV(high_em_rate_pct),1) AS peer_sd
  FROM  provider_em_rate
  GROUP BY specialty_group
)
-- Z-score: how many SDs above peer average. Flag > 2.0.
SELECT pe.rendering_npi, p.provider_full_name, p.specialty_group, p.county,
  pe.total_em, pe.high_em_rate_pct,
  pb.peer_avg AS peer_avg_pct,
  ROUND(pe.high_em_rate_pct - pb.peer_avg,1) AS deviation_from_peer,
  ROUND((pe.high_em_rate_pct - pb.peer_avg)/NULLIF(pb.peer_sd,0),2) AS z_score,
  CASE WHEN (pe.high_em_rate_pct-pb.peer_avg)/NULLIF(pb.peer_sd,0) > 2
    THEN 'FLAG — 2+ SD above peer: clinical review' ELSE 'Within range' END AS fwa_flag
FROM  provider_em_rate pe
JOIN  peer_benchmark pb ON pe.specialty_group = pb.specialty_group
JOIN  dim_providers p ON pe.rendering_npi = p.npi
ORDER BY z_score DESC;
```

20.3 NCCI Unbundling Detection

NCCI edits define code pairs that should not be billed together — one is included in the other. Unbundling = billing both when only the comprehensive code should be submitted. SQL: identify same-day claims from the same provider where the code pair appears in ref_ncci_edits.

ANSI SQL — 20.3: NCCI Unbundling Detection (Fully Annotated)

```
-- PURPOSE: Detect claims where two CPT codes billed on the same date by the
-- same provider form an NCCI edit pair -- potential unbundling.
-- Self-join creates all same-day code pairs; NCCI join identifies violations.
WITH same_day_lines AS (
  SELECT c.member_id, c.rendering_npi, c.service_date,
       c.procedure_code AS code_billed, c.allowed_amount, c.claim_id
  FROM  fact_medical_claims c
  WHERE c.claim_status = 'PAID'
   AND EXTRACT(YEAR FROM c.service_date) = EXTRACT(YEAR FROM CURRENT_DATE)
),
-- Self-join: create all pairs of codes billed together on the same date
code_pairs AS (
  SELECT a.rendering_npi, a.member_id, a.service_date,
       a.code_billed AS comprehensive_code, -- column 1 (inclusive)
       b.code_billed AS component_code,    -- column 2 (bundled)
       a.allowed_amount + b.allowed_amount AS combined_allowed
  FROM  same_day_lines a
  JOIN  same_day_lines b
    ON a.rendering_npi = b.rendering_npi AND a.member_id = b.member_id
   AND a.service_date = b.service_date
   AND a.claim_id < b.claim_id -- avoid duplicate (A,B) and (B,A) pairs
),
-- Match code pairs against CMS NCCI edit table
unbundled AS (
  SELECT cp.*, n.modifier_allowed, n.effective_date
  FROM  code_pairs cp
  JOIN  ref_ncci_edits n
    ON n.column1_code = cp.comprehensive_code AND n.column2_code = cp.component_code
```

```
    AND cp.service_date >= n.effective_date
    AND (n.deletion_date IS NULL OR cp.service_date < n.deletion_date)
)
-- Summary: count unbundled pairs by provider
SELECT rendering_npi, p.provider_full_name, p.specialty_group,
   COUNT(*) AS unbundled_pair_count,
   ROUND(SUM(combined_allowed),0) AS total_unbundled_allowed,
   COUNT(DISTINCT CASE WHEN modifier_allowed='0' THEN member_id END) AS never_modifier_count,
   CASE WHEN COUNT(DISTINCT CASE WHEN modifier_allowed='0' THEN member_id END)>=10
      THEN 'FLAG — systemic NCCI violation' ELSE 'Review' END AS fwa_flag
FROM  unbundled
JOIN  dim_providers p ON rendering_npi = p.npi
GROUP BY rendering_npi, p.provider_full_name, p.specialty_group
ORDER BY never_modifier_count DESC;
```

20.4 Opioid Diversion Detection

Opioid diversion detection identifies members obtaining controlled substances from 3+ prescribers or 3+ pharmacies within a rolling 90-day window — a pattern consistent with prescription diversion.

ANSI SQL — 20.4: Opioid Diversion — Multi-Prescriber Multi-Pharmacy (Fully Annotated)

```
-- PURPOSE: Identify members filling Schedule II/III opioids from multiple
-- prescribers AND multiple pharmacies within a 90-day rolling window.
-- 3+ prescribers OR 3+ pharmacies in 90 days = high-risk diversion flag.
WITH opioid_claims AS (
   SELECT p.member_id, p.prescribing_npi, p.dispensing_pharmacy_npi,
        p.dispensing_date, p.ndc_code, d.drug_name, p.days_supply
   FROM  fact_pharmacy_claims p
   JOIN  ref_drug_schedule d ON p.ndc_code = d.ndc_code
   WHERE d.dea_schedule IN ('CII','CIII') AND d.drug_class = 'OPIOID'
    AND p.claim_status = 'PAID'
    AND p.dispensing_date >= CURRENT_DATE - INTERVAL '12' MONTH
),
-- Rolling 90-day window: count unique prescribers and pharmacies per fill
rolling_window AS (
   SELECT a.member_id, a.dispensing_date,
        COUNT(DISTINCT b.prescribing_npi)        AS prescribers_90d,
        COUNT(DISTINCT b.dispensing_pharmacy_npi) AS pharmacies_90d,
        SUM(b.days_supply)                  AS days_supply_90d
   FROM  opioid_claims a
   -- b = all opioid fills within 90 days before each fill a
   JOIN  opioid_claims b
     ON b.member_id = a.member_id
    AND b.dispensing_date BETWEEN a.dispensing_date - 90 AND a.dispensing_date
   GROUP BY a.member_id, a.dispensing_date
),
-- Keep peak risk window (max prescribers and pharmacies) per member
member_peak AS (
   SELECT member_id,
        MAX(prescribers_90d) AS max_prescribers_90d,
        MAX(pharmacies_90d)  AS max_pharmacies_90d
   FROM  rolling_window GROUP BY member_id
)
SELECT mp.member_id, m.member_name, m.date_of_birth, m.county,
   mp.max_prescribers_90d, mp.max_pharmacies_90d,
   CASE
     WHEN mp.max_prescribers_90d>=3 AND mp.max_pharmacies_90d>=3
     THEN 'HIGH — multi-prescriber AND multi-pharmacy'
     WHEN mp.max_prescribers_90d>=3 THEN 'MODERATE — 3+ prescribers 90d'
     WHEN mp.max_pharmacies_90d>=3  THEN 'MODERATE — 3+ pharmacies 90d'
     ELSE 'Monitor'
```

```
    END AS diversion_risk_flag
FROM member_peak mp
JOIN dim_members m ON mp.member_id = m.member_id
WHERE mp.max_prescribers_90d>=3 OR mp.max_pharmacies_90d>=3
ORDER BY mp.max_prescribers_90d DESC, mp.max_pharmacies_90d DESC;
-- NOTE: All flags require clinical review before any member action.
```

Chapter 20 Review

Unit Test · Key Takeaways

Answer each question before reading the explanation.

Q1. An FWA statistical flag (Z-score > 2.0 above peer) means:

A. The provider has committed fraud and should be terminated

B. The billing pattern is statistically unusual — an investigative hypothesis requiring clinical record review, not a confirmed violation

C. The provider should be placed on immediate pre-payment review

D. The provider's claims should be automatically denied

Answer: B. *Z > 2.0 = statistically unusual within specialty. ~Top 2.3% of the distribution. Every flag requires: random sample of 20–30 records → clinical/coder review → decision tree (close / education / SIU). Never take adverse action based on the statistical flag alone.*

Q2. NCCI unbundling occurs when:

A. Two diagnosis codes are applied to one procedure

B. Two CPT codes on the same date form an NCCI edit pair — one code is defined as included in the other, but both are billed separately to collect higher combined payment

C. A procedure code is billed with an invalid modifier

D. The same CPT is billed on consecutive days without documentation

Answer: B. *NCCI Column 1 = comprehensive code. Column 2 = component that is bundled into Column 1. Self-join SQL creates all same-day code pairs; JOIN to ref_ncci_edits finds violations. a.claim_id < b.claim_id prevents counting each pair twice.*

Q3. The opioid diversion rolling 90-day window captures:

A. The entire prior year of opioid fills for pattern review

B. The sustained behavioral pattern of prescription shopping — a single multi-pharmacy fill may be coincidental, but 3+ prescribers or pharmacies over 90 days indicates a recurring behavior consistent with diversion

C. The 90-day supply limit on Schedule II prescriptions

D. The CMS Part D required monitoring window for all opioid prescriptions

Answer: B. *Rolling window self-join: JOIN b ON b.member_id = a.member_id AND b.dispensing_date BETWEEN a.dispensing_date - 90 AND a.dispensing_date. For each fill, count unique prescribing_npi and dispensing_pharmacy_npi in the 90 days before. MAX() across all windows per member = peak risk period.*

Q4. Z-score in upcoding detection measures:

A. The provider's overall quality rating

B. How many standard deviations the provider's high-complexity E&M rate is above the specialty peer average: (provider_rate - peer_avg) / peer_stddev. Z > 2.0 flags statistical outliers warranting review

C. The ratio of 99215 to total claims

D. The provider's percentile rank within their specialty group

Answer: B. *STDDEV in peer_benchmark CTE = population standard deviation across all providers in the specialty. Provider with high_em_rate_pct = 62%, peer_avg = 38%, peer_sd = 8%: Z = (62−38)/8 = 3.0 → significant flag. Pair with HAVING total_em >= 100 to avoid false positives from low-volume providers.*

Q5. Impossible billing detection focuses on:

A. Claims from providers who have not completed annual credentialing

B. Combinations physically or logically impossible: provider billing >24 hours in one day, same service at two facilities simultaneously for the same member, services after a member's death date, gender-inconsistent diagnosis codes

C. Claims with procedure codes that don't exist in the current CPT set

D. Claims submitted after the timely filing deadline

Answer: B. *Impossible billing SQL examples: (a) >24 hrs: SUM(units × minutes) > 1440 per provider per date. (b) Two facilities, same member, same date, same procedure: self-join WHERE rendering_npi_a <> rendering_npi_b. (c) After death: JOIN dim_members WHERE service_date > death_date. All require member/provider verification before adverse action.*

Q6. The NCCI self-join uses a.claim_id < b.claim_id to:

A. Select the higher-value claim in each pair

B. Prevent counting each pair twice — without this condition (A,B) and (B,A) would both appear, doubling the violation count

C. Order the pairs chronologically

D. Ensure the Column 1 (comprehensive) code always appears first

Answer: B. *Without the < condition: member M, date D, codes 99215 and 99213 produces both (99215,99213) and (99213,99215) as separate rows. Each matches the NCCI edit. Violation count doubles. Using claim_id < claim_id ensures each unordered pair is counted exactly once.*

Q7. Describe the complete FWA investigation workflow after the SQL flags a provider for upcoding. What must occur before adverse action?

(Short answer)

> **Sample Answer:**
> Step 1 — Preliminary data review: pull claim-level detail — all E&M visits for the year with dates, procedure codes, diagnoses, allowed amounts. Calculate 99215 rate by quarter — recent spike vs. sustained high rate? Step 2 — Specialty peer validation: confirm the benchmark used the correct specialty group. Pull 5 peer providers in same specialty and geography. Step 3 — Random record request: send Retrospective Medical Record Request (RMRR) for 20–30 flagged 99215 claims. Request progress note, HPI, and medical decision-making documentation. Step 4 — Clinical review: certified professional coder or physician reviewer evaluates whether documentation supports 99215 per CMS 1995/1997 guidelines. Step 5 — Decision: <10% support → systemic upcoding; refer to SIU, consider pre-payment review. 10–30% fail → education and corrective action plan. >70% support → false positive, close. Step 6 — Pre-payment review: only after documented fraud pattern and legal review. All claims require manual approval before payment. Reserve for confirmed fraud.

Q8. Write the SQL to identify providers billing more than 24 hours of service time in a single day.

(Short answer)

> **Sample Answer:**
> SELECT c.rendering_npi, p.provider_full_name, p.specialty_group, c.service_date, COUNT(DISTINCT c.claim_id) AS claim_count, SUM(c.units_of_service) AS total_units, SUM(c.units_of_service * COALESCE(ref.typical_minutes_per_unit,15)) AS estimated_total_minutes, ROUND(SUM(c.units_of_service * COALESCE(ref.typical_minutes_per_unit,15))/60.0,1) AS estimated_hours, CASE WHEN SUM(c.units_of_service*COALESCE(ref.typical_minutes_per_unit,15))>1440 THEN 'FLAG — exceeds 24 hours' WHEN SUM(c.units_of_service*COALESCE(ref.typical_minutes_per_unit,15))>960 THEN 'REVIEW — exceeds 16 hours' ELSE 'Within range' END AS billing_flag FROM fact_medical_claims c JOIN dim_providers p ON c.rendering_npi=p.npi JOIN ref_procedure_minutes ref ON c.procedure_code=ref.procedure_code WHERE c.claim_status='PAID' AND EXTRACT(YEAR FROM c.service_date)=EXTRACT(YEAR FROM CURRENT_DATE) GROUP BY c.rendering_npi, p.provider_full_name, p.specialty_group, c.service_date HAVING SUM(c.units_of_service*COALESCE(ref.typical_minutes_per_unit,15))>960 ORDER BY estimated_hours DESC. ref_procedure_minutes maps CPT codes to CMS-typical minutes: 99213≈20min, 99215≈40min, therapy codes 15 min/unit. > 24 hours = impossible billing. 16–24 hours = possible but unusual; verify with provider.

Q9. Describe the opioid diversion detection methodology and what constitutes a high-risk flag.

(Short answer)

> **Sample Answer:**
> Methodology: (1) Filter pharmacy claims to Schedule II/III opioid NDC codes via ref_drug_schedule. (2) For each fill, count unique prescribing_npi and dispensing_pharmacy_npi within rolling 90-day window using self-join. (3) MAX() per member = peak risk window. Flag HIGH = 3+ prescribers AND 3+ pharmacies in 90 days. MODERATE = either criterion alone. Additional signals: excessive days_supply (>90 in 30 days = overlapping fills), opioid + benzodiazepine combination (CDC warns against concurrent prescribing), multiple specialties with no apparent clinical rationale. Clinical response for HIGH: (a) Outreach to the member's PCP with full prescribing history — PCP may be unaware of other prescribers. (b) Case management referral for SUD support resources. (c) Add concurrent DUR edit alerting pharmacist when second opioid from different prescriber fills within 30 days. NEVER automatically restrict access without clinical review — some members have legitimate complex pain management from multiple specialists. The flag triggers clinical outreach, not automatic restriction.

Q10. Write the SQL to detect same-service, same-date, two-facility impossible billing.

(Short answer)

Sample Answer:
SELECT a.member_id, m.member_name, m.date_of_birth, a.service_date, a.procedure_code, r.procedure_description, a.rendering_npi AS facility_1_npi, p1.provider_full_name AS facility_1, b.rendering_npi AS facility_2_npi, p2.provider_full_name AS facility_2, a.allowed_amount AS f1_allowed, b.allowed_amount AS f2_allowed, a.allowed_amount+b.allowed_amount AS total_allowed FROM fact_medical_claims a JOIN fact_medical_claims b ON a.member_id=b.member_id AND a.service_date=b.service_date AND a.procedure_code=b.procedure_code AND a.rendering_npi<>b.rendering_npi AND a.claim_id<b.claim_id JOIN dim_members m ON a.member_id=m.member_id JOIN dim_providers p1 ON a.rendering_npi=p1.npi JOIN dim_providers p2 ON b.rendering_npi=p2.npi JOIN ref_procedure_codes r ON a.procedure_code=r.procedure_code WHERE a.claim_status='PAID' AND b.claim_status='PAID' AND EXTRACT(YEAR FROM a.service_date)=EXTRACT(YEAR FROM CURRENT_DATE) AND p1.provider_type<>'TELEHEALTH' AND p2.provider_type<>'TELEHEALTH' ORDER BY total_allowed DESC. Exclude telehealth + in-person same day (legitimate). Detects: (a) Same procedure, same member, two facilities — one is likely a duplicate or clone. (b) Member physically present at two inpatient facilities simultaneously. Administrative errors (wrong NPI on claim) produce false positives — always verify with provider before action.

Key Takeaways

What every analyst must remember from this chapter.

1. FWA flags are investigative hypotheses, not accusations. Z-score > 2.0 above specialty peer = statistical outlier. Always: random record pull (20–30 claims) → clinical/coder review → decision tree before any adverse action.

2. Upcoding SQL: high_em_rate_pct = COUNT(99215 or 99205)/COUNT(all E&M). Z-score = (provider_rate - peer_avg)/peer_stddev. Flag Z > 2.0. HAVING total_em >= 100. Benchmark must use correct specialty group.

3. NCCI unbundling: same-member, same-date, same-provider self-join + JOIN ref_ncci_edits. a.claim_id < b.claim_id prevents duplicate pairs. modifier_allowed = '0' = never permitted = requires recovery.

4. Opioid diversion: rolling 90-day self-join counting distinct prescribing_npi and dispensing_pharmacy_npi. Flag: 3+ prescribers OR 3+ pharmacies. HIGH = both. Clinical outreach first — never auto-restrict.

5. Impossible billing: >24 hrs in one day (SUM units × minutes > 1440); same procedure two facilities (self-join WHERE rendering_npi_a <> rendering_npi_b AND claim_id < claim_id); service after death_date. Verify before adverse action.

6. FWA investigation sequence: SQL flag → specialty peer validation → random medical record request → clinical review → decision: close / education / SIU / pre-payment review. Never skip clinical review.

7. Pre-payment review = all claims require manual approval before payment. Significant operational burden. Legal review required. Reserve for confirmed or near-confirmed fraud patterns only.

8. OIG exclusion = retrospective (Ch 16). FWA detection = prospective. Both run weekly. Neither replaces the other.

Chapter 21: Epidemiology & Population Health

Prevalence · Incidence · PQI avoidable admissions · Disease burden · SDOH in claims

21.1 Prevalence and Incidence

Prevalence = proportion of the population with a condition in the measurement period. Incidence = new cases only — members with the condition this year who did NOT have it in the prior year. Both use member months as the denominator, not claim counts.

> **Key Rule** Always use member months as denominator for population rates — never claim counts. A member enrolled for 3 months contributes 3 member months. Claim counts conflate frequency of utilization with population size.

ANSI SQL — 21.1: Prevalence and Incidence by Condition (Fully Annotated)

```
-- PURPOSE: Calculate period prevalence (any claim with condition this year)
-- and incidence (new cases: condition present this year but NOT last year)
-- for each chronic condition in ref_condition_definitions.
WITH current_year_cases AS (
  SELECT DISTINCT c.member_id, cd.condition_name
  FROM fact_medical_claims c
  JOIN ref_condition_definitions cd
    ON c.primary_diag LIKE cd.icd10_prefix || '%' -- match ICD-10 code family
  WHERE c.claim_status = 'PAID'
   AND EXTRACT(YEAR FROM c.service_date) = EXTRACT(YEAR FROM CURRENT_DATE)
),
-- Prior year cases: used to distinguish incidence from prevalence
prior_year_cases AS (
  SELECT DISTINCT c.member_id, cd.condition_name
  FROM fact_medical_claims c
  JOIN ref_condition_definitions cd
    ON c.primary_diag LIKE cd.icd10_prefix || '%'
  WHERE c.claim_status = 'PAID'
   AND EXTRACT(YEAR FROM c.service_date) = EXTRACT(YEAR FROM CURRENT_DATE) - 1
),
-- Total enrolled member months: the denominator for all population rates
enrolled_mm AS (
  SELECT SUM(member_months) AS total_mm
  FROM fact_member_months
  WHERE membership_year = EXTRACT(YEAR FROM CURRENT_DATE)
   AND line_of_business = 'COMMERCIAL'
)
SELECT cy.condition_name,
  COUNT(DISTINCT cy.member_id) AS prevalent_cases,
  -- Incidence: present this year AND NOT present last year
  COUNT(DISTINCT CASE WHEN py.member_id IS NULL THEN cy.member_id END) AS incident_cases,
  em.total_mm,
  ROUND(1000.0*COUNT(DISTINCT cy.member_id)/NULLIF(em.total_mm,0),2) AS prevalence_per_1k_mm,
  ROUND(1000.0*COUNT(DISTINCT CASE WHEN py.member_id IS NULL THEN cy.member_id END)
    /NULLIF(em.total_mm,0),2) AS incidence_per_1k_mm,
  -- Disease burden: total allowed cost for this condition per MM
  ROUND(SUM(c2.allowed_amount)/NULLIF(em.total_mm,0),2) AS condition_pmpm
FROM current_year_cases cy
LEFT JOIN prior_year_cases py
```

```sql
  ON cy.member_id = py.member_id AND cy.condition_name = py.condition_name
JOIN enrolled_mm em ON 1=1 -- deliberate single-row cross join for denominator
JOIN fact_medical_claims c2
  ON c2.member_id = cy.member_id AND c2.claim_status = 'PAID'
  AND EXTRACT(YEAR FROM c2.service_date) = EXTRACT(YEAR FROM CURRENT_DATE)
JOIN ref_condition_definitions cd2
  ON c2.primary_diag LIKE cd2.icd10_prefix || '%' AND cd2.condition_name = cy.condition_name
GROUP BY cy.condition_name, em.total_mm
ORDER BY prevalence_per_1k_mm DESC;
```

21.2 PQI — Prevention Quality Indicators

PQI are AHRQ measures of ambulatory care quality: hospital admissions for conditions that, with appropriate outpatient care, should rarely require hospitalization — diabetes, hypertension, CHF, COPD, asthma. High PQI rates indicate primary care access gaps or chronic disease management failures.

ANSI SQL — 21.2: PQI Avoidable Admission Rate (Fully Annotated)

```sql
-- PURPOSE: Calculate AHRQ Prevention Quality Indicator (PQI) avoidable
-- admission rates. TOB 11x = inpatient acute. Exclude obstetric DRGs.
-- Standard rate: per 100,000 member months.
WITH pqi_admissions AS (
   SELECT c.member_id, c.rendering_npi, c.service_date,
         c.primary_diag, p.pqi_condition, p.pqi_number, c.allowed_amount
   FROM fact_medical_claims c
   JOIN ref_pqi_diagnoses p ON c.primary_diag LIKE p.icd10_prefix || '%'
   WHERE c.type_of_bill LIKE '11%'  -- inpatient acute (UB-04 TOB 11x)
    AND c.claim_status = 'PAID'
    AND EXTRACT(YEAR FROM c.service_date) = EXTRACT(YEAR FROM CURRENT_DATE)
    -- Exclude obstetric/newborn DRGs per AHRQ PQI methodology
    AND c.primary_drg NOT BETWEEN '765' AND '782'
    AND c.primary_drg NOT BETWEEN '790' AND '795'
),
enrolled_mm AS (SELECT SUM(member_months) AS total_mm FROM fact_member_months
   WHERE membership_year = EXTRACT(YEAR FROM CURRENT_DATE))
SELECT pa.pqi_number, pa.pqi_condition,
   COUNT(DISTINCT pa.member_id) AS admission_count,
   ROUND(SUM(pa.allowed_amount),0) AS total_cost,
   ROUND(AVG(pa.allowed_amount),0) AS avg_cost_per_admit,
   em.total_mm,
   -- AHRQ standard: rate per 100,000 member months
   ROUND(100000.0*COUNT(DISTINCT pa.member_id)/NULLIF(em.total_mm,0),1) AS pqi_rate_per_100k_mm
FROM pqi_admissions pa
CROSS JOIN enrolled_mm em
GROUP BY pa.pqi_number, pa.pqi_condition, em.total_mm
ORDER BY pqi_rate_per_100k_mm DESC;
```

Chapter 21 Review

Unit Test · Key Takeaways

Answer each question before reading the explanation.

Q1. Incidence differs from prevalence in that:

A. Incidence uses claims denominator; prevalence uses member month denominator

B. Prevalence = all existing cases in the period. Incidence = new cases only — members with the condition this year who did NOT have it in the prior year. SQL: LEFT JOIN prior_year_cases WHERE prior.member_id IS NULL

C. Incidence is always lower than prevalence for chronic conditions

D. Prevalence is per 1,000 MM; incidence is per 100,000

Answer: B. *For chronic conditions (diabetes, CHF): prevalence grows each year accumulating all existing cases; incidence measures only newly diagnosed. For acute conditions (pneumonia): prevalence ≈ incidence in a 12-month window. The LEFT JOIN + IS NULL idiom is standard SQL for "exists this year, absent last year."*

Q2. PQI admissions filter to TOB LIKE '11%' because:

A. 11x is the HIPAA EDI code for inpatient claims

B. Type of bill 11x identifies inpatient acute hospital claims on the UB-04. PQI measures count inpatient acute admissions only — outpatient or ED encounters with the same diagnosis are NOT PQI events; they represent the appropriate care that should prevent PQI admissions

C. 11x identifies claims with 11+ diagnosis codes

D. Claims with TOB 11x are auto-validated against AHRQ PQI criteria

Answer: B. *UB-04 TOB structure: first two digits = facility type and bill classification. 11x = inpatient acute. 13x = outpatient. 23x = ambulatory surgery. 81x = hospice. A primary care visit for uncontrolled diabetes (TOB 13x) is excellent care — it is the opposite of a PQI admission.*

Q3. SDOH data can be approximated in claims analytics by:

A. Analyzing income fields in dim_members

B. Member ZIP → Area Deprivation Index (ADI), and ICD-10 Z-codes (Z55–Z65) documenting social determinants directly on claims

C. Calculating PMPM for members in low-income vs. high-income areas

D. Using plan type (Medicaid vs. commercial) as a proxy

Answer: B. *Two approaches: (1) Geographic proxy: ZIP → ref_adi_scores → ADI national rank. High ADI = high socioeconomic disadvantage. (2) Direct Z-codes: Z59 (housing instability), Z60 (social environment), Z62 (family stress), Z64. Z-codes are under-captured (<5% of visits) but highly actionable when present.*

Q4. Disease burden is measured as condition_pmpm because:

A. It is the total number of inpatient admissions for the condition

B. condition_pmpm = SUM(allowed_amount for condition) / total_member_months — quantifies the financial impact per enrolled member per month. Combines prevalence (how common) with unit cost (how expensive per episode) into a single actionable metric for program prioritization.

C. It is the ratio of condition prevalence to the national NHANES average

D. It represents the cost per affected member only

Answer: B. *condition_pmpm is more actionable than raw prevalence. A condition with 15% prevalence but $20 PMPM costs less than 2% prevalence at $800 PMPM. Always present both the population burden (prevalence_per_1k_mm) and financial burden (condition_pmpm) together for program prioritization.*

Q5. The PQI exclusion of DRGs 765–782 and 790–795 removes:

A. Pediatric admissions measured separately under PDI

B. Obstetric and newborn admissions — maternal delivery DRGs should not count as avoidable regardless of diagnosis code. A pregnant woman with gestational diabetes (ICD-10 O24.x) should not generate a PQI event for her delivery admission.

C. Mental health and SUD admissions

D. DRGs below 800 which are auto-excluded

Answer: B. *Without the DRG exclusion, a delivery admission with a gestational diabetes primary diagnosis would be counted as a PQI avoidable admission for diabetes — clinically incorrect. The exclusion removes all obstetric and newborn admissions from the PQI numerator regardless of primary diagnosis code.*

Q6. JOIN enrolled_mm ON 1=1 in the PQI query is:

A. A safety check preventing Cartesian product errors

B. A deliberate single-row CROSS JOIN — enrolled_mm has exactly one row (total member months). JOIN ON 1=1 attaches that single denominator value to every result row. Equivalent to CROSS JOIN enrolled_mm. CROSS JOIN keyword is clearer in production code.

C. A placeholder requiring the actual join key

D. A filter returning only rows where 1=1 is true

Answer: B. *When a CTE produces a single scalar value, it cannot be joined on a real business key. JOIN ON 1=1 and CROSS JOIN are equivalent — both perform a Cartesian product on a single-row table, producing one output row per left-table row with the denominator value appended. This is the correct and idiomatic SQL pattern for attaching a global denominator.*

Q7. Describe how PQI rates build a care gap prioritization matrix for the medical director.

(Short answer)

Sample Answer:

Step 1 — PQI rate table: run the PQI avoidable admission rate query for all conditions. Rank by pqi_rate_per_100k_mm descending. Top 5 = largest ambulatory care gaps. Step 2 — Geographic clustering: add GROUP BY county_fips. High-PQI counties = geographic access gaps or specific provider quality issues. Step 3 — PCP attribution: JOIN pqi_admissions back to dim_pcp_attribution. PCPs with 3× higher-than-average PQI rates for COPD = specific intervention targets. Step 4 — Cost justification: avg_cost_per_admit × admission_count = total_cost_of_pqi. Compare to estimated cost of care management intervention ($50/member/month × 12 months for high-risk members). If intervention prevents 20% of admissions: savings > program cost → proceed. Step 5 — Medical director matrix: rows = conditions, columns = current PQI rate | benchmark | gap | program cost | estimated savings. Makes the investment decision data-driven and defensible.

Q8. Write the SQL for SDOH scores by joining ZIP codes to the Area Deprivation Index.

(Short answer)

Sample Answer:

SELECT m.member_id, m.county_fips, m.zip_code, adi.adi_national_rank, CASE WHEN adi.adi_national_rank>=80 THEN 'HIGH DISADVANTAGE — Q5' WHEN adi.adi_national_rank>=60 THEN 'MODERATE-HIGH — Q4' WHEN adi.adi_national_rank>=40 THEN 'MODERATE — Q3' WHEN adi.adi_national_rank>=20 THEN 'LOW-MODERATE — Q2' ELSE 'LOW DISADVANTAGE — Q1' END AS adi_quintile, COUNT(DISTINCT CASE WHEN hg.gap_status='OPEN' THEN hg.measure_id END) AS open_hedis_gaps, ROUND(SUM(c.allowed_amount)/NULLIF(mm.member_months,0),2) AS pmpm FROM dim_members m JOIN ref_adi_scores adi ON m.zip_code=adi.zip_code JOIN fact_member_months mm ON m.member_id=mm.member_id AND mm.membership_year=EXTRACT(YEAR FROM CURRENT_DATE) LEFT JOIN fact_hedis_gaps hg ON m.member_id=hg.member_id AND hg.measurement_year=EXTRACT(YEAR FROM CURRENT_DATE) LEFT JOIN fact_medical_claims c ON m.member_id=c.member_id AND EXTRACT(YEAR FROM c.service_date)=EXTRACT(YEAR FROM CURRENT_DATE) AND c.claim_status='PAID' WHERE m.coverage_status='ACTIVE' GROUP BY m.member_id, m.county_fips, m.zip_code, adi.adi_national_rank ORDER BY adi.adi_national_rank DESC. Members in Q5 (ADI ≥ 80) with most open HEDIS gaps = priority for SDOH-informed outreach including transportation, food security, and social work referral.

Q9. Explain point prevalence vs. period prevalence. Give SQL for each.

(Short answer)

Sample Answer:

Point prevalence: proportion of members with the condition on a specific date. SQL: SELECT COUNT(DISTINCT c.member_id) FROM fact_medical_claims c WHERE c.primary_diag LIKE :prefix AND :measurement_date BETWEEN c.service_date AND c.service_date+30 AND c.claim_status='PAID'. Period prevalence: proportion with the condition at any point in the measurement period (usually 1 year). SQL: SELECT COUNT(DISTINCT c.member_id) FROM fact_medical_claims c WHERE c.primary_diag LIKE :prefix AND EXTRACT(YEAR FROM c.service_date)=:year AND c.claim_status='PAID'. Denominator for both: enrolled member months. In healthcare claims, period prevalence is preferred for chronic disease management — a diabetic member who had no diabetes-coded encounter in a narrow window would be missed by point prevalence but correctly captured by period prevalence. Period prevalence provides the complete census of the condition population for care management targeting.

Q10. Describe ICD-10 Z-codes and their role in SDOH analytics. Give five specific Z-codes and the operational action each triggers.

(Short answer)

Sample Answer:

Z-codes (Z00–Z99) are ICD-10 codes for factors influencing health status that are not diseases. Z55–Z65 document social determinants: Z59.0 = Homelessness → immediate social work referral, housing resource connection, complex care management enrollment. Z59.4 = Lack of adequate food → food bank referral, SNAP enrollment assistance, home meal delivery for high-risk. Z60.2 = Living alone → falls risk assessment, caregiver support, medication adherence monitoring. Z62.3 = Child scapegoating/hostility → mandatory reporting review with Compliance; document carefully per state law. Z63.4 = Death of family member → grief counseling, mental health gap closure, medication adherence monitoring during bereavement. Analyst note: Z-codes are severely under-documented (<5% of visits capture them even when the need is present). Report Z-code capture rates by provider to the medical director — low capture = documentation education opportunity. When present, Z-codes are highly actionable: the social need is explicitly identified and can be routed to the appropriate resource.

Key Takeaways

What every analyst must remember from this chapter.

1 Prevalence = all cases per 1,000 MM. Incidence = new cases only (LEFT JOIN prior year WHERE IS NULL) per 1,000 MM. Member months denominator always — never claim counts.

2 Disease burden = condition_pmpm = SUM(allowed) / total_MM. Prioritize programs by prevalence_per_1k_mm × condition_pmpm — invest where both are high.

3 PQI: TOB 11x, primary_diag in ref_pqi_diagnoses, EXCLUDE DRGs 765–782 and 790–795 (obstetric). Rate per 100,000 MM. High rates = primary care access gaps.

4 SDOH geographic: ZIP → ref_adi_scores. ADI national rank ≥ 80 = high disadvantage (Q5). SDOH direct: Z55–Z65. Z-codes under-captured; report capture rates to medical director.

5 Incidence SQL: LEFT JOIN prior_year_cases WHERE prior.member_id IS NULL. SELECT only rows present in current year but absent in prior year = new (incident) cases.

6 CROSS JOIN on single-row CTE: JOIN mm ON 1=1. Attaches total_mm denominator to every result row. Equivalent to CROSS JOIN enrolled_mm. Use CROSS JOIN keyword for clarity in production code.

7 PQI prioritization matrix: conditions × PQI rate × benchmark gap × prevention program cost × estimated savings. Makes intervention investment decision data-driven.

8 Condition PMPM is more actionable than raw prevalence. 15% prevalence at $20 PMPM < 2% prevalence at $800 PMPM. Present both population and financial burden together.

Chapter 22: Patient Risk Stratification

CCI scoring · Composite risk score · Trajectory prediction · Risk tier assignment

22.1 Risk Stratification Purpose

Risk stratification ranks members by probability of high future healthcare utilization — enabling care management to invest intervention resources where they will have the most impact. The model combines clinical complexity (CCI), cost trajectory, utilization patterns, pharmacy complexity, and SDOH risk.

22.2 Charlson Comorbidity Index

The Charlson Comorbidity Index assigns weights 1–6 to 17 chronic conditions. CCI 0 = no comorbidities; CCI ≥ 5 = severe burden. Key implementation detail: prevent double-counting by taking MAX weight per condition group before summing.

ANSI SQL — 22.2: Charlson Comorbidity Index Calculation (Fully Annotated)

```
-- PURPOSE: Calculate CCI for each member from ICD-10 diagnosis codes.
-- Weights: 1=mild (MI, CHF, COPD, dementia), 2=moderate (hemiplegia, cancer),
-- 3=severe liver disease, 6=HIV/AIDS, metastatic tumor.
-- Double-counting prevention: MAX weight per condition group before SUM.
WITH member_conditions AS (
  SELECT DISTINCT c.member_id, cci.condition_name, cci.cci_weight
  FROM  fact_medical_claims c
  -- Check primary AND secondary diagnosis fields for any CCI condition
  JOIN  ref_cci_weights cci
    ON c.primary_diag LIKE cci.icd10_prefix || '%'
    OR c.diag_2      LIKE cci.icd10_prefix || '%'
    OR c.diag_3      LIKE cci.icd10_prefix || '%'
  WHERE c.claim_status = 'PAID'
   AND EXTRACT(YEAR FROM c.service_date) = EXTRACT(YEAR FROM CURRENT_DATE)
),
-- Deduplicate: take highest weight per condition group per member.
-- Prevents counting both diabetes (CCI=1) and diabetes with complications (CCI=2)
member_cci AS (
  SELECT member_id, SUM(max_wt) AS cci_score
  FROM (
    SELECT member_id, condition_name, MAX(cci_weight) AS max_wt
    FROM  member_conditions
    GROUP BY member_id, condition_name  -- one row per condition per member
  ) deduped
  GROUP BY member_id
)
SELECT mc.member_id, m.member_name,
  DATEDIFF('year', m.date_of_birth, CURRENT_DATE) AS age,
  COALESCE(mc.cci_score,0) AS cci_score,
  CASE
    WHEN COALESCE(mc.cci_score,0) = 0   THEN 'No comorbidities'
    WHEN COALESCE(mc.cci_score,0) <= 2  THEN 'Mild (CCI 1-2)'
    WHEN COALESCE(mc.cci_score,0) <= 4  THEN 'Moderate (CCI 3-4)'
    ELSE 'Severe (CCI 5+)'
  END AS cci_severity,
  ROUND(ytd.ytd_allowed,0) AS ytd_allowed_cost
FROM  dim_members m
LEFT JOIN member_cci mc ON m.member_id = mc.member_id
LEFT JOIN (SELECT member_id, SUM(allowed_amount) AS ytd_allowed FROM fact_medical_claims
  WHERE claim_status='PAID' AND EXTRACT(YEAR FROM service_date)=EXTRACT(YEAR FROM CURRENT_DATE)
```

```
  GROUP BY member_id) ytd ON m.member_id = ytd.member_id
WHERE m.coverage_status = 'ACTIVE'
ORDER BY cci_score DESC NULLS LAST;
```

22.3 Composite Risk Score & Tier Assignment

Five dimensions: CCI (clinical), cost trajectory (year-over-year PMPM change), utilization (IP admissions, ED visits), pharmacy (polypharmacy flag), and SDOH (ADI quintile). Weighted sum → tier assignment: Tier 1 Low → Tier 4 Complex Care. Use LEFT JOIN + COALESCE(x,0) so healthy members with no claims remain in the model.

ANSI SQL — 22.3: Composite Risk Score and Tier Assignment (Fully Annotated)

```
-- PURPOSE: Build composite risk score combining clinical, financial, utilization,
-- pharmaceutical, and social dimensions for care management tier assignment.
-- LEFT JOIN + COALESCE(x,0) keeps all active members -- healthy ones score 0.
WITH cci_scores AS (
  SELECT member_id, COALESCE(SUM(max_wt),0) AS cci_score
  FROM (
    SELECT DISTINCT c.member_id, cci.condition_name, MAX(cci.cci_weight) AS max_wt
    FROM  fact_medical_claims c
    JOIN  ref_cci_weights cci ON c.primary_diag LIKE cci.icd10_prefix || '%'
    WHERE c.claim_status='PAID'
     AND EXTRACT(YEAR FROM c.service_date)=EXTRACT(YEAR FROM CURRENT_DATE)
    GROUP BY c.member_id, cci.condition_name
  ) x GROUP BY member_id
),
-- Cost trajectory: current PMPM minus prior year PMPM
cost_trajectory AS (
  SELECT cy.member_id,
       COALESCE(cy.pmpm,0) - COALESCE(py.pmpm,0) AS pmpm_change
  FROM (
    SELECT member_id,
         SUM(allowed_amount)/NULLIF(COUNT(DISTINCT DATE_TRUNC('month',service_date)),0) AS pmpm
    FROM fact_medical_claims WHERE claim_status='PAID'
     AND EXTRACT(YEAR FROM service_date)=EXTRACT(YEAR FROM CURRENT_DATE)
    GROUP BY member_id) cy
  LEFT JOIN (
    SELECT member_id,
         SUM(allowed_amount)/NULLIF(COUNT(DISTINCT DATE_TRUNC('month',service_date)),0) AS pmpm
    FROM fact_medical_claims WHERE claim_status='PAID'
     AND EXTRACT(YEAR FROM service_date)=EXTRACT(YEAR FROM CURRENT_DATE)-1
    GROUP BY member_id) py ON cy.member_id=py.member_id
),
-- Utilization: IP admissions and ED visits
util_flags AS (
  SELECT member_id,
       SUM(CASE WHEN type_of_bill LIKE '11%' THEN 1 ELSE 0 END) AS ip_admits,
       SUM(CASE WHEN revenue_code IN ('0450','0456','0459') THEN 1 ELSE 0 END) AS ed_visits
  FROM  fact_medical_claims WHERE claim_status='PAID'
   AND EXTRACT(YEAR FROM service_date)=EXTRACT(YEAR FROM CURRENT_DATE)
  GROUP BY member_id
),
-- Polypharmacy: 10+ unique drug NDC codes in the year
pharmacy_complexity AS (
  SELECT member_id,
       CASE WHEN COUNT(DISTINCT ndc_code)>=10 THEN 1 ELSE 0 END AS polypharmacy_flag
  FROM  fact_pharmacy_claims
  WHERE claim_status='PAID'
   AND EXTRACT(YEAR FROM dispensing_date)=EXTRACT(YEAR FROM CURRENT_DATE)
  GROUP BY member_id
),
-- SDOH risk score from ADI national rank
```

```
sdoh_risk AS (
  SELECT m.member_id,
       CASE WHEN adi.adi_national_rank>=80 THEN 2 – high disadvantage
          WHEN adi.adi_national_rank>=60 THEN 1 -- moderate
          ELSE 0 END AS sdoh_score
  FROM dim_members m
  LEFT JOIN ref_adi_scores adi ON m.zip_code = adi.zip_code
)
SELECT m.member_id, m.member_name, m.date_of_birth,
  COALESCE(cs.cci_score,0)*3
  + CASE WHEN COALESCE(ct.pmpm_change,0)>200 THEN 2 ELSE 0 END
  + COALESCE(uf.ip_admits,0)*4  – IP admission gets highest weight
  + COALESCE(uf.ed_visits,0)*2
  + COALESCE(pc.polypharmacy_flag,0)*2
  + COALESCE(sr.sdoh_score,0)  AS composite_risk_score,
  CASE
    WHEN COALESCE(cs.cci_score,0)*3+CASE WHEN COALESCE(ct.pmpm_change,0)>200 THEN 2 ELSE 0 END
      +COALESCE(uf.ip_admits,0)*4+COALESCE(uf.ed_visits,0)*2
      +COALESCE(pc.polypharmacy_flag,0)*2+COALESCE(sr.sdoh_score,0)>=20
    THEN 'TIER 4 — Complex Care'
    WHEN COALESCE(cs.cci_score,0)*3+CASE WHEN COALESCE(ct.pmpm_change,0)>200 THEN 2 ELSE 0 END
      +COALESCE(uf.ip_admits,0)*4+COALESCE(uf.ed_visits,0)*2
      +COALESCE(pc.polypharmacy_flag,0)*2+COALESCE(sr.sdoh_score,0)>=12
    THEN 'TIER 3 — High Risk'
    WHEN COALESCE(cs.cci_score,0)*3+CASE WHEN COALESCE(ct.pmpm_change,0)>200 THEN 2 ELSE 0 END
      +COALESCE(uf.ip_admits,0)*4+COALESCE(uf.ed_visits,0)*2
      +COALESCE(pc.polypharmacy_flag,0)*2+COALESCE(sr.sdoh_score,0)>=5
    THEN 'TIER 2 — Rising Risk'
    ELSE 'TIER 1 — Low Risk'
  END AS risk_tier
FROM dim_members m
LEFT JOIN cci_scores cs       ON m.member_id=cs.member_id
LEFT JOIN cost_trajectory ct  ON m.member_id=ct.member_id
LEFT JOIN util_flags uf       ON m.member_id=uf.member_id
LEFT JOIN pharmacy_complexity pc ON m.member_id=pc.member_id
LEFT JOIN sdoh_risk sr        ON m.member_id=sr.member_id
WHERE m.coverage_status='ACTIVE'
ORDER BY composite_risk_score DESC;
```

Chapter 22 Review

Unit Test · Key Takeaways

Answer each question before reading the explanation.

Q1. CCI assigns higher weights to:

A. Conditions with higher treatment costs

B. Conditions associated with higher 1-year mortality risk — HIV/AIDS and metastatic solid tumor receive weight 6; moderate-to-severe liver disease weight 3; diabetes without complications weight 1. Weights reflect mortality impact, not cost.

C. Conditions more prevalent in Medicaid

D. Conditions requiring specialty care

Answer: B. *CCI weight 1: MI, CHF, PVD, dementia, COPD, rheumatic disease, peptic ulcer, mild liver disease, diabetes without end-organ damage. Weight 2: hemiplegia, moderate-to-severe CKD, diabetes with end-organ damage, cancer. Weight 3: moderate-to-severe liver disease. Weight 6: HIV/AIDS, metastatic solid tumor.*

Q2. All dimension CTEs use LEFT JOIN (not INNER JOIN) because:

A. LEFT JOIN is always faster

B. Members with no claims, no CCI conditions, or no pharmacy fills would be dropped by INNER JOIN. LEFT JOIN + COALESCE(x,0) keeps all active members with zero scores for missing dimensions — correctly representing them as Tier 1 Low Risk.

C. LEFT JOIN allows NULL values needed for CCI

D. INNER JOIN double-counts members in multiple CTEs

Answer: B. *A healthy member with no claims has no rows in member_cci, util_flags, or pharmacy_complexity. INNER JOIN drops them from output. LEFT JOIN preserves them with null values; COALESCE(x,0) sets those nulls to zero. The member correctly appears in Tier 1 with composite_risk_score = 0.*

Q3. Polypharmacy is defined as 10+ unique NDC codes in the year because:

A. Any member on more than 3 medications simultaneously

B. 10+ unique drugs is a proxy for high pharmaceutical complexity, drug interaction risk, and adherence challenges. This flag adds weight to the composite score. For production, use unique drug classes (not NDC codes) to reduce false positives from multiple short-course antibiotics.

C. Any opioid + benzodiazepine combination

D. More than 12 prescription fills regardless of unique medications

Answer: B. *Clinical standard for polypharmacy: typically 5+ concurrent medications. Claims analytics uses 10+ unique NDC codes in the year as an approximation. Limitation: multiple short-course antibiotics can trigger the flag without true polypharmacy. Improvement: JOIN to ref_drug_class and count unique classes rather than unique NDC codes.*

Q4. Cost trajectory is included in the composite score because:

A. Rising costs indicate fraud

B. A member with moderate current cost trending rapidly upward is likely to become high-cost in the next 12 months. Trajectory captures acceleration — early identification enables preventive intervention before the trend culminates in an expensive admission.

C. CMS requires cost trajectory in all risk models

D. PMPM change is easier to calculate than absolute PMPM

Answer: B. *Predictive logic: a member with CCI=2 and PMPM rising from $200 to $600 (+$400) is at higher future risk than a member with CCI=4 and stable $400 PMPM. The trajectory signal identifies the rate of change, not just the current level. Care managers can intervene on a rising-trajectory member while the clinical situation is still manageable.*

Q5. IP admissions receive the highest weight (×4) because:

A. CMS requires IP weight = 4× in all risk models

B. A member with an inpatient admission has demonstrated the highest clinical acuity and is statistically at 3–4× higher risk of readmission and repeat high-cost utilization compared to members with only ED or outpatient visits

C. IP admissions cost more than ED visits per episode

D. Weight 4 ensures Tier 4 always includes at least one IP admission

Answer: B. *CMS risk adjustment research: prior inpatient admission is one of the strongest predictors of future high-cost utilization. CHF admission = 25–30% 30-day readmission risk. The high IP weight ensures these members float to the top of the care management worklist for intensive post-discharge follow-up.*

Q6. Risk tier thresholds (5, 12, 20) should be:

A. Fixed at these exact values for all plans

B. Plan-specific and calibrated annually so approximately 5% of members fall in Tier 4, 15% in Tier 3, 25% in Tier 2, 55% in Tier 1 — matching the care management program capacity. Thresholds in this chapter are illustrative.

C. Set equal to the CCI score thresholds

D. Approved by NCQA before use

Answer: B. *Calibration process: run the model on the full population, check the tier distribution. If 30% fall in Tier 4, the care management team cannot serve all of them. Adjust thresholds until the Tier 4 count ≈ care management capacity × (1/caseload per CM). Recalibrate annually.*

Q7. Explain the CCI double-counting prevention logic using GROUP BY member_id, condition_name with MAX(cci_weight).

(Short answer)

Sample Answer:

CCI assigns one weight per condition group, not per ICD-10 code. Example: diabetes without complications = E11.0 (weight 1), diabetes with end-organ damage = E11.21 (weight 2). Both are the same CCI condition group at different severity levels. A member with both codes should get CCI weight = 2 (the maximum for diabetes), not 2+1=3. Without GROUP BY condition_name + MAX: both codes produce separate rows in member_conditions, both with different weights. Summing all rows double-counts the diabetes condition. Fix: SELECT member_id, condition_name, MAX(cci_weight) AS max_wt FROM member_conditions GROUP BY member_id, condition_name. This produces one row per member per CCI condition group with the highest applicable weight. Then SUM(max_wt) in the outer query. Same logic applies to liver disease (mild=1, moderate/severe=3) and renal disease (mild=1, moderate/severe=2).

Q8. Describe a care management tier assignment workflow and what intervention is appropriate for each tier.

(Short answer)

Sample Answer:

Tier 4 — Complex Care (score ≥ 20, ~5% of population): dedicated complex care nurse, bi-weekly telephonic outreach, care conference with PCP and specialists, documented care plan, home visit if warranted. Caseload per nurse: 50–75 members. Tier 3 — High Risk (12–19, ~15%): monthly outreach, medication reconciliation, 30-day post-discharge follow-up calls, care gap closure support. Caseload: 150–200. Tier 2 – Rising Risk (5–11, ~25%): quarterly outreach, health coaching, preventive care reminders, HEDIS gap closure via mail or app. Population health approach, not 1:1. Tier 1 — Low Risk (0–4, ~55%): wellness programs, preventive care reminders, annual HRA mailings. No active care management. Delivery: daily ETL job sends updated tier assignments to the care management system. Care managers log in Monday morning to see their caseload sorted by composite_risk_score descending.

Q9. Write the SQL to identify members who escalated from Tier 1–2 to Tier 3–4 between this year and last year.

(Short answer)

Sample Answer:

WITH current_tiers AS (-- composite risk score query for current year → member_id, risk_tier, composite_risk_score, cci_score, ip_admits, cost_trajectory), prior_tiers AS (-- same query for prior year) SELECT ct.member_id, m.member_name, m.date_of_birth, pt.risk_tier AS prior_tier, ct.risk_tier AS current_tier, ct.composite_risk_score AS current_score, pt.composite_risk_score AS prior_score, ct.cci_score, ct.ip_admits FROM current_tiers ct JOIN prior_tiers pt ON ct.member_id=pt.member_id JOIN dim_members m ON ct.member_id=m.member_id WHERE pt.risk_tier IN ('TIER 1 — Low Risk','TIER 2 — Rising Risk') AND ct.risk_tier IN ('TIER 3 — High Risk','TIER 4 — Complex Care') ORDER BY ct.composite_risk_score DESC. This escalation cohort is the highest-ROI care management target: they have entered high complexity but haven't accumulated years of chronic disease history. Members escalating from Tier 2 to Tier 3 due to rising cost trajectory (no IP admission yet) are especially valuable — proactive intervention can prevent the first admission that would escalate them to Tier 4. Deliver this list to care management director weekly.

Q10. Explain trajectory prediction without ML. What indicators are used?

(Short answer)

Sample Answer:

(1) Rolling PMPM slope: calculate PMPM for each of the last 6 months using LAG(). AVG() the month-over-month change = slope. predicted_pmpm_12m = current_pmpm + slope × 12. Rising slope > $50/month = trajectory flag. (2) Admission prediction: member with any IP admission in the last 90 days has 25–35% 30-day readmission probability. SQL: WHERE ip_admits >= 1 AND MAX(ip_service_date) >= CURRENT_DATE - 90. (3) Condition escalation: new high-weight CCI condition (incident case for CCI weight ≥ 2) in the last 6 months = rapid cost escalation expected. SQL: present in current 6-month window, absent in prior year, for ref_cci_weights WHERE cci_weight >= 2. (4) Composite trajectory score: rising_cost_flag × 2 + new_high_weight_CCI × 3 + recent_IP × 4 + escalation_from_lower_tier × 2. Rule-based additive model achieves 60–70% positive predictive value for identifying top-decile future cost members — sufficient for care management targeting, fully explainable without ML black boxes.

Key Takeaways

What every analyst must remember from this chapter.

1 CCI = SUM of MAX weight per condition group. Weights: 1–6. GROUP BY member_id, condition_name before SUM to prevent double-counting. CCI ≥ 5 = severe; 3–4 = moderate; 1–2 = mild; 0 = no comorbidities.

2 Composite risk score: CCI×3 + cost_trajectory_flag×2 + IP_admits×4 + ED_visits×2 + polypharmacy×2 + SDOH×1. LEFT JOIN + COALESCE(x,0) for all dimensions to keep healthy members in the model.

3 Cost trajectory = current_pmpm - prior_pmpm. Rising trajectory (+$200 PMPM) signals a member trending toward high complexity. Early intervention before the first IP admission = highest ROI scenario.

4 Tier thresholds must be calibrated to care management capacity. Target: T4 ≈ 5%, T3 ≈ 15%, T2 ≈ 25%, T1 ≈ 55%. Recalibrate annually. Thresholds in this chapter are illustrative.

5 Polypharmacy flag: 10+ unique NDC codes. For production, use unique drug classes to reduce false positives from multiple short-course antibiotics.

6 Escalation cohort (T1–2 → T3–4): highest-ROI care management target. Early intervention prevents the first admission that escalates a member to T4.

7 Tier interventions: T4 = dedicated nurse, bi-weekly, caseload 50–75. T3 = monthly outreach, medication reconciliation, caseload 150–200. T2 = population programs, quarterly. T1 = wellness, preventive reminders.

8 Simple trajectory prediction: rolling 6-month PMPM slope + IP_admission_flag (last 90 days) + new_high_weight_CCI. Rule-based additive model, ~65% PPV for top-decile future cost. Explainable to medical director without ML.

Chapter 23: Health Equity Analytics

Stratified HEDIS · Wilson confidence intervals · Disparity gap scoring · CMS Health Equity Index

23.1 Health Equity Framework

Health equity analytics measures disparities in care quality, access, and outcomes across demographic groups — race, ethnicity, language, disability, and socioeconomic factors. The CMS Health Equity Index (HEI) rewards plans that improve performance for historically underserved members. The analyst's role: stratify all quality metrics by equity dimensions, quantify gaps, and identify actionable drivers.

> **Data Completeness** Race/ethnicity data completeness in commercial claims is typically < 40%. Best sources: (1) Self-reported enrollment. (2) BISG (Bayesian Improved Surname Geocoding). (3) Geography-based proxy. Always document completeness before interpreting stratified results.

ANSI SQL — 23.1: Stratified HEDIS with Disparity Gap and Wilson CI (Fully Annotated)

```
-- PURPOSE: Calculate HEDIS measure rates by race/ethnicity with Wilson 95% CI.
-- Disparity gap = stratum rate minus plan average. Flag >5pp below = disparity.
-- Used for CMS Health Equity Index (HEI) reporting.
WITH hedis_stratified AS (
  SELECT hg.measure_id, hg.measure_description,
       COALESCE(m.race_ethnicity_self_reported, m.race_ethnicity_bisg,
              'Unknown/Unreported') AS race_ethnicity,
       COUNT(DISTINCT hg.member_id) AS denominator,
       COUNT(DISTINCT CASE WHEN hg.gap_status='CLOSED' THEN hg.member_id END) AS numerator
  FROM  fact_hedis_gaps hg
  JOIN  dim_members m ON hg.member_id = m.member_id
  WHERE hg.measurement_year = EXTRACT(YEAR FROM CURRENT_DATE)
   AND hg.denominator_eligible = 'Y'
  GROUP BY hg.measure_id, hg.measure_description,
        COALESCE(m.race_ethnicity_self_reported, m.race_ethnicity_bisg, 'Unknown/Unreported')
  HAVING COUNT(DISTINCT hg.member_id) >= 30  -- minimum for reportable stratum
),
-- Wilson 95% CI: performs better near 0% and 100%, and with small denominators.
-- Normal approximation fails (produces impossible CIs) for small strata.
-- Wilson formula uses z=1.96; in SQL: 1.92 ≈ z²/2, 3.84 ≈ z².
rates_with_ci AS (
  SELECT measure_id, measure_description, race_ethnicity, denominator, numerator,
       ROUND(100.0*numerator/NULLIF(denominator,0),1) AS rate_pct,
       ROUND(100.0*((numerator+1.92)-1.96*SQRT(numerator*(1.0-numerator/NULLIF(denominator,0.0))+0.96))
         /NULLIF(denominator+3.84,0),1) AS wilson_ci_lower,
       ROUND(100.0*((numerator+1.92)+1.96*SQRT(numerator*(1.0-numerator/NULLIF(denominator,0.0))+0.96))
         /NULLIF(denominator+3.84,0),1) AS wilson_ci_upper
  FROM  hedis_stratified
),
-- Plan-wide overall rate as the disparity benchmark
overall_rate AS (
  SELECT measure_id,
       ROUND(100.0*SUM(numerator)/NULLIF(SUM(denominator),0),1) AS overall_rate_pct
  FROM  hedis_stratified GROUP BY measure_id
)
SELECT rc.measure_id, rc.measure_description, rc.race_ethnicity,
```

```
    rc.denominator, rc.numerator, rc.rate_pct,
    rc.wilson_ci_lower, rc.wilson_ci_upper,
    ov.overall_rate_pct,
    ROUND(rc.rate_pct - ov.overall_rate_pct,1) AS gap_vs_plan_avg,
    -- Disparity flag: >5pp below plan average
    CASE WHEN rc.rate_pct < ov.overall_rate_pct - 5
        THEN 'DISPARITY — >5pp below plan average'
        ELSE 'Within 5pp of plan average' END AS disparity_flag
FROM rates_with_ci rc
JOIN overall_rate ov ON rc.measure_id = ov.measure_id
ORDER BY rc.measure_id, rc.rate_pct ASC;
```

Chapter 23 Review

Unit Test · Key Takeaways

Answer each question before reading the explanation.

Q1. Wilson CI is preferred over normal approximation for stratified HEDIS because:

A. Wilson CI is required by NCQA for all stratified reporting

B. Normal approximation (p ± 1.96×SE) performs poorly when proportions are near 0% or 100% or with small denominators — which are common in racial/ethnic subgroups. Wilson CI remains well-behaved across the full 0–100% range.

C. Wilson CI always produces narrower intervals

D. Normal approximation cannot be computed in SQL

Answer: B. *Normal approximation with n=30, rate=100%: $\sqrt{(1\times 0/30)} = 0 \rightarrow$ CI collapses to [100%, 100%] — falsely implying perfect certainty. Wilson CI handles this correctly. SQL implementation: $1.92 \approx z^2/2$, $3.84 \approx z^2$. The formula shifts the proportion center by $z^2/2$ to stay within [0%,100%].*

Q2. Race/ethnicity data completeness in commercial claims is typically:

A. > 90% — required by ACA Section 4302

B. < 40% — not required on CMS 1500 or UB-04 claim forms. Best sources: self-reported enrollment (20–40% complete), BISG using surname + ZIP (60–75% effective completeness), geographic proxy for area-level only.

C. > 75% for Medicare Advantage

D. Exactly 100% — required field on the 837

Answer: B. *Race/ethnicity is voluntary on enrollment applications. Commercial populations: typically 20–40%. BISG (Bayesian Improved Surname Geocoding) probabilistically assigns race/ethnicity from surname + ZIP using Census data, improving effective completeness to 60–75%. Always report data completeness alongside stratified results.*

Q3. The CMS Health Equity Index rewards plans that:

A. Have highest overall HEDIS performance

B. Show improvement in HEDIS performance specifically for members from historically underserved populations (Black, Hispanic, AIAN, NHOPI, dual-eligible, LTSS, disabled) — separate from overall Stars score

C. Submit complete race/ethnicity data for >80% of members

D. Maintain network adequacy in high-ADI counties

Answer: B. *HEI was introduced in MA Star Ratings to create direct financial incentives for reducing health disparities. A plan earns HEI credit by improving breast cancer screening rates for Black women or diabetes care for Hispanic members. Plans should target gap closure efforts specifically to underserved populations, not just the overall denominator.*

Q4. A disparity gap of −12 percentage points means:

A. The group has 12 fewer members in the HEDIS denominator

B. That group's HEDIS rate is 12 percentage points below the plan average — a significant disparity requiring targeted gap closure outreach. Plan average 68%, Hispanic subgroup 56%: gap = 56% - 68% = -12pp.

C. The group has 12 more open gaps per member

D. Wilson CI lower bound is 12 points below the estimate

Answer: B. *Disparity flags: 5pp below plan average = moderate disparity. 10+pp = significant, requiring a formal improvement plan. CMS HEI uses lowest-performing group vs. highest-performing group gap. Identifying both the gap AND the root cause (language barrier, access issue, documentation gap) makes the finding actionable.*

Q5. BISG improves race/ethnicity data completeness by:

A. Sending member surveys through the portal

B. Using surname + ZIP to probabilistically estimate race/ethnicity via Bayesian statistics and Census Bureau surname/geographic race distributions

C. Importing race/ethnicity from EHR via FHIR

D. Applying national prevalence rates to fill in missing values uniformly

Answer: B. *BISG: posterior = P(surname|race) × P(race|ZIP) / normalizing constant. Outputs probability vector across racial/ethnic categories. Assign highest-probability category. Accuracy: ~82% Black, ~79% Hispanic, ~65% AIAN, ~55% NHOPI. BISG was developed by RAND Corporation.*

Q6. HAVING COUNT(DISTINCT hg.member_id) >= 30 ensures:

A. Meets NCQA minimum denominator for Stars

B. Statistical reliability — strata with < 30 members have too-wide CIs to distinguish a true disparity from random variation. With n=10 at 80%: Wilson CI ≈ [44%, 96%] — 52pp wide, not actionable. At n=30: ≈ [62%, 91%] — 29pp wide. Label sub-30 as "insufficient data."

C. Prevents Wilson CI divide-by-zero

D. Only active members at measurement date are included

Answer: B. *NCQA minimum for HEDIS stratification: 11 members. CMS HEI: 30+. For internal analytics, 30 is the appropriate minimum for reporting a disparity flag. Below threshold: label "insufficient data" and do not suppress silently — include the count in a data quality footnote.*

Q7. Describe the CMS Health Equity Index methodology and how to build the HEI calculation in SQL.

(Short answer)

Sample Answer:

CMS HEI (MA Star Ratings): calculates the plan's HEDIS rate for the disadvantaged subpopulation and rewards year-over-year improvement. SQL Step 1 — Define disadvantaged: SELECT DISTINCT member_id FROM dim_members WHERE dual_eligible_flag='Y' OR lis_flag='Y' OR disability_flag='Y' OR race_ethnicity_bisg IN ('Black','Hispanic','AIAN','NHOPI'). Step 2 — Calculate rates: SELECT COALESCE(d.disadvantaged_flag,0) AS disadvantaged, measure_id, COUNT(DISTINCT hg.member_id) AS denom, ROUND(100.0*COUNT(DISTINCT CASE WHEN gap_status='CLOSED' THEN hg.member_id END)/COUNT(DISTINCT hg.member_id),1) AS rate_pct FROM fact_hedis_gaps hg LEFT JOIN (SELECT member_id, 1 AS disadvantaged_flag FROM disadvantaged_pop) d ON hg.member_id=d.member_id GROUP BY COALESCE(d.disadvantaged_flag,0), measure_id. Step 3 — Year-over-year improvement: JOIN current to prior year rates WHERE disadvantaged=1; calculate rate_change. HEI credit = improvement. Step 4 — Gap closure prioritization: for each HEI measure, sort by (gap_size × denominator_size) = maximum HEI impact per intervention dollar.

Q8. A plan finds a 15pp disparity in breast cancer screening for Black women. Describe the investigation and intervention SQL.

(Short answer)

Sample Answer:

Investigation: Step 1 — Confirm statistical significance: Wilson CI for Black women stratum. If CI does not overlap plan average CI, the gap is statistically significant. Step 2 — Access vs. quality: GROUP BY attributed_pcp_npi where m.race_ethnicity_bisg='Black' AND m.gender='F' for BCS measure. Are low rates concentrated in specific PCPs or counties? Step 3 — Outreach channel: what % have valid phone, email, mailing address? Step 4 — Language: what % prefer non-English? Intervention list SQL: SELECT m.member_id, m.member_name, m.preferred_language, m.phone, m.address FROM dim_members m JOIN fact_hedis_gaps hg ON m.member_id=hg.member_id WHERE hg.measure_id='BCS' AND hg.gap_status='OPEN' AND m.race_ethnicity_bisg='Black' AND m.gender='F'. Route to community health workers fluent in the member's language. Partner with community organizations (churches, community centers) in high-ADI ZIP codes for trusted messenger outreach.

Q9. Explain the Wilson CI formula and why it handles small denominators better than normal approximation.

(Short answer)

Sample Answer:

Normal approximation: $p \pm 1.96\times\sqrt{p(1-p)/n}$. Failure at extreme proportions: p=100%, n=30 → $\sqrt{1\times0/30}=0$ → CI collapses to [100%,100%] — falsely implying perfect certainty. Wilson CI formula: lower = $(n\times p + z^2/2 - z\times\sqrt{n\times p\times(1-p) + z^2/4}) / (n+z^2)$. Upper = same with + instead of −. The formula centers on a shifted proportion (numerator + $z^2/2$)/(denominator + z^2), expanding the interval appropriately when p is near 0 or 1. SQL approximation: $1.92 \approx z^2/2$ ($1.96^2/2 = 1.9208$), $3.84 \approx z^2$ ($1.96^2 = 3.8416$). At n=30, p=100%: Wilson CI upper ≈ 99.5% — does not collapse to 100%. The interval correctly reflects uncertainty from small n.

Q10. Describe the three data sources for race/ethnicity and how to document and report data quality.

(Short answer)

Sample Answer:
Source 1 — Self-reported enrollment: voluntary at enrollment. Completeness: 20–40% commercial, 60–70% Medicaid. Documentation SQL: SELECT race_ethnicity_self_reported, COUNT(*) AS count, ROUND(100.0*COUNT(*)/SUM(COUNT(*)) OVER(),1) AS pct FROM dim_members WHERE coverage_status='ACTIVE' GROUP BY race_ethnicity_self_reported. Report: XX% self-reported; YY% Unknown. Source 2 — BISG: probabilistic from surname + ZIP. Accuracy: ~80% Black/Hispanic; ~65% AIAN/NHOPI. Report % of members with BISG confidence score ≥ 0.70 as "high confidence." Source 3 — Geographic proxy: member ZIP → Census tract → ACS race/ethnicity distribution. Least accurate; appropriate only for area-level analysis, not individual assignment. Data quality statement (required in every stratified report): "Race/ethnicity data source: self-reported (XX%), BISG (YY%), geographic proxy (ZZ%), unknown (WW%)." Never present stratified results without completeness caveat. CMS and NCQA regulatory submissions require data completeness documentation.

Key Takeaways

What every analyst must remember from this chapter.

1. Stratify all quality measures by race/ethnicity, language, dual eligibility, disability, and ADI quintile. Disparity flag: rate > 5pp below plan average. Significant: > 10pp. CMS HEI rewards improvement for disadvantaged members.

2. Race/ethnicity completeness: self-reported < 40%, BISG 60–75%, geographic proxy area-level only. Document and report completeness alongside every stratified result.

3. Wilson CI: $1.92 = z^2/2$, $3.84 = z^2$. Handles near-0% and near-100% rates and small n without producing impossible values. Use for all stratified HEDIS reporting.

4. Minimum stratum: 30 for internal, 11 per NCQA, 30+ per CMS HEI. Label sub-threshold as "insufficient data" — never suppress silently.

5. Disparity investigation: (1) Confirm with Wilson CI. (2) PCP/geographic clustering. (3) Outreach channel availability. (4) Language preference. Targeted intervention: community health workers, trusted messenger outreach.

6. BISG: P(surname|race) × P(race|ZIP) / normalizing constant. Outputs probability vector. Best accuracy: Black (~82%), Hispanic (~79%). Lower: AIAN (~60%), NHOPI (~55%).

7. CMS HEI SQL: disadvantaged = dual_eligible OR LIS OR disability OR BISG race. Calculate year-over-year rate improvement. Prioritize by gap_size × denominator_size.

8. Language barriers are often the root cause of HEDIS gaps for non-English speakers. Join preferred_language to outreach lists. Route to language-matched community health workers.

Chapter 24: Prior Authorization Analytics

72-hr turnaround · MHPAEA parity · Gold carding · CMS 2026 PA rule

24.1 PA Framework & CMS 2026 Rule

Prior authorization analytics tracks: (1) Turnaround time compliance (CMS: ≤72 hours urgent, ≤7 days standard). (2) Denial rate by service type. (3) MHPAEA parity (BH PA requirements not more restrictive than medical/surgical). (4) Gold carding eligibility (providers with high approval rates exempted).

> **CMS 2026 PA Rule** CMS Interoperability and PA Final Rule (CMS-0057-F): MA plans, Medicaid, and CHIP must implement PA APIs, respond to urgent PAs within 72 hours, standard within 7 calendar days, and publish PA reason codes electronically. Analytics must track all turnaround requirements.

ANSI SQL — 24.1: PA Turnaround Time Compliance (Fully Annotated)

```sql
-- PURPOSE: Measure PA processing time against CMS requirements.
-- Urgent ≤72 hours. Standard ≤7 calendar days.
-- Track denial rates and identify worst-compliance service types.
WITH pa_metrics AS (
  SELECT pa.auth_id, pa.member_id, pa.requesting_npi,
      pa.service_category, pa.urgency_flag,
      pa.request_date, pa.decision_date, pa.decision,
      pa.denial_reason_code,
      DATEDIFF('hour',pa.request_date,pa.decision_date) AS processing_hours,
      DATEDIFF('day', pa.request_date,pa.decision_date) AS processing_days,
      CASE
        WHEN pa.urgency_flag='URGENT'
         AND DATEDIFF('hour',pa.request_date,pa.decision_date)<=72
        THEN 'COMPLIANT — urgent within 72 hrs'
        WHEN pa.urgency_flag='URGENT'
         AND DATEDIFF('hour',pa.request_date,pa.decision_date)>72
        THEN 'VIOLATION — urgent exceeded 72 hrs'
        WHEN pa.urgency_flag='STANDARD'
         AND DATEDIFF('day',pa.request_date,pa.decision_date)<=7
        THEN 'COMPLIANT — standard within 7 days'
        ELSE 'VIOLATION — standard exceeded 7 days'
      END AS compliance_status
  FROM  fact_prior_auth pa
  WHERE pa.request_date >= CURRENT_DATE - INTERVAL '90' DAY
   AND pa.decision IN ('APPROVED','DENIED')
)
SELECT service_category, urgency_flag,
  COUNT(*) AS total_requests,
  ROUND(100.0*SUM(CASE WHEN compliance_status LIKE 'COMPLIANT%' THEN 1 ELSE 0 END)
    /COUNT(*),1) AS compliance_rate_pct,
  ROUND(100.0*SUM(CASE WHEN decision='DENIED' THEN 1 ELSE 0 END)/COUNT(*),1) AS denial_rate_pct,
  ROUND(AVG(processing_hours),1) AS avg_processing_hours,
  ROUND(PERCENTILE_CONT(0.90) WITHIN GROUP (ORDER BY processing_hours),1) AS p90_processing_hours,
  MAX(processing_hours) AS max_processing_hours
FROM  pa_metrics
GROUP BY service_category, urgency_flag
ORDER BY compliance_rate_pct ASC; -- worst compliance first
```

24.2 MHPAEA Parity Analytics

MHPAEA prohibits prior authorization requirements for BH/SUD that are more restrictive than those for comparable medical/surgical services. Compare PA denial rates and processing times across BH vs. medical/surgical — BH significantly worse = potential NQTL parity violation.

ANSI SQL — 24.2: MHPAEA PA Parity Comparison (Fully Annotated)

```
-- PURPOSE: Compare PA denial rates and processing times BH/SUD vs Medical/Surgical.
-- BH denial rate significantly higher than Medical = potential MHPAEA violation.
WITH parity_comparison AS (
  SELECT
    CASE WHEN pa.service_category IN
          ('Mental Health Outpatient','Mental Health Inpatient',
           'SUD Outpatient','SUD Residential','SUD Detox')
       THEN 'BH/SUD' ELSE 'Medical/Surgical' END AS benefit_classification,
    pa.urgency_flag, pa.auth_id, pa.member_id, pa.decision,
    DATEDIFF('hour',pa.request_date,pa.decision_date) AS processing_hours
  FROM  fact_prior_auth pa
  WHERE pa.request_date >= CURRENT_DATE - INTERVAL '12' MONTH
   AND pa.decision IN ('APPROVED','DENIED')
)
SELECT benefit_classification, urgency_flag,
  COUNT(*) AS total_pa_requests,
  ROUND(100.0*SUM(CASE WHEN decision='DENIED' THEN 1 ELSE 0 END)/COUNT(*),1) AS denial_rate_pct,
  ROUND(AVG(processing_hours),1) AS avg_processing_hours,
  ROUND(PERCENTILE_CONT(0.90) WITHIN GROUP (ORDER BY processing_hours),1) AS p90_processing_hours,
  COUNT(DISTINCT member_id) AS unique_members
FROM  parity_comparison
GROUP BY benefit_classification, urgency_flag
ORDER BY benefit_classification, urgency_flag;
-- PARITY VIOLATION INDICATORS:
-- BH denial_rate_pct significantly > Medical denial_rate_pct (same urgency)
-- BH avg/p90 processing hours significantly > Medical
-- "Significantly" = 5+ pp or 24+ hrs difference, or chi-square test result.
```

Chapter 24 Review

Unit Test · Key Takeaways

Answer each question before reading the explanation.

Q1. CMS regulatory turnaround time for urgent PA is:

A. 24 hours
B. 48 hours
C. 72 hours — CMS Interoperability and PA Final Rule (CMS-0057-F). Standard (non-urgent): ≤7 calendar days. Applies to MA, Medicaid, CHIP.
D. 7 calendar days

Answer: C. *SQL: DATEDIFF('hour', request_date, decision_date) <= 72 for urgent; DATEDIFF('day', ...) <= 7 for standard. Violations = regulatory exposure. Monitor DAILY for PAs approaching the deadline (flag urgent PAs at 48 hours still pending).*

Q2. MHPAEA parity is violated when:

A. A plan charges higher copays for BH than primary care
B. PA requirements, treatment limitations, or NQTLs applied to BH/SUD are more restrictive than those applied to substantially all medical/surgical benefits in the same classification
C. A plan does not cover 30 days of inpatient BH
D. More than 20% of BH PAs are denied in a quarter

Answer: B. *MHPAEA prohibits more restrictive quantitative limits (day/visit) AND non-quantitative limits (PA requirements, step therapy) for BH/SUD vs. medical/surgical. If BH denial rate is significantly higher for the same urgency level, this is a potential NQTL violation requiring MHPAEA compliance team investigation.*

Q3. Gold carding exempts providers from PA for specific services when:

A. They are Board certified in their specialty

B. Their demonstrated historical PA approval rate meets or exceeds the plan's threshold (typically 90%+) over 12 months with minimum volume (≥20 requests) — adding administrative burden with essentially no clinical benefit for these providers

C. They are credentialed at a Tier 1 hospital

D. CMS mandates gold carding for providers with > 10 years in network

Answer: B. *Gold carding acknowledges that PA targeting inappropriate services has zero utility for a provider with 98% approval rate. Most state gold carding laws set threshold at 90%+. Eligibility SQL: GROUP BY requesting_npi × service_category, HAVING total_requests >= 20 AND approval_rate >= 90%. Review quarterly — revoke if rate drops below threshold.*

Q4. P90 processing time is a better compliance metric than average because:

A. P90 is required by CMS in PA compliance reports

B. Average can mask a long tail: if 80% of PAs complete in 2 hours but 10% take 120+ hours, the average appears compliant while 10% of members experienced regulatory violations. P90 reveals the experience of those waiting longest.

C. P90 is easier to calculate

D. CMS defines compliance using P90

Answer: B. *PERCENTILE_CONT(0.90) WITHIN GROUP (ORDER BY processing_hours). A P90 of 92 hours for urgent PAs means 10% of urgent requests took longer than 72 hours — all regulatory violations. Present: compliance_rate_pct + avg_processing_hours + p90_processing_hours together for complete picture.*

Q5. Step therapy (fail-first) is MHPAEA-relevant because:

A. It adds CPT codes qualifying as quantitative limits

B. Requiring BH/SUD patients to fail a first-line treatment before approving second-line is an NQTL. If required for BH but NOT for comparable medical conditions, it creates an asymmetric administrative burden — a parity violation.

C. Step therapy applies only to pharmacy

D. Step therapy is exempt under MHPAEA safe harbor

Answer: B. *Common MHPAEA NQTL violations: step therapy for SUD medications (e.g., buprenorphine) not required for comparable medical biologics; PA required for all BH inpatient but only specific medical conditions; PA trigger after Day 7 for BH inpatient vs. Day 14 for medical. SQL: compare PA_required_flag and step_therapy_required_flag for BH vs. medical across all service categories.*

Q6. PA denial reason codes are important analytically because:

A. Required by CMS on all denied PAs

B. Each denial code identifies the specific clinical or administrative basis — allowing the analyst to determine whether denials are from missing documentation, medical necessity criteria, experimental/investigational, or network issues — routing each to a different operational fix.

C. They determine the appeal rights timeline

D. Denial codes are the primary input for MHPAEA calculation

Answer: B. *Denial reason categories and fixes: Missing documentation → provider documentation checklist. Medical necessity not met → review clinical criteria vs. accepted guidelines. Experimental/investigational → verify current guideline status. OON provider → direct to in-network alternative. Analyze denial reasons by service category to identify the primary operational failure driving the denial rate.*

Q7. Build a gold carding eligibility analysis. Write the SQL.

(Short answer)

Sample Answer:

SELECT pa.requesting_npi, p.provider_full_name, p.specialty_group, pa.service_category, COUNT(*) AS total_pa, SUM(CASE WHEN pa.decision='APPROVED' THEN 1 ELSE 0 END) AS approvals, ROUND(100.0*SUM(CASE WHEN pa.decision='APPROVED' THEN 1 ELSE 0 END)/COUNT(*),1) AS approval_rate_pct, CASE WHEN COUNT(*)>=20 AND ROUND(100.0*SUM(CASE WHEN pa.decision='APPROVED' THEN 1 ELSE 0 END)/COUNT(*),1)>=90 THEN 'GOLD CARD ELIGIBLE' ELSE 'Standard PA required' END AS gold_card_status FROM fact_prior_auth pa JOIN dim_providers p ON pa.requesting_npi=p.npi WHERE pa.request_date>=CURRENT_DATE-INTERVAL '12' MONTH AND pa.decision IN ('APPROVED','DENIED') GROUP BY pa.requesting_npi, p.provider_full_name, p.specialty_group, pa.service_category HAVING COUNT(*)>=20 ORDER BY approval_rate_pct DESC. Minimum 20 requests for statistical reliability. Operationally: adjudication system bypasses PA for claims from gold-card-eligible providers for the exempted service type. Review quarterly. Provider whose rate drops below threshold loses gold card status.

Q8. Write the SQL to identify PA denials overturned on appeal. What does this pattern tell the UM director?

(Short answer)

Sample Answer:
SELECT pa.auth_id, pa.member_id, pa.requesting_npi, pa.service_category, pa.decision AS initial_decision, pa.denial_reason_code, r.carc_description, ap.appeal_decision, DATEDIFF('day',pa.decision_date,ap.appeal_decision_date) AS days_to_overturn FROM fact_prior_auth pa JOIN fact_pa_appeals ap ON pa.auth_id=ap.auth_id AND ap.appeal_decision='OVERTURNED' JOIN ref_pa_denial_codes r ON pa.denial_reason_code=r.code WHERE pa.decision='DENIED' AND pa.request_date>=CURRENT_DATE-INTERVAL '12' MONTH ORDER BY pa.service_category, pa.denial_reason_code. Interpretation: (1) High overturn rate for specific denial code = initial criteria too restrictive or inconsistently applied. 60% overturn rate on "medical necessity not met" for BH inpatient → criteria need revision. (2) High overturn rate for specific service type = criteria misaligned with current clinical evidence. 70% overturn on genetic testing → outdated coverage policy. (3) High overturn rate for specific provider = they learned what documentation to submit on appeal; work with them to get it right on initial submission. (4) Long days_to_overturn (>30) = members waited unnecessarily. Regulatory and clinical implications, especially for urgent services.

Q9. Describe how the CMS 2026 PA Final Rule changes analytics requirements.

(Short answer)

Sample Answer:
CMS-0057-F effective 2026: (1) PA API: MA, Medicaid, CHIP must implement FHIR-based PA API. Analyst requirement: all PA requests captured in structured database — paper PAs digitized and tracked. Complete database: auth_id, request_date, decision_date, decision, denial_reason_code for every request. (2) Turnaround: urgent ≤72 hrs, standard ≤7 days. Analytics: DAILY automated compliance report; alert system for PAs approaching deadline (flag urgent at 48 hours pending). (3) Denial reason codes: must align with published clinical criteria using CMS-standardized codes — ad hoc internal codes insufficient. (4) Annual public reporting: approval rates, denial rates, overturn rates, avg processing times by service category. Analyst builds regulatory reporting tables with data quality certification. (5) Gold carding: state laws triggered by CMS rule require gold carding programs. Analyst SQL runs quarterly and feeds directly into adjudication exemption list.

Q10. BH inpatient PA denial rate = 28% vs. medical/surgical 9%. Walk through the MHPAEA compliance investigation.

(Short answer)

Sample Answer:
Step 1 — Statistical significance: chi-square test or Fisher's exact on denial counts. Large volumes → 19pp gap almost certainly significant. Document calculation. Step 2 — Decompose by denial reason: SELECT benefit_classification, denial_reason_code, COUNT(*) GROUP BY both WHERE decision='DENIED'. Is the gap driven by one code (operational issue) or broadly distributed (criteria-level issue)? Step 3 — Compare criteria: pull BH inpatient criteria and medical/surgical criteria side-by-side. Any additional BH requirement = potential NQTL. Step 4 — Reviewer qualifications: are BH PAs reviewed by licensed mental health professionals? Reviewer qualification is itself an NQTL under MHPAEA. Step 5 — Document: MHPAEA comparative analysis showing criteria comparison, statistical denial rate gap, denial reason distribution for both benefit types. Present to Compliance Officer and CMO. Step 6 — Remediation: if criteria-level violation confirmed, plan must revise BH criteria to match comparable medical criteria. Cannot lower medical criteria instead to close the gap.

Key Takeaways

What every analyst must remember from this chapter.

1 PA turnaround: urgent ≤72 hours, standard ≤7 days (CMS 2026 rule). DATEDIFF('hour', request_date, decision_date) <= 72 for urgent. Monitor DAILY. Flag urgent PAs at 48 hours still pending.

2 MHPAEA: compare denial_rate_pct and avg/p90_processing_hours for BH/SUD vs. Medical/Surgical. BH significantly worse = potential NQTL violation → escalate to Compliance and CMO.

3 Gold carding: GROUP BY requesting_npi × service_category, approval_rate_pct over 12 months. HAVING total >= 20. ≥90% = GOLD CARD ELIGIBLE. Review quarterly; revoke if rate drops.

4 PA denial root cause: GROUP BY denial_reason_code × service_category. High overturn rate = criteria too restrictive or inconsistently applied. Route fixes to specific operational teams.

5 P90 (PERCENTILE_CONT(0.90)) reveals the tail — the 10% who waited longest. Present with avg and compliance_rate_pct for complete picture. P90 > 72 hours for urgent = regulatory violations in the tail.

6 Step therapy as NQTL: if required for BH/SUD but not comparable medical → parity violation. Also check: PA after Day 7 BH inpatient vs. Day 14 medical; PA for all BH outpatient vs. limited medical outpatient.

7 CMS 2026 analytics requirements: complete PA database, daily turnaround monitoring, CMS-standardized denial codes, annual public reporting, quarterly gold card eligibility refresh.

8 Overturn rate > 20% for any denial code = initial criteria may be wrong. Report: "We denied X BH inpatient PAs; Y% overturned on appeal. We are delaying care with no clinical benefit."

Chapter 25: RAPS/EDPS Risk Adjustment Submission

HCC capture gaps · RAPS vs. EDPS · Submission windows · Revenue optimization

25.1 Risk Adjustment Overview

Medicare Advantage plans receive risk-adjusted capitation from CMS based on the Hierarchical Condition Categories (HCC) of enrolled members. Higher HCC risk scores = higher capitation. Accurate and complete HCC submission is both a compliance and a revenue function. The analyst identifies HCC capture gaps and validates submission accuracy.

> **RAPS vs. EDPS** RAPS = legacy CMS submission format (encounter summary records). EDPS = current required format using complete 837 encounter data with all claim lines and diagnosis codes. CMS phased out RAPS and moved to EDPS from 2016. All encounter data must be submitted through EDPS for risk adjustment credit.

ANSI SQL — 25.1: HCC Capture Gap Analysis (Fully Annotated)

```
-- PURPOSE: Identify members with HCC-qualifying diagnoses in claims
-- that were NOT submitted to CMS via EDPS = capture gap = missed revenue.
-- ref_hcc_crosswalk maps ICD-10 codes to CMS HCC model v28 codes.

-- STEP 1: All HCC-qualifying diagnoses in MA claims this year.
-- Search primary AND secondary diagnosis fields for any HCC code.
WITH claimed_hccs AS (
  SELECT DISTINCT c.member_id, hcc.hcc_code, hcc.hcc_description,
       hcc.raf_increment, -- additional RAF score this HCC adds
       c.rendering_npi, c.service_date, c.primary_diag
  FROM  fact_medical_claims c
  JOIN  ref_hcc_crosswalk hcc
    ON c.primary_diag = hcc.icd10_code
    OR c.diag_2     = hcc.icd10_code
    OR c.diag_3     = hcc.icd10_code
  WHERE c.claim_status = 'PAID'
   AND c.line_of_business = 'MEDICARE_ADVANTAGE'
   -- CMS uses prior year diagnoses to set current year payments
   AND EXTRACT(YEAR FROM c.service_date) = EXTRACT(YEAR FROM CURRENT_DATE) - 1
),
-- STEP 2: HCCs actually submitted and accepted through EDPS
submitted_hccs AS (
  SELECT DISTINCT member_id, hcc_code
  FROM  fact_edps_submissions
  WHERE submission_status = 'ACCEPTED'
   AND data_year = EXTRACT(YEAR FROM CURRENT_DATE) - 1
),
-- Current RAF score per member from CMS payment file
current_raf AS (
  SELECT member_id, total_raf_score
  FROM  raf_scores
  WHERE payment_year = EXTRACT(YEAR FROM CURRENT_DATE)
)
-- STEP 3: LEFT JOIN: NULL submission = HCC in claims but NOT submitted = gap.
SELECT ch.member_id, m.member_name, m.date_of_birth,
  cr.total_raf_score AS current_raf,
  ch.hcc_code, ch.hcc_description,
  ch.raf_increment,  -- RAF the plan is losing by not submitting this HCC
  ch.rendering_npi, p.provider_full_name,
  ch.service_date, ch.primary_diag,
  -- Estimated annual revenue gap: raf_increment × monthly rate × 12 months
```

```
  ROUND(ch.raf_increment * cr_rate.monthly_capitation_rate * 12,0) AS est_annual_revenue_gap
FROM  claimed_hccs ch
LEFT JOIN submitted_hccs sh ON ch.member_id=sh.member_id AND ch.hcc_code=sh.hcc_code
JOIN  dim_members m ON ch.member_id=m.member_id
LEFT JOIN current_raf cr ON ch.member_id=cr.member_id
JOIN  ref_county_rates cr_rate
  ON m.county_fips=cr_rate.county_fips AND cr_rate.payment_year=EXTRACT(YEAR FROM CURRENT_DATE)
WHERE sh.member_id IS NULL  -- HCC exists in claims but NOT in EDPS submission
 AND m.coverage_status = 'ACTIVE'
ORDER BY ch.raf_increment DESC, est_annual_revenue_gap DESC;
-- IMPORTANT: Validate every gap with clinical coders before submitting.
-- Submit corrected encounters within the CMS submission window.
```

Chapter 25 Review

Unit Test · Key Takeaways

Answer each question before reading the explanation.

Q1. EDPS replaced RAPS because:

A. RAPS was too accurate

B. EDPS uses complete 837 encounter data (all claim lines with all diagnosis codes) rather than just encounter summary records. EDPS gives CMS a more accurate and complete view of member clinical conditions for risk score calibration and RADV audit validation.

C. RAPS had higher per-transaction cost

D. EDPS is required for Medicaid but not MA

Answer: B. *RAPS accepted simplified encounter summaries with limited diagnosis codes. EDPS requires the complete 837 — equivalent to the full medical claim with all diagnosis fields. This enables CMS to validate HCC assignments more accurately and detect inflated risk scores. RADV audits can now cross-reference submitted diagnoses against encounter data.*

Q2. An HCC capture gap means:

A. Member's HCC score is lower than their clinical complexity

B. An HCC-qualifying diagnosis is documented in claims but NOT submitted to CMS via EDPS — resulting in a lower RAF score and therefore lower capitation than the member's actual health status warrants. The LEFT JOIN + IS NULL identifies the missing HCCs.

C. An HCC was submitted but rejected by EDPS

D. The plan coded more HCCs than diagnoses support

Answer: B. *The gap analysis uses LEFT JOIN claimed_hccs to submitted_hccs WHERE sh.member_id IS NULL — the same "find records in A not in B" pattern used throughout this book. raf_increment × monthly_capitation × 12 = annual revenue the plan is not receiving. This is legitimate revenue recovery — clinical documentation exists, it was just not submitted.*

Q3. RADV audits verify:

A. Whether the plan's network meets adequacy standards

B. Whether submitted HCC diagnoses are supported by clinical documentation in the medical record. Randomly selected members — auditors request records confirming each submitted HCC. Unsupported HCCs = payment clawbacks extrapolated to the entire contract.

C. Whether the EDPS submission file is correctly formatted

D. Whether the plan's capitation rates are correctly applied by CMS

Answer: B. *RADV readiness: for every submitted HCC, pre-locate the supporting clinical documentation. Check: (a) face-to-face encounter with qualified provider, (b) diagnosis in body of note (not just problem list), (c) licensed provider of record signed the note, (d) ICD-10 specificity supports the HCC. Revenue recovery without RADV readiness creates False Claims Act risk.*

Q4. HCC data year for risk adjustment is:

A. Current calendar year

B. Prior calendar year — diagnoses from year Y → EDPS submission → CMS calculates RAF → drives capitation in year Y+1. Missed HCCs in Y reduce payments in Y+1.

C. Most recent two years combined

D. The Medicare enrollment year

Answer: B. *Timeline: service_date in year Y → claimed in year Y → submit via EDPS → CMS closes submission window (typically mid-year Y+1) → RAF score calculated → drives capitation for months of year Y+1. SQL: WHERE EXTRACT(YEAR FROM c.service_date) = EXTRACT(YEAR FROM CURRENT_DATE) - 1 for the gap analysis.*

Q5. raf_increment in the capture gap query represents:

A. Increase in member risk score if the plan adds any new HCC

B. The additional RAF score coefficient that each specific HCC adds to the member's total score. Multiply by monthly_capitation × 12 = annual revenue the plan is not receiving. HCC 85 (CHF) raf_increment ≈ 0.331 in CMS v28.

C. Difference between current RAF and national average

D. CMS-assigned payment weight for each HCC model version

Answer: B. *Example: raf_increment = 0.331, monthly_capitation = $1,000 → annual_revenue_gap = 0.331 × $1,000 × 12 = $3,972 per member per year for this missing HCC. A large MA plan with hundreds of such gaps across its population can have millions in recoverable annual revenue.*

Q6. HCCs are "hierarchical" because:

A. HCCs are ranked by cost

B. Within each disease family, only the highest-severity HCC is credited — having both CHF (HCC 85) and a lower-ranked cardiac condition in the same hierarchy group earns credit only for CHF. Different disease families (CHF + diabetes) each earn their own credit independently.

C. HCCs must be documented in hierarchical order on the claim

D. The first HCC submitted in the data year takes precedence

Answer: B. *Hierarchy prevents double-counting within related condition groups. CMS v28 hierarchy groups: within each group, only the highest-ranked HCC code is credited to the RAF score. ref_hcc_crosswalk should include hierarchy_group field. Submitting two competing HCCs in the same hierarchy group does not earn both increments — only the higher-ranked one is credited.*

Q7. Describe the complete HCC capture gap workflow from data analysis to revenue recovery. What validation must occur before submitting?

(Short answer)

Sample Answer:
Step 1 — Run gap query: identify all member × HCC in claimed_hccs but absent from submitted_hccs (LEFT JOIN + IS NULL). Step 2 — Prioritize by est_annual_revenue_gap DESC. Top gaps = largest revenue recovery. Step 3 — Clinical documentation validation: before submitting any corrected encounter, coding team verifies: (a) Diagnosis documented in provider's note for that date of service — not inferred from lab results. (b) Documented by licensed provider of record (MD, DO, NP, PA) — not by nurse alone. (c) Encounter was face-to-face or telehealth equivalent. (d) ICD-10 specificity supports the HCC (e.g., CHF documented as "congestive heart failure" — shorthand alone may be insufficient). Step 4 — Corrected encounter submission: submit corrected 837 through EDPS within CMS submission window (typically closes mid-year for prior data year). Step 5 — Track acceptance: monitor fact_edps_submissions. If EDPS rejects: investigate rejection reason (not enrolled, invalid NPI, date out of range). Step 6 — RADV readiness: maintain digital copy of supporting documentation for every submitted HCC. CMS RADV audit response window: 30–45 days. Revenue recovery without documentation readiness = False Claims Act risk.

Q8. Explain HCC model v24 vs. v28. Why does the model version matter for analytics?

(Short answer)

Sample Answer:
CMS HCC v24 (through 2023): 86 HCC codes, calibrated to 2012–2014 Medicare FFS data. CMS HCC v28 (phased in 2024+): 115 HCC codes, recalibrated to more recent experience, revised ICD-10 mappings reflecting ICD-10 coding evolution, eliminates some groups that were difficult to validate clinically. Why it matters: (1) ICD-10 to HCC crosswalk changes — a code mapping to HCC X in v24 may map differently in v28. Always use model_version matching the payment year: WHERE model_version = :payment_year_version. (2) RAF increment coefficients change — same HCC may be worth a different RAF in v28. Revenue projections using v24 coefficients will be wrong for v28 years. (3) New HCCs in v28 = new capture gap opportunities. (4) CMS transition blend: 2024 = 67% v28 + 33% v24; 2025 = 33% v28 + 67% v24; 2026 = 100% v28. Apply correct blend ratio in revenue projections during transition years. SQL: JOIN ref_hcc_crosswalk WHERE model_version = :blended_year_version (or apply weighted average of both v24 and v28 results).

Q9. Write the SQL to calculate the total annual revenue impact of all HCC capture gaps for the MA book of business.

(Short answer)

Sample Answer:
WITH capture_gaps AS (-- HCC capture gap query: member_id, hcc_code, raf_increment), member_gaps AS (SELECT cg.member_id, SUM(cg.raf_increment) AS total_gap_raf FROM capture_gaps cg GROUP BY cg.member_id), revenue_impact AS (SELECT mg.member_id, m.county_fips, mg.total_gap_raf, cr.monthly_capitation_rate, ROUND(mg.total_gap_raf * cr.monthly_capitation_rate * 12,0) AS annual_revenue_gap FROM member_gaps mg JOIN dim_members m ON mg.member_id=m.member_id JOIN ref_county_rates cr ON m.county_fips=cr.county_fips AND cr.payment_year=EXTRACT(YEAR FROM CURRENT_DATE)) SELECT SUM(annual_revenue_gap) AS

total_portfolio_revenue_gap, COUNT(DISTINCT member_id) AS members_with_gaps, ROUND(AVG(annual_revenue_gap),0) AS avg_gap_per_member, MAX(annual_revenue_gap) AS max_single_member_gap FROM revenue_impact. Segment by county: GROUP BY county_fips, county_name ORDER BY county_gap DESC. Typical finding: top 10% of members with gaps account for 50–60% of total gap revenue. Focus clinical documentation improvement on highest-gap members first. Present total_portfolio_revenue_gap to CFO and VP Clinical Quality as the annual HCC improvement program business case.

Q10. Describe the RADV audit process and how the analyst prepares the plan for response.

(Short answer)

Sample Answer:

RADV process: CMS randomly selects ~200 MA members per contract. For each, CMS requests the medical record supporting every submitted HCC. Plan has 30–45 days to produce records. Independent medical record reviewer (MRR) codes records to determine whether each HCC is supported. Unsupported HCCs = payment clawbacks + extrapolated adjustment to entire contract. RADV preparation SQL: SELECT m.member_id, m.member_name, es.hcc_code, hcc.hcc_description, hcc.raf_increment, es.service_date, es.rendering_npi, p.provider_full_name FROM fact_edps_submissions es JOIN dim_members m ON es.member_id=m.member_id JOIN ref_hcc_crosswalk hcc ON es.hcc_code=hcc.hcc_code JOIN dim_providers p ON es.rendering_npi=p.npi WHERE es.data_year=EXTRACT(YEAR FROM CURRENT_DATE)-1 AND es.submission_status='ACCEPTED' ORDER BY m.member_id, hcc.raf_increment DESC. Use as RADV audit prep index. Pre-locate and digitize supporting documentation for every submitted HCC for the highest-RAF members. RADV readiness checklist per HCC: (a) Face-to-face encounter with qualified provider type. (b) Licensed provider of record signed the note. (c) Diagnosis in body of note — not just problem list or medication list. (d) Diagnosis consistent with clinical picture documented. (e) ICD-10 code specificity meets CMS v28 guidelines. Plans with robust RADV readiness have faster response times, fewer unsupported HCCs, and lower audit clawback risk.

Key Takeaways

What every analyst must remember from this chapter.

1 HCC capture gap: LEFT JOIN claimed_hccs to submitted_hccs WHERE sh.member_id IS NULL. Revenue impact = raf_increment × monthly_capitation × 12. Prioritize by revenue impact. Validate with clinical coders before submitting.

2 EDPS replaced RAPS: submit complete 837 with all diagnosis codes. RAPS accepted summaries; EDPS requires full claim. All CMS risk adjustment credit flows through accepted EDPS submissions.

3 CMS HCC data year: diagnoses from year Y → EDPS → RAF score → capitation in Y+1. Submit corrections before submission window closes (typically mid-year Y+1).

4 RADV readiness: digital index of all submitted HCCs mapped to supporting encounter. Pre-locate records for highest-RAF members. Response window: 30–45 days. Robust readiness reduces clawback risk.

5 Validate before submitting HCC corrections: face-to-face encounter, licensed provider of record, diagnosis in body of note, ICD-10 specificity meets v28 guidelines. Submit only supported diagnoses.

6 HCC hierarchy: within disease family, only highest-ranked HCC credited. JOIN ref_hcc_crosswalk with hierarchy_group to identify competing HCCs. Submitting competing HCCs does not earn both increments.

7 HCC model versions: v24 (86 HCCs) vs. v28 (115 HCCs). Always use model_version matching the payment year. CMS blended v24/v28 in 2024–2025 transition. Revenue projections must use correct blend ratio.

8 HCC improvement ROI: top 10% of members with gaps account for 50–60% of total gap revenue. Focus clinical documentation programs on highest-gap members and provider groups.

Chapter 26:Care Management & Predictive Modeling

Risk targeting · Intervention assignment · Program ROI · Admission prediction · 30-day readmission

26.1 Care Management Framework

Care management programs intervene on high-risk members to prevent avoidable admissions, improve medication adherence, close care gaps, and connect members to community resources. Analytics supports three functions: (1) Identifying the right members for each program. (2) Measuring whether interventions are working. (3) Calculating program ROI for CMO and CFO.

26.2 30-Day Readmission Prevention Worklist

The post-discharge readmission worklist identifies members discharged from inpatient in the last 7 days who have NOT yet been contacted by a care manager. Post-discharge follow-up within 2 business days reduces 30-day readmission by an estimated 20–30%.

ANSI SQL — 26.2: Post-Discharge Readmission Risk Worklist (Fully Annotated)

```
-- PURPOSE: Identify recently discharged members not yet contacted by a care manager.
-- Prioritize by readmission risk factors for same-day care manager outreach.
-- Run every morning at 7 AM. Deliver to care manager worklist.

-- STEP 1: Inpatient discharges in the last 7 days.
WITH recent_discharges AS (
  SELECT c.member_id, c.rendering_npi AS discharging_facility,
       MAX(c.service_date) AS discharge_date,
       c.primary_drg, c.primary_diag,
       MAX(c.service_date) - MIN(c.service_date) + 1 AS length_of_stay
  FROM fact_medical_claims c
  WHERE c.type_of_bill LIKE '11%'      -- inpatient acute TOB
   AND c.claim_status = 'PAID'
   AND c.discharge_status_code <> '20' -- exclude members who died (status 20)
   AND c.service_date >= CURRENT_DATE - 7
  GROUP BY c.member_id, c.rendering_npi, c.primary_drg, c.primary_diag
),
-- STEP 2: Post-discharge care manager contacts in the last 7 days.
-- NULL in cc.member_id after LEFT JOIN = not yet contacted = action required.
cm_contacts AS (
  SELECT DISTINCT member_id
  FROM fact_cm_contacts
  WHERE contact_date >= CURRENT_DATE - 7
   AND contact_type IN ('POST_DISCHARGE_CALL','POST_DISCHARGE_VISIT')
   AND contact_outcome = 'REACHED'
),
-- STEP 3: CCI scores for readmission risk stratification
cci AS (
  SELECT member_id, COALESCE(SUM(max_wt),0) AS cci_score
  FROM (
    SELECT DISTINCT c.member_id, cci.condition_name, MAX(cci.cci_weight) AS max_wt
    FROM fact_medical_claims c
    JOIN ref_cci_weights cci ON c.primary_diag LIKE cci.icd10_prefix || '%'
    WHERE c.claim_status='PAID'
     AND EXTRACT(YEAR FROM c.service_date)=EXTRACT(YEAR FROM CURRENT_DATE)
    GROUP BY c.member_id, cci.condition_name
  ) x GROUP BY member_id
)
-- STEP 4: Flag high-readmission-risk diagnoses.
-- CHF (I50%), COPD (J44%), Sepsis (A41%) have 15-25% 30-day readmission rates.
```

```sql
SELECT rd.member_id, m.member_name, m.date_of_birth, m.phone,
   m.preferred_language,
   rd.discharge_date,
   DATEDIFF('day',rd.discharge_date,CURRENT_DATE) AS days_since_discharge,
   rd.primary_drg, rd.primary_diag, rd.length_of_stay,
   COALESCE(ci.cci_score,0) AS cci_score,
   attr.attributed_pcp_npi,
   p.provider_full_name AS attributed_pcp,
   CASE
      WHEN rd.primary_diag LIKE 'I50%'   -- CHF
        OR rd.primary_diag LIKE 'J44%'   -- COPD
        OR rd.primary_diag LIKE 'A41%'   -- Sepsis
      THEN 'HIGH — 20%+ 30-day readmission rate'
      WHEN COALESCE(ci.cci_score,0) >= 4
      THEN 'MODERATE-HIGH — high comorbidity burden'
      ELSE 'STANDARD — follow protocol'
   END AS readmission_risk
FROM  recent_discharges rd
LEFT JOIN cm_contacts cc ON rd.member_id = cc.member_id
JOIN  dim_members m ON rd.member_id = m.member_id
LEFT JOIN cci ci ON rd.member_id = ci.member_id
LEFT JOIN dim_pcp_attribution attr ON rd.member_id = attr.member_id
LEFT JOIN dim_providers p ON attr.attributed_pcp_npi = p.npi
WHERE cc.member_id IS NULL  -- only members NOT yet contacted
ORDER BY readmission_risk, days_since_discharge ASC;
```

26.3 Care Management Program ROI

Program ROI requires difference-in-differences: compare cost change for enrolled members against a matched comparison group. Pre/post design without a comparison group overstates ROI by attributing natural regression-to-the-mean cost decline to the program.

ANSI SQL — 26.3: Care Management ROI — Difference-in-Differences (Fully Annotated)

```sql
-- PURPOSE: Compare pre/post PMPM change for CM enrollees vs. matched comparison.
-- Difference-in-differences isolates program effect from regression-to-mean.
-- net_program_effect_pmpm = enrollee_change - comparison_group_change.

-- Pre-enrollment cost: 12 months BEFORE CM start date
WITH cm_enrollees AS (
   SELECT member_id, MIN(enrollment_date) AS cm_start_date, program_name
   FROM  fact_cm_enrollments
   WHERE enrollment_status='ACTIVE' AND program_name=:program_name
   GROUP BY member_id, program_name
),
pre_cost AS (
   SELECT e.member_id,
        ROUND(SUM(c.allowed_amount)/NULLIF(SUM(mm.member_months),0),2) AS pre_pmpm
   FROM  cm_enrollees e
   JOIN  fact_medical_claims c ON e.member_id=c.member_id
   JOIN  fact_member_months mm ON e.member_id=mm.member_id
   WHERE c.claim_status='PAID'
    AND c.service_date BETWEEN e.cm_start_date-365 AND e.cm_start_date-1
   GROUP BY e.member_id
),
-- Post-enrollment cost: 12 months AFTER CM start date
post_cost AS (
   SELECT e.member_id,
        ROUND(SUM(c.allowed_amount)/NULLIF(SUM(mm.member_months),0),2) AS post_pmpm
   FROM  cm_enrollees e
   JOIN  fact_medical_claims c ON e.member_id=c.member_id
```

```
    JOIN fact_member_months mm ON e.member_id=mm.member_id
    WHERE c.claim_status='PAID'
     AND c.service_date BETWEEN e.cm_start_date AND e.cm_start_date+365
    GROUP BY e.member_id
),
-- Same pre/post change for the matched comparison group (not enrolled in CM)
comparison_delta AS (
    SELECT ROUND(AVG(post_pmpm - pre_pmpm),2) AS comparison_group_change
    FROM fact_cm_comparison_group cg
    JOIN (SELECT member_id, SUM(allowed_amount)/12.0 AS pre_pmpm FROM fact_medical_claims
        WHERE claim_status='PAID' GROUP BY member_id) pre ON cg.member_id=pre.member_id
    JOIN (SELECT member_id, SUM(allowed_amount)/12.0 AS post_pmpm FROM fact_medical_claims
        WHERE claim_status='PAID' GROUP BY member_id) post ON cg.member_id=post.member_id
)
-- Final ROI: net program effect and return on investment percentage
SELECT
    COUNT(DISTINCT pc.member_id)                AS enrollee_count,
    ROUND(AVG(prc.pre_pmpm),2)                  AS avg_pre_pmpm,
    ROUND(AVG(pc.post_pmpm),2)                  AS avg_post_pmpm,
    ROUND(AVG(pc.post_pmpm - prc.pre_pmpm),2)         AS enrollee_pmpm_change,
    cd.comparison_group_change,
    -- Difference-in-differences: program effect net of natural cost trend
    ROUND(AVG(pc.post_pmpm-prc.pre_pmpm)-cd.comparison_group_change,2) AS net_program_effect_pmpm,
    -- Annualized savings (negative net_effect = costs fell more than comparison)
    ROUND((AVG(pc.post_pmpm-prc.pre_pmpm)-cd.comparison_group_change)
      * COUNT(DISTINCT pc.member_id)*12,0)          AS annualized_savings,
    :program_cost_pmpm                          AS program_cost_pmpm,
    -- ROI = (gross_savings/program_cost - 1) × 100
    ROUND(ABS(AVG(pc.post_pmpm-prc.pre_pmpm)-cd.comparison_group_change)*12
      /NULLIF(:program_cost_pmpm*12,0)*100-100,1)       AS program_roi_pct
FROM  post_cost pc
JOIN  pre_cost prc ON pc.member_id=prc.member_id
CROSS JOIN comparison_delta cd;
```

Chapter 26 Review

Unit Test · Key Takeaways

Answer each question before reading the explanation.

Q1. The readmission worklist filters WHERE cc.member_id IS NULL because:

A. NULL member_id indicates un-enrolled members

B. LEFT JOIN between recent_discharges and cm_contacts returns NULL in cc.member_id when no matching post-discharge contact record exists — the member has been discharged but not yet reached by a care manager. These are the action items needing a call today.

C. Members with NULL contacts are excluded from care management

D. NULL indicates the member is deceased

Answer: B. *LEFT JOIN + IS NULL: all recent discharges appear in the left table. Members WITH a post-discharge contact show cc.member_id = a value. Members WITHOUT a contact show cc.member_id = NULL. WHERE cc.member_id IS NULL selects only un-contacted members. Identical pattern to HCC capture gap (Ch 25) and NCCI unbundling (Ch 20): find records in A not in B.*

Q2. Discharge status code 20 is excluded because:

A. Members discharged to SNF should not receive calls

B. Member expired (died) during the inpatient stay. These members cannot be readmitted or contacted. Attempting to call a deceased member causes distress to their family.

C. Status 20 indicates the member was transferred to another acute facility

D. Status 20 means the member is still hospitalized

Answer: B. *Standard UB-04 discharge status codes: 01 = home, 02 = home with home health, 03 = SNF, 20 = expired/died during stay, 30 = still patient, 41 = court/law enforcement. Also exclude 51 and 61–66 (transferred to other acute) when building the readmission worklist — these are not true community discharges and will not be readmitted to the same hospital from home.*

Q3. Difference-in-differences is required for program ROI because:

A. CMS requires it for all care management ROI reports

B. Members enrolled in care management are high-risk by selection. Even without the program, their costs will likely decline (regression-to-mean) after the acute episode resolves. Subtracting the comparison group's cost change removes the natural trend, isolating only the change attributable to the program.

C. Pre/post design without comparison is not permitted by NCQA

D. Difference-in-differences eliminates all statistical bias from ROI

Answer: B. *Regression-to-mean example: CHF admission costs $8,000 in month of admission, then naturally declines to $900/month as the patient stabilizes. Pre-period PMPM = $2,800 (inflated by admission). Post-period = $900. Pre/post ROI would credit $1,900/month to the CM program — mostly natural recovery. Comparison group with same pattern: if they also show -$1,400/month without the program, net program effect = only -$500/month. Much more honest.*

Q4. Post-discharge contact within 2 business days is targeted because:

A. CMS requires contact within 2 days for Stars credit

B. The first 48–72 hours post-discharge is the highest-risk window for complications, medication errors, and care confusion. Contact within 2 business days reduces 30-day readmission by 20–30% (evidence base for TCM CPT codes 99495/99496 and CMS FUH HEDIS measure).

C. MHPAEA requires 2-day contact for BH discharges

D. 2-day aligns with the 48-hour medication reconciliation requirement

Answer: B. *The worklist runs daily at 7 AM, sorted by days_since_discharge ASC — members discharged yesterday appear at the top. HIGH-risk diagnoses (CHF, COPD, sepsis) receive same-day contact. For members unreachable on first attempt: retry within 24 hours. Three unsuccessful attempts in 3 days → escalate to social worker for home visit.*

Q5. Program ROI 150% means:

A. The plan recovered $150 for every $100 in claims cost

B. For every $100 invested in the program, the plan saved $250 in claims — a net return of $150 above the investment. ROI formula: (gross_savings/program_cost - 1) × 100 = ($250/$100 - 1) × 100 = 150%.

C. The program reduced costs by 150% of baseline PMPM

D. The program served 150% more members than planned

Answer: B. *SQL formula: ABS(enrollee_pmpm_change - comparison_pmpm_change) × 12 / (program_cost_pmpm × 12) × 100 - 100. ABS() takes the absolute value of net savings (negative in the formula since cost fell). Subtract 100 to express as return above the investment. ROI > 100% = program pays for itself. Typical complex CM programs: 150–300% ROI.*

Q6. The matched comparison group should be matched on:

A. Age and gender only

B. Prior PMPM (12-month pre-period), CCI score, and prior IP admission flag — the strongest predictors of future cost. Ensures the comparison group would have experienced similar cost trajectory as the enrolled group without intervention.

C. Enrollment duration and plan type

D. Geographic region and attributed PCP

Answer: B. *Without proper matching, the comparison group may be systematically healthier. Propensity score matching or stratified matching on prior_pmpm decile + CCI severity band + IP_admission_flag (prior year) creates a comparable baseline risk group. Goal: if you gave 1,000 matched comparison members the same program, would they have had the same pre-period cost pattern? If yes, the match is valid.*

Q7. Describe the complete 30-day readmission prevention workflow from SQL alert to clinical intervention.

(Short answer)

Sample Answer:

Step 1 — Daily 7 AM worklist: run post-discharge query. Deliver to CM system worklist. Sort: HIGH risk first, then days_since_discharge ASC. Step 2 — CM assignment: assign each member to the care manager responsible for that PCP region. Unassigned members → worklist manager → next available CM. Step 3 — Outreach script: call covers: current medications (all discharge prescriptions filled?), PCP follow-up appointment (scheduled within 7 days?), warning signs requiring 911 or nurse line, transportation assistance. Step 4 — Contact logging: record outcome in fact_cm_contacts: REACHED, VOICEMAIL, NO_ANSWER, UNABLE_TO_REACH. Voicemail → retry within 24 hours. Three failed attempts in 3 days → escalate to social worker for home visit. Step 5 — Follow-up: if member has PCP appointment, confirm attendance. If not, contact PCP office to schedule. Step 6 — 30-day readmission tracking: at 30 days post-discharge, query fact_medical_claims for IP admission within 30 days (member_id, service_date BETWEEN discharge_date+1 AND discharge_date+30, TOB 11x). Report monthly to CMO: contacted vs. not-contacted readmission rates, and 2-business-day contact compliance rate.

Q8. Explain regression-to-the-mean and how difference-in-differences corrects for it.

(Short answer)

Sample Answer:
Regression-to-mean: extreme values tend to be followed by less extreme values due to random variation — not because of intervention. In care management: enrolled members had a high-cost event (hospital admission). In the pre-period, costs are elevated by the acute episode. Post-period, costs naturally decline as the episode resolves — even WITHOUT the program. Without DiD: a member admitted for CHF at $8,000/month naturally stabilizes to $900/month post-discharge. Pre-PMPM (including admission) = $2,800. Post-PMPM = $900. Naive ROI credits $1,900/month to the program — mostly natural recovery. Difference-in-differences fix: apply same pre/post to a matched comparison group NOT enrolled in CM. If comparison group also shows $1,400/month decline (RTM without program), net program effect = -$1,900 - (-$1,400) = -$500/month. SQL: net_program_effect_pmpm = enrollee_pmpm_change - comparison_group_change. This is the critical adjustment separating a legitimate from an inflated ROI analysis.

Q9. Write the SQL to calculate 30-day readmission rate by discharge diagnosis vs. national benchmarks.

(Short answer)

Sample Answer:
WITH index_admissions AS (SELECT c.member_id, MAX(c.service_date) AS discharge_date, c.primary_drg, c.primary_diag FROM fact_medical_claims c WHERE c.type_of_bill LIKE '11%' AND c.claim_status='PAID' AND c.discharge_status_code NOT IN ('20','30','51') AND EXTRACT(YEAR FROM c.service_date)=EXTRACT(YEAR FROM CURRENT_DATE) GROUP BY c.member_id, c.primary_drg, c.primary_diag), readmissions AS (SELECT ia.member_id, ia.discharge_date, 1 AS readmitted FROM index_admissions ia JOIN fact_medical_claims ra ON ra.member_id=ia.member_id AND ra.type_of_bill LIKE '11%' AND ra.claim_status='PAID' AND ra.service_date BETWEEN ia.discharge_date+1 AND ia.discharge_date+30) SELECT ia.primary_diag, dr.diagnosis_description, COUNT(DISTINCT ia.member_id) AS index_admits, COUNT(DISTINCT ra.member_id) AS readmitted_count, ROUND(100.0*COUNT(DISTINCT ra.member_id)/NULLIF(COUNT(DISTINCT ia.member_id),0),1) AS readmission_rate_pct, nb.national_benchmark_pct, ROUND(COUNT(DISTINCT ra.member_id)*100.0/NULLIF(COUNT(DISTINCT ia.member_id),0) - nb.national_benchmark_pct,1) AS gap_vs_national FROM index_admissions ia LEFT JOIN readmissions ra ON ia.member_id=ra.member_id AND ia.discharge_date=ra.discharge_date JOIN ref_diagnosis_codes dr ON ia.primary_diag=dr.icd10_code JOIN ref_readmission_benchmarks nb ON ia.primary_diag LIKE nb.icd10_prefix||'%' GROUP BY ia.primary_diag, dr.diagnosis_description, nb.national_benchmark_pct HAVING COUNT(DISTINCT ia.member_id)>=25 ORDER BY readmission_rate_pct DESC. Benchmarks: CHF ≈23–25%, COPD ≈19–22%, pneumonia ≈17–19%. Sort by gap_vs_national DESC to identify diagnoses where the plan most exceeds national benchmarks.

Q10. Describe three data science techniques beyond SQL for care management predictive modeling.

(Short answer)

Sample Answer:
Technique 1 — Logistic Regression: predicts probability of binary outcome (30-day readmission: yes/no) from multiple predictors. Appropriate when: binary outcome, interpretable model needed (coefficients have clear meanings for clinicians), moderate sample sizes (thousands of members). SQL-compatible: scores stored in a member risk table and joined to care management worklists. Limitation: assumes linear relationship between predictors and log-odds. Technique 2 — Gradient Boosting (XGBoost/LightGBM): ensemble of decision trees handling non-linear interactions and missing data. Higher predictive accuracy than logistic regression for complex healthcare outcomes. Appropriate when: 50,000+ members, many features, accuracy is primary goal. Use SHAP values for feature importance interpretation — required to explain "black box" decisions to clinicians. Technique 3 — Survival Analysis (Cox Proportional Hazards): models time-to-event outcomes (time to first admission, time to disease onset). Appropriate when: the question is not just "will the event happen?" but "when?" — and the population has varying follow-up lengths. Handles censoring (members who disenroll before the event occurs) correctly. SQL use: hazard ratio per member stored in risk table. Care manager sees "45% probability of admission within 60 days" — more actionable than a decile score. Decision rule: start with rule-based SQL scores for immediate deployment. Invest in ML models when sample sizes and infrastructure support them and when clinicians can be educated on the model's outputs.

Key Takeaways

What every analyst must remember from this chapter.

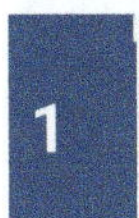
1 Post-discharge readmission worklist: recent IP discharges (last 7 days) LEFT JOIN cm_contacts WHERE cc.member_id IS NULL = un-contacted. Exclude discharge_status 20 (expired). Priority: CHF (I50%), COPD (J44%), Sepsis (A41%) = HIGH 30-day readmission risk.

2 2-business-day post-discharge contact standard reduces 30-day readmission by 20–30%. Run worklist daily at 7 AM. Sort HIGH risk first, days_since_discharge ASC. Log every attempt in fact_cm_contacts.

3 Discharge status exclusions: 20 (expired), 30 (still patient), 51/61–66 (transferred to other acute). Include true discharges only.

4 Care management ROI = difference-in-differences: net_program_effect_pmpm = enrollee_pmpm_change - comparison_group_change. Match comparison group on prior_pmpm decile + CCI + prior_IP_admission.

5 ROI formula: (ABS(net_effect_pmpm) × 12 / (program_cost_pmpm × 12)) × 100 - 100. ROI > 100% = program pays for itself. Typical complex CM: 150–300% ROI.

6 30-day readmission rate SQL: index admissions (TOB 11x, exclude death/still patient) LEFT JOIN readmissions WHERE service_date BETWEEN discharge+1 AND discharge+30. HAVING COUNT >= 25. Compare to benchmarks: CHF ~23%, COPD ~21%, pneumonia ~18%.

7 Regression-to-mean: high-cost members' costs naturally decline after acute episode resolves without intervention. DiD design removes this natural decline, isolating only the intervention effect.

8 Predictive modeling progression: rule-based SQL → logistic regression (interpretable) → gradient boosting (higher accuracy) → survival analysis (time-to-event, handles censoring). Start SQL; invest in ML when data and infrastructure are ready.

Part VIII — Quality Programs & Regulatory Mastery

Chapters 27–30

HEDIS · CMS/NCQA/CAHPS/HOS · Star Ratings Pipeline · Data Quality & Governance

A health plan's quality analytics function is simultaneously a performance measurement discipline, a regulatory compliance obligation, and a strategic competitive lever. Part VIII covers the four pillars that define how plans are evaluated, accredited, and rewarded by regulators, employers, and consumers.

Chapter 27 opens with HEDIS — the Healthcare Effectiveness Data and Information Set — the de facto standard for measuring quality of care and service across the US health insurance industry. Maintained by the National Committee for Quality Assurance (NCQA), HEDIS comprises more than 90 measures spanning prevention, chronic disease management, behavioral health, and patient experience. Every measure has a precisely specified eligible population (denominator), numerator criteria, and exclusion logic. The analyst's role is to implement these specifications faithfully in SQL: first construct the denominator from enrollment and claims data, then identify numerator events, then compute the gap closure list that care managers use for outreach. The chapter covers measure domains, the administrative vs. hybrid distinction, denominator construction for the CDC Comprehensive Diabetes Care measure, HbA1c numerator logic, and the multi-measure Stars-aligned quality dashboard.

Chapter 28 maps the full quality ecosystem that surrounds HEDIS: CMS's role as the federal regulator for Medicare Advantage and Medicaid managed care; NCQA accreditation — the gold standard for health plan credentialing sought by most commercial and government plans; CAHPS (Consumer Assessment of Healthcare Providers and Systems), the standardized survey instrument that measures member experience of care; and HOS (Health Outcomes Survey), which tracks functional health status and physical and mental health outcomes for Medicare Advantage members over time. Understanding how these programs interconnect — and how each feeds into the CMS Star Ratings calculation — is essential context for every quality analyst.

Chapter 29 delivers an end-to-end CMS Star Ratings pipeline. Star Ratings determine whether a Medicare Advantage plan receives quality bonus payments (QBP) — worth up to 5% of benchmark revenue — and affect enrollment growth through CMS's public plan finder ratings. The chapter covers the full calculation architecture: measure collection, cut-point determination, domain weighting, summary score computation, and gap closure simulation. The analyst learns to build a score simulator that forecasts what the plan's Star Rating will be under different gap closure scenarios — enabling the VP of Quality to make data-driven prioritization decisions.

Chapter 30 closes Part VIII with data quality and governance — the foundation on which every other analytic in this book rests. A claims database with missing NPIs, duplicate member records, inconsistent diagnosis coding, or stale reference tables will produce incorrect HEDIS rates, wrong risk scores, and flawed financial projections. The chapter introduces a six-dimension data quality framework (completeness, validity, timeliness, consistency, uniqueness, and accuracy), implements an automated DQ dashboard with threshold-based gates, and provides SQL for NPI validation, duplicate member detection, and claims anomaly monitoring. Without rigorous data governance, none of the analytics in Parts I through VII can be trusted.

Together, Chapters 27–30 give the healthcare data analyst the technical and conceptual toolkit to support a plan's quality improvement program from denominator build to Stars simulation, from CAHPS survey analysis to data quality certification. The SQL patterns in this section are production-ready — they follow the same annotated, modular CTE structure used throughout this book, and every query is designed to feed directly into a care management worklist, a regulatory submission, or an executive dashboard.

Chapter 27: HEDIS & Quality Measures

Measure domains · Stars alignment · Denominator/numerator SQL · Administrative vs. hybrid

27.1 HEDIS Architecture

HEDIS (Healthcare Effectiveness Data and Information Set), maintained by NCQA, contains 90+ measures across six domains: Effectiveness of Care, Access/Availability, Experience of Care, Utilization, Health Plan Descriptive Information, and ECDS (Electronic Clinical Data Systems). Each measure has a precisely defined Eligible Population (denominator), numerator criteria, and exclusion logic. NCQA publishes updated technical specifications each fall for the following measurement year. The analyst's job is to implement those specifications faithfully in SQL.

> **Administrative vs. Hybrid** Administrative measures use claims data only. Hybrid measures supplement claims with medical record data to capture events never billed to the plan (e.g., a mammogram at an employer health fair, blood pressure readings documented in the office note). Hybrid rates consistently run 5–10 percentage points higher than administrative-only. Hybrid requires medical record abstraction resources.

27.2 Denominator (Eligible Population) Construction

The denominator is always constructed first — the numerator is a subset of it. Common criteria: age range as of December 31 of the measurement year, continuous enrollment (≥11 of 12 months), line of business, and absence of specified exclusions. The two-claim rule for chronic conditions (two outpatient claims OR one inpatient/ED claim) provides confidence the condition is established, not just screened for.

ANSI SQL — 27.2: HEDIS CDC Denominator — Comprehensive Diabetes Care (Fully Annotated)

```
-- PURPOSE: Build the HEDIS CDC (Comprehensive Diabetes Care) eligible population.
-- CDC denominator = members 18–75 WITH diabetes AND continuously enrolled ≥11/12 months.
-- This denominator is shared by all CDC sub-measures:
-- HbA1c control, BP control, eye exam, kidney health, statin therapy.

-- STEP 1: Age 18–75 as of December 31 of the measurement year.
WITH age_eligible AS (
  SELECT m.member_id, m.date_of_birth,
       DATEDIFF('year', m.date_of_birth,
         DATE(:meas_year || '-12-31')) AS age_at_year_end
  FROM  dim_members m
  WHERE m.line_of_business IN ('COMMERCIAL','MEDICARE_ADVANTAGE')
    AND m.coverage_status IN ('ACTIVE','TERMED')
    AND DATEDIFF('year', m.date_of_birth,
      DATE(:meas_year || '-12-31')) BETWEEN 18 AND 75
),

-- STEP 2: Continuous enrollment = member enrolled for at least 11 of 12 months.
-- NCQA allows one gap of ≤45 days. Simplified: SUM(member_months) >= 11.
continuous_enrolled AS (
  SELECT member_id, SUM(member_months) AS enrolled_months
  FROM  fact_member_months
  WHERE membership_year = :meas_year
```

```
    GROUP BY member_id
    HAVING SUM(member_months) >= 11
),

-- STEP 3: Diabetes identification using NCQA two-claim rule.
-- Two or more outpatient visits with diabetes dx (E08–E13)
-- OR one acute inpatient / ED claim with diabetes dx.
-- ICD-10 range E08–E13 covers all diabetes types except gestational (O24.4).
diabetes_dx AS (
    SELECT c.member_id
    FROM  fact_medical_claims c
    WHERE EXTRACT(YEAR FROM c.service_date) = :meas_year
      AND c.claim_status = 'PAID'
      AND c.primary_diag BETWEEN 'E08' AND 'E13z'
    GROUP BY c.member_id
    HAVING
        -- Two or more outpatient diabetes claims
        COUNT(DISTINCT CASE
            WHEN c.type_of_bill NOT LIKE '11%'  -- not inpatient
            THEN c.claim_id END) >= 2
        OR
        -- OR at least one inpatient/ED diabetes claim (higher clinical confidence)
        MAX(CASE WHEN c.type_of_bill LIKE '11%' THEN 1 ELSE 0 END) = 1
),

-- STEP 4: Exclusions per NCQA CDC spec.
-- Exclude: gestational diabetes only (O24.4x), ESRD/dialysis, members who died.
exclusions AS (
    SELECT DISTINCT c.member_id
    FROM  fact_medical_claims c
    WHERE EXTRACT(YEAR FROM c.service_date) = :meas_year
      AND c.claim_status = 'PAID'
      AND (
          c.primary_diag LIKE 'O24.4%'  -- gestational diabetes only
          OR c.procedure_code IN ('90935','90937','90945','90947','90999')  -- dialysis
      )
)
-- STEP 5: Final denominator = age AND enrollment AND diabetes MINUS exclusions.
SELECT ae.member_id, ae.age_at_year_end,
    m.member_name, m.date_of_birth, ce.enrolled_months,
    attr.attributed_pcp_npi,
    p.provider_full_name AS attributed_pcp
FROM  age_eligible ae
JOIN  continuous_enrolled ce ON ae.member_id = ce.member_id
JOIN  diabetes_dx dd        ON ae.member_id = dd.member_id
LEFT JOIN exclusions ex      ON ae.member_id = ex.member_id
JOIN  dim_members m          ON ae.member_id = m.member_id
LEFT JOIN dim_pcp_attribution attr ON ae.member_id = attr.member_id
LEFT JOIN dim_providers p   ON attr.attributed_pcp_npi = p.npi
WHERE ex.member_id IS NULL  -- remove members meeting any exclusion criterion
ORDER BY attr.attributed_pcp_npi, ae.member_id;
```

27.3 Numerator: CDC HbA1c Control (<8%) with Gap Flag

For each CDC-eligible member, determine whether any HbA1c lab result with a numeric value < 8.0% was documented during the measurement year. Members with no result are the most urgent gap — they need a lab order, not just a follow-up visit. Members with a result ≥ 8.0% need clinical intensification. NULLS FIRST in the sort ensures no-result members surface at the top of the care manager worklist.

ANSI SQL — 27.3: CDC HbA1c Control Numerator & Gap Closure List (Fully Annotated)

```sql
-- PURPOSE: For each CDC-eligible member, check whether an HbA1c < 8.0%
-- was documented during the measurement year.
-- Gap status drives the care management outreach action.
-- LOINC codes for HbA1c: 4548-4, 4549-2, 17856-6, 59261-8.

WITH hba1c_results AS (
  SELECT lr.member_id,
      lr.result_date,
      lr.numeric_result,
      CASE WHEN lr.numeric_result < 8.0 THEN 1 ELSE 0 END AS meets_threshold
  FROM  fact_lab_results lr
  WHERE lr.loinc_code IN ('4548-4','4549-2','17856-6','59261-8')
   AND EXTRACT(YEAR FROM lr.result_date) = :meas_year
   AND lr.result_status = 'FINAL' -- only finalized lab results, not pending
),

-- Aggregate per member: best result, most recent date, numerator met flag
member_hba1c AS (
  SELECT cdc.member_id,
      MIN(hr.numeric_result)  AS best_hba1c,
      MAX(hr.result_date)     AS most_recent_result_date,
      -- 1 if ANY result in the year is < 8.0%, else 0
      MAX(hr.meets_threshold) AS numerator_met
  FROM  cdc_denominator cdc  -- denominator CTE from Section 27.2
  LEFT JOIN hba1c_results hr ON cdc.member_id = hr.member_id
  GROUP BY cdc.member_id
)
SELECT mh.member_id, m.member_name, m.phone, m.preferred_language,
  m.date_of_birth, mh.best_hba1c,
  mh.most_recent_result_date,
  attr.attributed_pcp_npi,
  p.provider_full_name AS attributed_pcp,
  -- Gap status classification drives care management action
  CASE
    WHEN mh.numerator_met = 1   THEN 'CLOSED — HbA1c < 8.0%'
    WHEN mh.best_hba1c >= 9.0   THEN 'OPEN — HbA1c ≥ 9.0% (very poor control)'
    WHEN mh.best_hba1c >= 8.0   THEN 'OPEN — HbA1c ≥ 8.0% (poor control)'
    WHEN mh.best_hba1c IS NULL  THEN 'OPEN — No HbA1c result this year'
  END AS gap_status,
  CASE
    WHEN mh.best_hba1c IS NULL  THEN 'Order HbA1c lab — no result this year'
    WHEN mh.best_hba1c >= 9.0   THEN 'Urgent: intensify therapy, schedule within 2 wks'
    WHEN mh.best_hba1c >= 8.0   THEN 'Schedule follow-up — HbA1c above target'
    ELSE                        'No action — numerator met'
  END AS recommended_action
FROM  member_hba1c mh
JOIN  dim_members m ON mh.member_id = m.member_id
LEFT JOIN dim_pcp_attribution attr ON mh.member_id = attr.member_id
LEFT JOIN dim_providers p ON attr.attributed_pcp_npi = p.npi
WHERE mh.numerator_met = 0 OR mh.numerator_met IS NULL
ORDER BY mh.best_hba1c DESC NULLS FIRST; -- no-result members at top = most urgent
```

27.4 Multi-Measure Quality Dashboard with Stars Weighting

ANSI SQL — 27.4: HEDIS Rate Summary — All Measures with Stars Weight (Fully Annotated)

```sql
-- PURPOSE: Monthly quality dashboard showing all HEDIS measure rates,
-- flagged with Stars domain and weight, and open gap counts.
-- Stars-weighted measures sorted first: highest financial impact.
SELECT
  hg.measure_id,
```

```
    hg.measure_description,
    COALESCE(sm.stars_domain, 'HEDIS Only') AS stars_domain,
    COALESCE(sm.stars_weight, 0)          AS stars_weight,
    COUNT(DISTINCT hg.member_id)          AS denominator,
    COUNT(DISTINCT CASE WHEN hg.gap_status='CLOSED'
      THEN hg.member_id END)            AS numerator,
    ROUND(100.0*COUNT(DISTINCT CASE WHEN hg.gap_status='CLOSED'
      THEN hg.member_id END)
      /NULLIF(COUNT(DISTINCT hg.member_id),0),1) AS rate_pct,
    sm.ncqa_national_avg_pct,
    -- Positive = above national average (favorable)
    ROUND(100.0*COUNT(DISTINCT CASE WHEN hg.gap_status='CLOSED'
      THEN hg.member_id END)
      /NULLIF(COUNT(DISTINCT hg.member_id),0),1)
      - sm.ncqa_national_avg_pct        AS gap_vs_national,
    COUNT(DISTINCT CASE WHEN hg.gap_status='OPEN'
      THEN hg.member_id END)            AS open_gaps
FROM  fact_hedis_gaps hg
LEFT JOIN ref_stars_measures sm ON hg.measure_id = sm.measure_id
WHERE hg.measurement_year = :meas_year
  AND hg.denominator_eligible = 'Y'
GROUP BY hg.measure_id, hg.measure_description,
       sm.stars_domain, sm.stars_weight, sm.ncqa_national_avg_pct
ORDER BY sm.stars_weight DESC NULLS LAST, open_gaps DESC;
-- Sort: highest Stars weight first, then by most open gaps -- maximize ROI
```

Chapter 27 Review

Unit Test · Key Takeaways

Answer each question before reading the explanation.

Q1. The CDC denominator requires two outpatient diabetes claims because:

A. One claim may be a data entry error

B. Two outpatient claims provide confidence the condition is established — one claim may represent a rule-out or screening visit. One inpatient or ED claim is sufficient alone because inpatient diagnoses are confirmed to a higher clinical standard.

C. Two claims satisfy the continuous enrollment criterion

D. ICD-10 diabetes codes require two qualifying codes to activate

Answer: B. *The two-claim rule prevents false inclusion of members who were screened for or ruled out of a diabetes diagnosis. Example: a non-diabetic member tested for diabetes who has one E11.9 on the visit claim would not qualify — they need a second claim with the code. The exception for inpatient/ED: these settings presuppose a more rigorous clinical evaluation.*

Q2. Hybrid HEDIS rates are higher than administrative-only because:

A. Hybrid uses a smaller denominator

B. Medical records capture clinical events that never generate a claim — blood pressure readings in the office note, mammograms at employer health fairs, lab results from reference labs not billing the plan. Hybrid supplementation closes these gaps, improving the numerator rate by 5–10 percentage points on average.

C. Hybrid measures have a less strict numerator definition

D. NCQA awards bonus points for hybrid submission

Answer: B. *BCS example: a mammogram at a community screening event, billed only to the patient's deductible account rather than to the plan, produces no plan claim. Administrative data misses this event. Hybrid review of the PCP's chart finds the result documented. Rate improvement for BCS from hybrid: typically 5–8pp. Plans with medical record abstraction programs consistently outperform administrative-only plans on hybrid measures.*

Q3. The HbA1c Control numerator is met when:

A. The member has an HbA1c test ordered during the year

B. ANY documented HbA1c result with a numeric value < 8.0% during the measurement year qualifies. MAX(meets_threshold) across all results: 1 if any result < 8.0%. One qualifying result is sufficient — the member does not need consistent good control throughout the year.

C. **The member's average HbA1c across all tests is < 8.0%**

D. The member has an HbA1c test AND a follow-up visit

Answer: C. *The HEDIS CDC specification for HbA1c Control (<8%) is point-in-time: any result below the threshold in the measurement year meets the numerator. A member with results of 8.4% in January and 7.8% in September meets the numerator because of the September result. The gap query uses MAX(meets_threshold) across all results to capture this logic correctly.*

Q4. ORDER BY best_hba1c DESC NULLS FIRST prioritizes:

A. Members with the best HbA1c control at the top

B. Members with NO HbA1c result (NULL) at the very top — the most urgent care gap. Below them: members with the worst HbA1c values descending. This ensures care managers see the highest-need members first, not the lowest.

C. Members enrolled most recently

D. Members with the highest number of open gaps

Answer: B. *NULLS FIRST in a DESC sort inverts the default behavior (which would put NULLs last). The logic: a member with no HbA1c result at all is more clinically urgent than a member with a result of 9.2% — at least the 9.2% member has been tested. No result = zero monitoring of diabetes. NULLS FIRST keeps those members at the top of every care manager's worklist.*

Q5. The continuous enrollment criterion SUM(member_months) >= 11 is a simplification because:

A. The exact rule requires 12 months of enrollment

B. NCQA's full rule allows one gap in coverage of ≤45 days. A member enrolled Jan–Mar, then Apr 16–Dec (one 15-day gap in April) qualifies. The simplified SUM(member_months) >= 11 approximates this by requiring at least 11 calendar months and is appropriate for monthly monitoring, though the exact gap logic should be used for formal HEDIS submission.

C. Member months are counted differently for Medicaid vs. commercial

D. The simplification applies only to administrative measures, not hybrid

Answer: B. *Full NCQA continuous enrollment logic requires: identify all enrollment segments, calculate gaps between segments, fail the member if any single gap exceeds 45 days or if the total enrolled months < 11. The exact SQL involves a LAG() window function to calculate gap days between consecutive enrollment end and start dates. Simplified SUM(member_months) >= 11 misses a member who has two 30-day gaps (total = 60 days) but still has 10 months of enrollment — they fail the full rule but pass the simplified rule.*

Q6. Stars measures are sorted by stars_weight DESC in the quality dashboard because:

A. Stars measures are always easier to improve

B. Stars weights (1, 2, or 3) determine each measure's contribution to the overall Star Rating score. A 1-percentage-point improvement on a triple-weighted measure contributes 3× more to the Stars score than the same improvement on a single-weighted measure. Sorting by weight focuses team effort where financial impact is greatest.

C. Stars measures have larger denominators than non-Stars measures

D. NCQA requires Stars-weighted measures to appear first in HEDIS reports

Answer: B. *Quality Bonus Payment (QBP) logic: plans with Stars ≥ 4.0 receive up to 5% bonus on their benchmark revenue. For a plan with $500M in MA revenue, one Star Rating point difference can mean $25M+ annually. Prioritizing triple-weighted Stars measures in the gap closure program maximizes the ROI on each care management outreach dollar invested.*

Q7. Walk through the complete denominator construction logic for the HEDIS BCS (Breast Cancer Screening) measure. What are the key differences from CDC?

(Short answer)

Sample Answer:

BCS denominator: (1) Age: women 52–74 as of December 31 of the measurement year. (2) Continuous enrollment: enrolled for at least 11 of 12 months in the measurement year OR the year prior — BCS uses a 27-month look-back for the numerator, so enrollment continuity spans two years. (3) Line of business: commercial or MA. (4) Exclusions: members with a bilateral mastectomy at any time prior to the end of the measurement year (CPT 19180 + 19180 bilaterally, or 19305/19306 bilaterally, or unilateral mastectomy ×2); members who died during the year. Key differences from CDC: (a) BCS is female-only — filter: WHERE m.gender = 'F'. (b) BCS age window is narrower (52–74 vs. 18–75). (c) BCS uses a 27-month look-back for the numerator (mammogram any time in the 27 months ending December 31 of the measurement year), not just the current year. (d) BCS has a life-event exclusion (mastectomy) that must be searched across all historical claims, not just the measurement year. SQL: the mastectomy exclusion requires: SELECT DISTINCT member_id FROM fact_medical_claims WHERE procedure_code IN (:bilateral_mast_codes) AND service_date <= DATE(:meas_year||'- 12-31') — no year filter, because the exclusion is permanent once it occurs.

Q8. Describe how to build a HEDIS gap closure prioritization score for the care management team. What inputs are combined and why?

(Short answer)

Sample Answer:
A gap closure prioritization score ranks open gaps by the combination of Stars impact, clinical urgency, and closability. Components: (1) Stars weight (1–3): a triple-weighted measure gap is worth 3× a single-weighted gap. (2) Days until measurement snapshot: gaps that can still be closed before the measurement year ends are worth more than those already past the deadline. SQL: DATEDIFF('day', CURRENT_DATE, DATE(:meas_year||'- 12-31')). (3) Clinical urgency: HbA1c ≥ 9.0 is more urgent than HbA1c 8.1; no result at all is most urgent. (4) Closability: some gaps close with a phone call (medication adherence reminders); others require an office visit (eye exam, HbA1c draw). Phone-closable gaps have higher conversion rates and lower per-closure cost. Composite score SQL: SELECT member_id, measure_id, COALESCE(sm.stars_weight,1)*10 + CASE WHEN DATEDIFF('day',CURRENT_DATE,DATE(:meas_year||'- 12-31'))>90 THEN 5 ELSE 2 END + CASE WHEN measure_closability='PHONE' THEN 3 ELSE 1 END AS priority_score FROM fact_hedis_gaps hg LEFT JOIN ref_stars_measures sm ON hg.measure_id=sm.measure_id LEFT JOIN ref_measure_closability mc ON hg.measure_id=mc.measure_id WHERE hg.gap_status='OPEN' ORDER BY priority_score DESC. Deliver this sorted list to care managers weekly — the top of the list maximizes Stars impact per intervention dollar.

Q9. Explain the NCQA HEDIS audit process and what data the analyst must prepare to support an audit response.

(Short answer)

Sample Answer:
NCQA HEDIS Compliance Audit: NCQA-certified auditors verify that the plan's HEDIS rates are accurately calculated per published technical specifications. Process: (1) Documentation review: auditors examine the plan's source system documentation, ETL logic, and measure algorithms. Every SQL query used to build the denominator and numerator must be documented with the specific NCQA specification page it implements. (2) Data integrity: auditors pull random samples of denominator-eligible members and verify their claims data matches what was used in the calculation. The analyst must be able to reproduce the denominator and numerator for any individual member on demand. (3) Hybrid record review: for hybrid measures, auditors review a random sample of medical records to verify that abstracted data was correctly recorded and credited to the numerator. (4) Numerator validation: auditors verify that only qualifying events (correct LOINC code, correct date range, result status = FINAL) were counted in the numerator. Common audit findings: claims included with wrong date ranges, LOINC codes not matching the NCQA value set, continuous enrollment calculated incorrectly, exclusions not applied. Analyst preparation: maintain a member-level audit trail table: SELECT member_id, measure_id, denominator_flag, exclusion_flag, exclusion_reason, numerator_event_date, numerator_event_code, gap_status FROM hedis_audit_trail. This lets auditors drill down to any member and verify each decision point in the algorithm.

Q10. Write the SQL for the Medication Adherence for Diabetes Medications (MDD) HEDIS measure. Explain the PDC (Proportion of Days Covered) calculation.

(Short answer)

Sample Answer:
MDD measures whether members with diabetes who are on oral antidiabetic medications have a PDC ≥ 80% during the measurement year. PDC = days covered by medication / days in measurement period. SQL: WITH rx_fills AS (SELECT p.member_id, p.dispensing_date, p.days_supply, p.ndc_code FROM fact_pharmacy_claims p JOIN ref_drug_schedule d ON p.ndc_code=d.ndc_code WHERE d.drug_class='ORAL_ANTIDIABETIC' AND p.claim_status='PAID' AND EXTRACT(YEAR FROM p.dispensing_date)=:meas_year), -- Build coverage intervals: each fill covers dispensing_date through dispensing_date+days_supply-1 coverage_days AS (SELECT member_id, dispensing_date AS start_day, dispensing_date + days_supply - 1 AS end_day FROM rx_fills), -- Count distinct covered days (overlapping fills should not be double-counted) -- Standard approach: generate a calendar of the measurement year and flag covered days covered_calendar AS (SELECT member_id, cal.cal_date, MAX(CASE WHEN cal.cal_date BETWEEN cd.start_day AND cd.end_day THEN 1 ELSE 0 END) AS covered FROM coverage_days cd JOIN ref_calendar cal ON cal.cal_date BETWEEN DATE(:meas_year||'-01-01') AND DATE(:meas_year||'-12-31') GROUP BY member_id, cal.cal_date) SELECT cc.member_id, m.member_name, 365 AS measurement_days, SUM(cc.covered) AS days_covered, ROUND(100.0*SUM(cc.covered)/365.0,1) AS pdc_pct, CASE WHEN SUM(cc.covered)/365.0 >= 0.80 THEN 'CLOSED — PDC >= 80%' ELSE 'OPEN — PDC below 80%' END AS gap_status FROM covered_calendar cc JOIN dim_members m ON cc.member_id=m.member_id GROUP BY cc.member_id, m.member_name ORDER BY pdc_pct ASC. PDC key rule: overlapping fills are not double-counted — a member who refills early has their overlap period counted only once. The calendar join approach handles this correctly by flagging each calendar day as covered/not covered, then summing.

Key Takeaways

What every analyst must remember from this chapter.

1 HEDIS denominator first: age range (as of Dec 31), continuous enrollment (≥11/12 months), condition identification (two-claim rule for chronic conditions), minus exclusions. Numerator is always a subset of the denominator.

2 Two-claim rule: two outpatient claims with condition dx OR one inpatient/ED claim. Prevents false inclusion of rule-out or screening visits as confirmed diagnoses.

3 HbA1c Control (<8%) numerator: MAX(meets_threshold) across all LOINC-coded lab results in the year. One result < 8.0% is sufficient. NULLS FIRST in sort: no-result members at top — they need a lab order, the most urgent gap.

4 Administrative vs. hybrid: administrative uses claims only. Hybrid supplements with medical records. Hybrid rates run 5–10pp higher. Invest in hybrid abstraction for high-weight Stars measures with significant denominator populations.

5 Gap closure prioritization: Stars weight × clinical urgency × closability × days remaining. Triple-weighted Stars measures with phone-closable gaps and >90 days remaining = highest ROI per outreach dollar.

6 Stars weights (1–3) determine each measure's contribution to the summary score. Sorting the quality dashboard by stars_weight DESC focuses team effort where financial impact is greatest. A 1pp improvement on a triple-weighted measure = 3× the Stars impact.

7 PDC (Proportion of Days Covered) for adherence measures: calendar-join approach avoids double-counting overlapping fills. PDC ≥ 80% = numerator met. Sort by PDC_pct ASC to prioritize the least adherent members for pharmacy outreach.

8 HEDIS audit readiness: maintain a member-level audit trail table for every measure. Every algorithm decision (denominator flag, exclusion reason, numerator event code, gap status) must be reproducible for any individual member on demand.

Chapter 28:CMS, NCQA, CAHPS & HOS

Quality ecosystem · HEDIS deep dive · CAHPS survey analytics · NCQA accreditation · HOS outcomes

28.1 The Quality Ecosystem

Four organizations define the quality measurement landscape for US health plans: (1) CMS: the federal regulator for Medicare Advantage, Medicaid managed care, and ACA marketplace plans. CMS administers Star Ratings, HEDIS reporting requirements, and plan audits. (2) NCQA: the independent accreditation body that certifies plan quality through HEDIS submission, CAHPS administration, and the Health Plan Accreditation program. (3) CAHPS (Consumer Assessment of Healthcare Providers and Systems): the standardized member experience survey administered annually. (4) HOS (Health Outcomes Survey): a two-year longitudinal survey for MA members measuring functional health status and physical and mental health outcomes.

> **NCQA Accreditation Levels** Excellent (highest) · Commendable · Accredited · Provisional · Denied. Commercial employers increasingly require NCQA accreditation as a plan selection criterion. MA plans with NCQA accreditation receive automatic deemed status for certain CMS requirements, reducing regulatory burden.

28.2 CAHPS Survey Analytics

CAHPS surveys measure member experience across composites: Getting Care Quickly, Getting Needed Care, How Well Doctors Communicate, Customer Service, Rating of Health Plan, and Rating of Personal Doctor. Each composite is scored 0–100. The analyst receives survey microdata and must calculate composite scores, stratify by demographic group, and track year-over-year trends. CMS uses CAHPS scores in Stars calculations (weighted equally with clinical measures in some domains).

ANSI SQL — 28.2: CAHPS Composite Score Calculation (Fully Annotated)

```
-- PURPOSE: Calculate CAHPS composite scores from survey microdata.
-- Each respondent answers multiple questions; questions roll up to composites.
-- Composite score = average of question-level "Always/Usually" rates.
-- CMS CAHPS scoring: Always=100, Usually=67, Sometimes=33, Never=0.

-- STEP 1: Score each individual survey question response.
-- Convert 4-point scale to 0-100 numeric for composite averaging.
WITH question_scores AS (
  SELECT
    s.survey_id,
    s.member_id,
    s.survey_year,
    s.question_id,
    q.composite_name,       -- e.g., 'Getting Care Quickly'
    q.composite_weight,     -- CMS-specified weight within composite
    -- Convert Likert response to 0-100 CMS scoring scale
    CASE s.response_value
      WHEN 'Always'    THEN 100
      WHEN 'Usually'   THEN 67
      WHEN 'Sometimes' THEN 33
      WHEN 'Never'     THEN 0
      -- Rating questions (1-10 scale): 9-10 = positive response
      WHEN '9'         THEN 100
      WHEN '10'        THEN 100
      ELSE             33  -- catch-all for middle ratings
    END AS question_score
```

```
    FROM fact_cahps_responses s
    JOIN ref_cahps_questions q ON s.question_id = q.question_id
    WHERE s.survey_year = :survey_year
      AND s.response_value IS NOT NULL  -- exclude non-respondents
      AND s.question_id NOT IN (        -- exclude screener / skip questions
        SELECT question_id FROM ref_cahps_questions
        WHERE question_type = 'SCREENER')
),

-- STEP 2: Roll up question scores to composite level per respondent.
respondent_composites AS (
    SELECT survey_id, member_id, composite_name,
           ROUND(AVG(question_score),1) AS respondent_composite_score
    FROM question_scores
    GROUP BY survey_id, member_id, composite_name
),

-- STEP 3: Calculate plan-level composite score and case mix adjustment.
-- Case mix adjustment removes demographic effects (age, education, health status)
-- so plan scores reflect care quality, not member population differences.
plan_composites AS (
    SELECT composite_name,
           COUNT(DISTINCT member_id)                  AS respondent_count,
           ROUND(AVG(respondent_composite_score),1)  AS unadjusted_score,
           -- Case-mix adjusted score stored in ref_cahps_adjustments
           -- (pre-calculated by the CAHPS vendor using regression)
           ca.adjusted_score
    FROM respondent_composites rc
    LEFT JOIN ref_cahps_adjustments ca
      ON rc.composite_name = ca.composite_name
     AND ca.survey_year = :survey_year
    GROUP BY composite_name, ca.adjusted_score
)
-- STEP 4: Compare to national mean and prior year for trending.
SELECT pc.composite_name,
    pc.respondent_count,
    pc.unadjusted_score,
    pc.adjusted_score,
    nm.national_mean_score,
    -- Positive = above national mean (favorable)
    ROUND(pc.adjusted_score - nm.national_mean_score,1) AS vs_national_mean,
    py.adjusted_score                        AS prior_year_score,
    ROUND(pc.adjusted_score - py.adjusted_score,1) AS year_over_year_change,
    COALESCE(sm.stars_weight,0)              AS stars_weight
FROM plan_composites pc
LEFT JOIN ref_cahps_national_means nm
   ON pc.composite_name = nm.composite_name AND nm.survey_year = :survey_year
LEFT JOIN plan_composites py
   ON pc.composite_name = py.composite_name  -- self-join for prior year
   -- Note: py uses survey_year = :survey_year - 1 in a separate CTE in production
LEFT JOIN ref_stars_measures sm ON pc.composite_name = sm.measure_description
ORDER BY sm.stars_weight DESC NULLS LAST, vs_national_mean ASC;
```

28.3 HOS — Health Outcomes Survey Analytics

HOS is a two-year longitudinal survey: Cohort 1 members are surveyed in Year 1 (baseline) and again two years later (follow-up). The measure compares the physical and mental health component scores (PCS and MCS from the VR-12 or SF-36 instrument) at follow-up vs. what would be expected based on baseline characteristics and age. Plans are scored on whether their members' functional health maintained or improved beyond the expected trajectory.

ANSI SQL — 28.3: HOS Cohort Matching and Year-over-Year Outcome Tracking (Fully Annotated)

```
-- PURPOSE: Match HOS respondents across the two survey years.
-- Calculate change in Physical Component Score (PCS) and
-- Mental Component Score (MCS) from baseline to follow-up.
-- Plans are scored on members who maintained or improved beyond expected.

-- STEP 1: Baseline survey scores (Year 1 of the HOS cohort).
WITH hos_baseline AS (
  SELECT h.member_id,
      h.survey_cohort_id,
      h.survey_year               AS baseline_year,
      h.pcs_score                 AS baseline_pcs, -- Physical Component Score
      h.mcs_score                 AS baseline_mcs, -- Mental Component Score
      h.age_at_survey,
      h.self_reported_health_status   -- 'Excellent','Very Good','Good','Fair','Poor'
  FROM  fact_hos_responses h
  WHERE h.survey_wave = 'BASELINE'
   AND h.survey_year = :cohort_baseline_year
   AND h.response_complete = 'Y'
),

-- STEP 2: Follow-up survey scores (two years later).
hos_followup AS (
  SELECT h.member_id, h.survey_cohort_id,
      h.pcs_score  AS followup_pcs,
      h.mcs_score  AS followup_mcs
  FROM  fact_hos_responses h
  WHERE h.survey_wave = 'FOLLOWUP'
   AND h.survey_year = :cohort_baseline_year + 2
   AND h.response_complete = 'Y'
)
-- STEP 3: Match baseline to follow-up on member_id and cohort.
-- Calculate actual vs. expected score change.
-- Expected change comes from CMS-supplied regression equations
-- based on baseline score, age, and self-reported health status.
SELECT b.member_id, m.member_name,
  b.baseline_pcs, f.followup_pcs,
  ROUND(f.followup_pcs - b.baseline_pcs,1)    AS pcs_change,
  b.baseline_mcs, f.followup_mcs,
  ROUND(f.followup_mcs - b.baseline_mcs,1)    AS mcs_change,
  -- Expected change from CMS regression model (stored in ref table)
  exp.expected_pcs_change, exp.expected_mcs_change,
  -- Maintained/improved: actual change >= expected change
  CASE WHEN f.followup_pcs - b.baseline_pcs >= exp.expected_pcs_change
    THEN 'MAINTAINED/IMPROVED PCS'
    ELSE 'DECLINED PCS' END             AS pcs_outcome,
  CASE WHEN f.followup_mcs - b.baseline_mcs >= exp.expected_mcs_change
    THEN 'MAINTAINED/IMPROVED MCS'
    ELSE 'DECLINED MCS' END             AS mcs_outcome
FROM  hos_baseline b
JOIN  hos_followup f   ON b.member_id = f.member_id
           AND b.survey_cohort_id = f.survey_cohort_id
JOIN  dim_members m   ON b.member_id = m.member_id
LEFT JOIN ref_hos_expected_change exp
  ON exp.baseline_pcs_quintile = NTILE(5) OVER (ORDER BY b.baseline_pcs)
 AND exp.age_band = CASE WHEN b.age_at_survey < 70 THEN '<70'
            WHEN b.age_at_survey < 80 THEN '70-79'
            ELSE '80+' END
ORDER BY pcs_change ASC; -- members with largest PCS decline at top for review
```

Chapter 28 Review

Unit Test · Key Takeaways

Answer each question before reading the explanation.

Q1. NCQA accreditation benefits a health plan because:

A. NCQA accreditation replaces all state licensure requirements

B. NCQA Excellent or Commendable status signals verified quality to employers and members, is required by many employer purchasers as a plan selection criterion, and provides deemed status for certain CMS requirements in MA — reducing regulatory burden.

C. Plans with NCQA accreditation pay lower HEDIS submission fees

D. NCQA accreditation guarantees a plan at least 4 Stars in CMS ratings

Answer: B. *NCQA accreditation is a market-access credential as much as a quality signal. Large self-insured employers — particularly those with multi-state workforces — typically require NCQA accreditation at the "Accredited" level or above as a precondition for plan inclusion in their benefits portfolio. Losing accreditation can trigger contract terminations with major employer groups.*

Q2. CAHPS composite scores are case-mix adjusted because:

A. CMS requires case-mix adjustment for all survey scores

B. Different plans serve populations with different demographic characteristics — older, sicker, less educated members tend to report lower experience scores independent of care quality. Case-mix adjustment removes these demographic effects so plan scores reflect true care quality differences, not population differences.

C. Case-mix adjustment inflates scores to be more comparable to HEDIS rates

D. Case-mix adjustment is required only for MA plans, not commercial

Answer: B. *Case-mix adjustment variables in CAHPS: member age, education level, self-reported health status (Excellent/Very Good/Good/Fair/Poor), and number of chronic conditions. A plan serving a predominantly low-income, chronically ill population will have lower unadjusted scores than a plan serving a young, healthy workforce — even if care quality is identical. The adjusted score removes these structural differences, enabling fair plan-to-plan comparison.*

Q3. HOS measures functional health outcomes over two years because:

A. Two years is the minimum period required by HEDIS specifications

B. Functional health status changes too slowly to measure meaningfully in a single year. The two-year longitudinal design captures whether care management programs are maintaining or improving members' physical and mental function over a clinically meaningful timeframe. The plan is scored against the expected trajectory, not an absolute threshold.

C. Two-year surveys are more cost-effective than annual surveys

D. CAHPS covers year-one outcomes; HOS covers years two and beyond

Answer: B. *HOS scoring logic: CMS regression equations predict the expected PCS and MCS score change for each member based on their baseline score, age, and initial health status. A member who starts with low baseline PCS has a different expected trajectory than a member who starts with high PCS. Plans are scored on the percentage of members who maintained or improved relative to their individual expected trajectory — not against a fixed cutpoint.*

Q4. The CAHPS "Getting Care Quickly" composite measures:

A. How quickly members receive their membership cards

B. Whether members could get an appointment as soon as they needed one (urgent and non-urgent) and how quickly they got care. Key questions: "In the last 6 months, when you needed care right away, how often did you get care as soon as you needed?" and "How often did you get an appointment for a check-up or routine care as soon as you needed?"

C. Whether care managers responded to member calls within 24 hours

D. The number of days from diagnosis to first specialist appointment

Answer: B. *Getting Care Quickly is consistently one of the lowest-scoring CAHPS composites nationally. Operational drivers: primary care appointment availability (especially for new patients), after-hours access, and telehealth availability for urgent needs. Plans that score poorly on this composite typically have network access issues — too few PCPs accepting new patients, or insufficient after-hours coverage.*

Q5. CAHPS response rates matter for Stars calculations because:

A. CMS requires a minimum 30% response rate for scores to count

B. Low response rates increase sampling variability and confidence interval width, making plan-to-plan comparisons less reliable. CMS applies a minimum case requirement; plans with too few respondents have their CAHPS score statistically adjusted or imputed rather than directly measured.

C. Response rates above 60% trigger a bonus adjustment in the Stars formula

D. Low response rates indicate that members are dissatisfied with the plan

Answer: B. *CAHPS response rates nationally average 35–45%. Plans invest in response rate optimization: multiple survey waves (mail + phone + web), reminder postcards, pre-notification letters in the member's preferred language, and stratified sampling to ensure demographic representation. A 5-percentage-point improvement in response rate typically reduces the confidence interval around composite scores by 15–20%, making the scores more stable year-over-year.*

Q6. The HOS PCS outcome "MAINTAINED/IMPROVED" is defined as:

A. The member's follow-up PCS score is higher than their baseline score

B. The member's actual PCS change (followup_pcs - baseline_pcs) is greater than or equal to the CMS regression-model expected change for a member with those baseline characteristics. A member expected to decline by 2 points who actually declines by only 1 point has "maintained" — because their outcome exceeded the prediction.

C. The member reported "Excellent" or "Very Good" health status at follow-up

D. The member's PCS score is in the top quartile of the plan's follow-up distribution

Answer: B. *This is the key conceptual distinction in HOS: the standard is relative to expected trajectory, not absolute. An 85-year-old member with very poor baseline physical function who loses only 1 point of PCS over two years may have "maintained" if the regression model predicted a 3-point decline for someone with those characteristics. The plan is rewarded for slowing the rate of functional decline in high-need members, not just for serving already-healthy members.*

Q7. Describe the NCQA Health Plan Accreditation process and how the analyst supports the accreditation submission.

(Short answer)

> **Sample Answer:**
> NCQA Health Plan Accreditation evaluates plans across six standards: Quality Management and Improvement (QI), Population Health Management (PHM), Network Management (NM), Utilization Management (UM), Credentialing and Recredentialing (CR), and Members Rights and Responsibilities (MR). Process: (1) Application: the plan submits an application specifying which accreditation level it seeks (Excellent, Commendable, Accredited, Provisional). (2) Document review: NCQA reviewers examine policies, procedures, and program descriptions for each standard. (3) Data submission: the plan submits HEDIS rates (for commercial plans) or HEDIS + CAHPS + HOS (for MA plans). (4) Audit: for Excellent or Commendable status, NCQA auditors conduct an on-site or virtual audit. Analyst support: (a) HEDIS rate production: run all applicable HEDIS measures with full audit trails. (b) QI program documentation: provide data showing the plan's quality improvement activities — member count, gap closure rates, year-over-year improvement trends. (c) PHM program data: risk stratification tier distributions (from Ch 22), care management program enrollment rates, high-risk member outreach rates. (d) UM documentation: PA turnaround times (Ch 24), denial rates, appeal overturn rates. Each data point must link to a specific NCQA standard element. The analyst provides the data; the QM director writes the narrative.

Q8. Write the SQL to stratify CAHPS composite scores by dual-eligible vs. non-dual-eligible members and identify the largest experience disparities.

(Short answer)

> **Sample Answer:**
> SELECT q.composite_name, CASE WHEN m.dual_eligible_flag='Y' THEN 'Dual Eligible' ELSE 'Non-Dual' END AS member_segment, COUNT(DISTINCT rc.member_id) AS respondent_count, ROUND(AVG(rc.respondent_composite_score),1) AS composite_score, ROUND(STDDEV(rc.respondent_composite_score),1) AS score_stddev FROM respondent_composites rc JOIN dim_members m ON rc.member_id=m.member_id JOIN ref_cahps_questions q ON rc.composite_name=q.composite_name WHERE rc.survey_year=:survey_year GROUP BY q.composite_name, CASE WHEN m.dual_eligible_flag='Y' THEN 'Dual Eligible' ELSE 'Non-Dual' END HAVING COUNT(DISTINCT rc.member_id)>=30 ORDER BY q.composite_name, member_segment. Then compute disparity: pivot to get dual and non-dual scores side by side, calculate the gap. Common finding: dual-eligible members score 8–15 points lower on "Getting Needed Care" and "Customer Service" composites — consistent with access barriers for this population. Action: route dual-eligible members with low Getting Care Quickly scores to the member advocacy team for appointment scheduling assistance. Report disparity gaps to CMO alongside CMS HEI analysis from Ch 23 — the same population driving HEDIS disparities is often driving CAHPS disparities.

Q9. Describe HOS data linkage to clinical analytics. How does the analyst connect HOS outcomes to care management program data?

(Short answer)

> **Sample Answer:**
> HOS data linkage: join fact_hos_responses to dim_members on member_id, then to care management program data (fact_cm_enrollments) to compare outcomes between enrolled and not-enrolled members. Key linkage: WITH hos_outcomes

AS (-- HOS PCS/MCS maintained/improved flags from Section 28.3), cm_enrollment AS (SELECT member_id, program_name, enrollment_date FROM fact_cm_enrollments WHERE enrollment_status='ACTIVE' AND program_name IN ('COMPLEX_CARE','CHRONIC_DISEASE_MGMT')), linked AS (SELECT h.member_id, h.pcs_outcome, h.mcs_outcome, CASE WHEN c.member_id IS NOT NULL THEN 'CM Enrolled' ELSE 'Not Enrolled' END AS cm_status FROM hos_outcomes h LEFT JOIN cm_enrollment c ON h.member_id=c.member_id) SELECT cm_status, COUNT(*) AS members, ROUND(100.0*SUM(CASE WHEN pcs_outcome='MAINTAINED/IMPROVED PCS' THEN 1 ELSE 0 END)/COUNT(*),1) AS pcs_maintained_pct, ROUND(100.0*SUM(CASE WHEN mcs_outcome='MAINTAINED/IMPROVED MCS' THEN 1 ELSE 0 END)/COUNT(*),1) AS mcs_maintained_pct FROM linked GROUP BY cm_status. If CM enrolled members have materially higher maintained/improved rates, this supports the program's ROI narrative for the CMO. Important caveat: CM-enrolled members are higher-risk by selection — raw comparison overstates the program effect. Apply the same difference-in-differences adjustment as in Ch 26: compare CM enrolled vs. a matched non-enrolled comparison group with similar baseline PCS/MCS scores and health status.

Q10. Describe three CAHPS composite improvement strategies and the SQL that supports each.

(Short answer)

Sample Answer:

Strategy 1 — Getting Care Quickly: low scores indicate access barriers. SQL: SELECT attr.attributed_pcp_npi, p.provider_full_name, COUNT(DISTINCT rc.member_id) AS respondents, ROUND(AVG(CASE WHEN rc.composite_name='Getting Care Quickly' THEN rc.respondent_composite_score END),1) AS gcq_score FROM respondent_composites rc JOIN dim_pcp_attribution attr ON rc.member_id=attr.member_id JOIN dim_providers p ON attr.attributed_pcp_npi=p.npi GROUP BY attr.attributed_pcp_npi, p.provider_full_name HAVING COUNT(DISTINCT rc.member_id)>=15 ORDER BY gcq_score ASC. Low-scoring PCPs receive a Provider Relations visit to address appointment availability and after-hours access. Strategy 2 — How Well Doctors Communicate: low scores indicate communication quality gaps. SQL: same structure, filter composite_name='How Well Doctors Communicate'. Route low-scoring providers to communication skills training programs or patient advisory committee engagement. Strategy 3 — Customer Service (plan-level): measures member service center interactions. SQL: link CAHPS respondents to fact_member_service_calls on member_id. Compare composite scores for members who called member services in the 6 months before the survey vs. those who did not. If callers score lower: identify the top call reasons (denials, billing, prior auth) and route to process improvement. If non-callers also score low: the issue is broader than service center quality — survey the full member experience. Present all three strategies with SQL evidence to the VP of Quality as the annual CAHPS improvement action plan.

Key Takeaways

What every analyst must remember from this chapter.

1 Quality ecosystem: CMS (regulator, Stars), NCQA (accreditor, HEDIS/CAHPS/HOS standards), CAHPS (member experience survey), HOS (two-year longitudinal functional outcomes). All four feed into the CMS Star Ratings for MA plans.

2 NCQA accreditation levels: Excellent → Commendable → Accredited → Provisional → Denied. Employer purchasers require Accredited or above. MA plans with NCQA accreditation receive deemed CMS status, reducing regulatory burden.

3 CAHPS composite scoring: Always=100, Usually=67, Sometimes=33, Never=0. Case-mix adjust for age, education, and self-reported health status before plan-to-plan comparison. Unadjusted scores favor plans serving healthier, more educated populations.

4 CAHPS improvement tactics: Getting Care Quickly → PCP appointment availability and after-hours access. How Well Doctors Communicate → provider communication skills programs. Customer Service → member service center process improvement.

5 HOS scoring: compare actual PCS/MCS change to CMS regression-model expected change. Maintained/improved = actual change ≥ expected change. A member who declines less than expected has "maintained." Plans are rewarded for slowing functional decline in high-need populations.

6 HOS-to-CM linkage: join HOS outcomes to care management enrollment. Compare maintained/improved rates for CM-enrolled vs. not-enrolled members. Apply difference-in-differences adjustment (Ch 26) to remove selection bias before claiming program credit.

7 CAHPS response rate optimization: multiple survey waves, reminder postcards, pre-notification letters in preferred language, stratified sampling for demographic representation. Higher response rate → narrower confidence intervals → more stable year-over-year scores.

8 NCQA audit support: HEDIS rate production with full member-level audit trail, QI program data (gap closure rates, year-over-year trends), PHM tier distributions, UM turnaround times and denial rates. Every data point links to a specific NCQA standard element.

Chapter 29:CMS Star Ratings — End-to-End Pipeline

Measure collection · Cut-point methodology · Domain weighting · Score simulation · Gap closure ROI

29.1 Star Ratings Architecture

CMS calculates MA Star Ratings annually for each plan contract (H-number). The rating aggregates up to 50+ measures across five domains: Staying Healthy (screenings, tests, vaccines), Managing Chronic Conditions, Plan Responsiveness and Care, Member Complaints and Appeals, and Health Plan Administrative Measures. Each measure is rated 1–5 stars based on national cut-points. Measures are weighted (1–3) within domains; domains are combined into a Part C Summary Rating. A ≥ 4.0 Star plan receives a Quality Bonus Payment (QBP) worth up to 5% of benchmark.

Cut-Point Methodology CMS uses clustering algorithms (k-means or hierarchical) to set measure-level cut-points that divide all MA plans into five equal groups. Cut-points are not fixed year-to-year — they shift as the industry improves. A plan that achieved 4 Stars last year at 72% may need 75% next year to remain at 4 Stars if the national distribution improved.

29.2 Measure-Level Star Score Assignment

ANSI SQL — 29.2: Assign Star Score per Measure Using Cut-Points (Fully Annotated)

```
-- PURPOSE: Assign a 1–5 star score to each measure based on the plan's
-- calculated rate and CMS-published cut-points for that measurement year.
-- cut-points stored in ref_star_cutpoints per measure_id and star_year.

-- STEP 1: Calculate plan-level rates for all Stars-eligible measures.
WITH plan_rates AS (
  SELECT
    hg.measure_id,
    hg.measure_description,
    COUNT(DISTINCT hg.member_id)                AS denominator,
    COUNT(DISTINCT CASE WHEN hg.gap_status = 'CLOSED'
      THEN hg.member_id END)                   AS numerator,
    ROUND(100.0 * COUNT(DISTINCT CASE WHEN hg.gap_status = 'CLOSED'
      THEN hg.member_id END)
      / NULLIF(COUNT(DISTINCT hg.member_id),0), 2)  AS rate_pct
  FROM  fact_hedis_gaps hg
  WHERE hg.measurement_year = :meas_year
   AND hg.denominator_eligible = 'Y'
  GROUP BY hg.measure_id, hg.measure_description
),

-- STEP 2: Join plan rates to CMS-published cut-points.
-- Cut-points: cut1 = top of 1-Star range, cut2 = top of 2-Star, etc.
-- A plan's star score = the lowest cut-point its rate does NOT exceed.
star_assignment AS (
  SELECT pr.measure_id, pr.measure_description,
     pr.denominator, pr.numerator, pr.rate_pct,
     cp.cut1, cp.cut2, cp.cut3, cp.cut4,
     sm.stars_weight,
     sm.stars_domain,
     -- Assign star score by comparing rate to each cut-point
     CASE
       WHEN pr.rate_pct >= cp.cut4 THEN 5
       WHEN pr.rate_pct >= cp.cut3 THEN 4
       WHEN pr.rate_pct >= cp.cut2 THEN 3
```

```
            WHEN pr.rate_pct >= cp.cut1 THEN 2
            ELSE 1
        END AS measure_star_score
    FROM  plan_rates pr
    JOIN  ref_star_cutpoints cp
      ON cp.measure_id  = pr.measure_id
     AND cp.star_year   = :meas_year
    JOIN  ref_stars_measures sm ON pr.measure_id = sm.measure_id
)
-- STEP 3: Show rate vs. cut-points and how close to the next star threshold.
SELECT measure_id, measure_description, stars_domain, stars_weight,
    denominator, numerator, rate_pct,
    measure_star_score,
    cut4,
    -- Points needed to reach the next star threshold
    CASE
      WHEN measure_star_score = 5 THEN 0
      WHEN measure_star_score = 4 THEN ROUND(cut4 - rate_pct,2)
      WHEN measure_star_score = 3 THEN ROUND(cp.cut3 - rate_pct,2)
      WHEN measure_star_score = 2 THEN ROUND(cp.cut2 - rate_pct,2)
      ELSE ROUND(cut1 - rate_pct,2)
    END AS pct_pts_to_next_star
FROM  star_assignment
JOIN  ref_star_cutpoints cp ON star_assignment.measure_id=cp.measure_id AND cp.star_year=:meas_year
ORDER BY measure_star_score ASC, pct_pts_to_next_star ASC;
-- Lowest stars first, then closest to next threshold = highest uplift opportunity
```

29.3 Domain and Summary Score Calculation

ANSI SQL — 29.3: Domain Score and Part C Summary Star Rating Simulation (Fully Annotated)

```
-- PURPOSE: Aggregate measure-level star scores to domain scores,
-- then to the overall Part C Summary Rating.
-- This is the plan's simulated Star Rating based on current performance.
-- Use it to model gap closure scenarios: "If we improve X to 4 Stars,
-- what happens to the Summary Rating?"

-- STEP 1: Weighted measure score per domain.
-- Each measure's contribution = star_score × stars_weight.
WITH weighted_measures AS (
    SELECT
      stars_domain,
      measure_id,
      measure_description,
      measure_star_score,
      stars_weight,
      -- Weighted contribution of this measure to its domain
      measure_star_score * stars_weight        AS weighted_score
    FROM  star_assignment   -- from Section 29.2
),

-- STEP 2: Domain-level weighted average score.
-- Domain score = SUM(measure_star_score × weight) / SUM(weights) per domain.
domain_scores AS (
    SELECT stars_domain,
        SUM(weighted_score)        AS total_weighted_score,
        SUM(stars_weight)          AS total_weight,
        -- Weighted average star score for the domain
        ROUND(SUM(weighted_score * 1.0)
          / NULLIF(SUM(stars_weight),0), 2) AS domain_star_score
    FROM  weighted_measures
```

```
    GROUP BY stars_domain
),

-- STEP 3: Part C Summary Rating.
-- Summary = weighted average of domain scores, each domain weighted equally
-- in CMS methodology (unless plan is under a special adjustment).
summary_rating AS (
    SELECT
        ROUND(AVG(domain_star_score),2) AS raw_summary_score,
        -- CMS rounds to the nearest 0.5 for the displayed Star Rating
        ROUND(AVG(domain_star_score) * 2) / 2.0 AS displayed_star_rating
    FROM domain_scores
)
-- STEP 4: Show full detail plus summary.
SELECT 'Domain' AS level, ds.stars_domain AS label,
    ds.total_weight, ds.domain_star_score AS score,
    NULL AS displayed_rating
FROM domain_scores ds
UNION ALL
SELECT 'SUMMARY', 'Part C Overall Rating',
    NULL, sr.raw_summary_score, sr.displayed_star_rating
FROM summary_rating sr
ORDER BY level DESC, score ASC;
```

29.4 Gap Closure Simulation — "What-If" Score Projector

The gap closure simulator answers the question: "If we close all open gaps for measure X (moving it from 3 Stars to 4 Stars), what happens to our Summary Rating?" This is the most valuable analytics output the quality team can produce — it converts clinical gap closure work into a projected Stars score change and a dollar estimate of the QBP impact.

ANSI SQL — 29.4: Stars Gap Closure Scenario Simulator (Fully Annotated)

```
-- PURPOSE: Simulate the Stars Rating impact of closing all open gaps
-- for each measure. Shows which measures, if improved to the next star
-- threshold, would move the overall Summary Rating.
-- Output: the strategic gap closure priority list for the VP of Quality.

-- STEP 1: For each measure at 1-3 Stars, calculate what rate is needed
-- to reach the next cut-point, and how many gaps must close to get there.
WITH improvement_scenarios AS (
    SELECT
        sa.measure_id, sa.measure_description,
        sa.stars_domain, sa.stars_weight,
        sa.denominator, sa.numerator, sa.rate_pct,
        sa.measure_star_score AS current_star,
        -- Target rate = just above the cut-point for the next star
        CASE
            WHEN sa.measure_star_score = 4 THEN cp.cut4
            WHEN sa.measure_star_score = 3 THEN cp.cut4 -- jump to 5 Stars
            WHEN sa.measure_star_score = 2 THEN cp.cut3
            ELSE cp.cut2
        END AS target_rate,
        -- Gaps to close = members needed in numerator to hit target rate
        CEIL((
            CASE
                WHEN sa.measure_star_score = 4 THEN cp.cut4
                WHEN sa.measure_star_score = 3 THEN cp.cut4
                WHEN sa.measure_star_score = 2 THEN cp.cut3
                ELSE cp.cut2
            END / 100.0 * sa.denominator) - sa.numerator
```

```
    ) AS gaps_to_close_for_next_star
  FROM  star_assignment sa
  JOIN  ref_star_cutpoints cp
    ON cp.measure_id = sa.measure_id AND cp.star_year = :meas_year
  WHERE sa.measure_star_score < 5
),

-- STEP 2: Calculate the Summary Rating impact of each improvement scenario.
-- Recompute domain score and summary with the improved measure.
simulated_impact AS (
  SELECT
    is_tbl.measure_id,
    is_tbl.measure_description,
    is_tbl.stars_domain,
    is_tbl.stars_weight,
    is_tbl.current_star,
    is_tbl.current_star + 1 AS simulated_star,
    is_tbl.gaps_to_close_for_next_star,
    -- Current domain score
    ds_current.domain_star_score AS current_domain_score,
    -- Simulated domain score with this measure improved by 1 star
    ROUND((
      ds_current.total_weighted_score
      - is_tbl.current_star * is_tbl.stars_weight  -- remove current contribution
      + (is_tbl.current_star + 1) * is_tbl.stars_weight  -- add improved contribution
    ) / NULLIF(ds_current.total_weight,0), 2)       AS simulated_domain_score
  FROM  improvement_scenarios is_tbl
  JOIN  domain_scores ds_current ON is_tbl.stars_domain = ds_current.stars_domain
)
-- STEP 3: Show the full priority list with simulated summary rating impact.
SELECT
  si.measure_id, si.measure_description,
  si.stars_domain, si.stars_weight,
  si.current_star, si.simulated_star,
  si.gaps_to_close_for_next_star,
  ROUND(si.current_domain_score,2)    AS current_domain_score,
  ROUND(si.simulated_domain_score,2)  AS simulated_domain_score,
  -- Estimated QBP revenue impact (each 0.5 star improvement ≈ plan-specific $)
  ROUND((si.simulated_domain_score - si.current_domain_score)
    * :annual_benchmark_revenue * 0.01, 0) AS est_qbp_revenue_impact,
  -- ROI: revenue impact per gap closed
  ROUND(ROUND((si.simulated_domain_score-si.current_domain_score)
    * :annual_benchmark_revenue * 0.01,0)
    / NULLIF(si.gaps_to_close_for_next_star,0), 0)  AS revenue_per_gap_closed
FROM  simulated_impact si
WHERE si.gaps_to_close_for_next_star > 0
ORDER BY revenue_per_gap_closed DESC NULLS LAST;
-- Highest revenue per gap closed = best investment for the quality team
```

Chapter 29 Review

Unit Test · Key Takeaways

Answer each question before reading the explanation.

Q1. CMS uses clustering algorithms for Star Rating cut-points because:

A. Fixed cut-points are simpler to administer

B. Clustering ensures cut-points reflect the actual distribution of national plan performance — they shift each year as the industry improves, preventing grade inflation. A fixed 70% threshold for 4 Stars becomes meaningless if 90% of plans exceed 70%.

C. CMS is required by ACA to use statistical methods for cut-points

D. Clustering rewards plans that improve most, regardless of their absolute level

Answer: B. *CMS historically used k-means clustering (or CAHPs-specific hierarchical clustering) to divide all MA plan rates into five clusters representing Stars 1–5. The key implication: a plan that maintains 72% on a measure where the national mean is rising from 70% to 77% could drop from 4 Stars to 3 Stars without making any errors — because the cut-points shifted. Plans must benchmark not just against last year's cut-points but against projected industry trends.*

Q2. The Quality Bonus Payment (QBP) for plans with ≥ 4.0 Stars is significant because:

A. QBP funds are used to pay HEDIS auditors

B. Plans rated ≥ 4.0 Stars receive up to 5% of their CMS benchmark revenue as a quality bonus, which can fund lower member premiums, enhanced benefits, and higher provider rates — directly improving competitive position. For a plan with $500M in MA revenue, 5% = $25M annually.

C. QBP is the only funding source for NCQA accreditation activities

D. 4-Star plans are exempt from CMS RADV audits

Answer: B. *The QBP financial mechanism: CMS multiplies the plan's benchmark by the quality bonus percentage. Plans use this additional revenue to offer zero-premium plans, supplemental benefits (dental, vision, over-the-counter allowances), lower cost-sharing, or higher provider payment rates. These features attract enrollment — creating a virtuous cycle where more Stars = more enrollment = larger scale = better negotiating leverage. Plans below 3.0 Stars for three consecutive years face contract termination.*

Q3. The pct_pts_to_next_star field in the star assignment query identifies:

A. How many members need to be enrolled to improve the denominator

B. How many percentage points the plan's current rate must increase to reach the next Star threshold. Combined with the denominator, this translates directly into: gaps_to_close = CEIL(pct_pts_to_next_star/100 × denominator). Measures with small gaps-to-close and high Stars weight are the highest ROI targets.

C. The year-over-year improvement needed to maintain the current star score

D. The difference between the plan rate and the NCQA national average

Answer: B. *Example: BCS at 72.3% on a 3-Star rating; cut4 (4-Star threshold) = 75.0%. pct_pts_to_next_star = 75.0 - 72.3 = 2.7pp. With denominator = 800 women: gaps_to_close = CEIL(2.7/100 × 800) = CEIL(21.6) = 22 additional mammograms needed. At an outreach cost of $50 per closed gap: total program cost = 22 × $50 = $1,100 to potentially improve a triple-weighted measure from 3 to 4 Stars.*

Q4. Domain score is calculated as a weighted average because:

A. All measures within a domain have equal clinical importance

B. Measures within each domain carry different Stars weights (1–3) reflecting CMS's assessment of their relative importance to member outcomes. Weighting ensures that measures more predictive of health outcomes and member experience contribute more to the domain score than administrative or reporting measures.

C. CMS requires equal weighting within domains but differential weighting across domains

D. Weighted averages produce more stable scores year-over-year

Answer: B. *Domain score formula: SUM(measure_star_score × stars_weight) / SUM(stars_weight). A domain with three measures at weights 3, 2, and 1, with star scores of 4, 3, and 5 respectively: weighted sum = 4×3 + 3×2 + 5×1 = 12+6+5 = 23. Total weight = 6. Domain score = 23/6 = 3.83. The triple-weighted measure (HbA1c testing) contributes half the domain weight — improving it from 4 to 5 Stars moves the domain from 3.83 to 4.17.*

Q5. The revenue_per_gap_closed field in the simulation query is the key prioritization metric because:

A. It measures member satisfaction per gap closure

B. It converts the Stars impact of each gap closure scenario into a financial return per individual gap closed — enabling the VP of Quality to compare investments across measures with very different denominators. A measure where each gap closure is worth $800 in QBP revenue deserves more resources than one where each gap is worth $50.

C. It is required by CMS in the annual quality attestation

D. It replaces the need for gap closure ROI analysis from Chapter 26

Answer: B. *Revenue per gap closed example: a triple-weighted measure with 30 gaps to close, where closing them would improve the Summary Rating by 0.25 Stars = approximately 0.25% QBP uplift on $400M benchmark = $1M additional QBP revenue. Revenue per gap = $1M / 30 = ~$33,333 per gap. A care management outreach program that costs $200 per closed gap generates $33,133 net per gap — extraordinary ROI. This calculation transforms quality improvement from a compliance exercise into a capital allocation decision.*

Q6. CMS displays Stars ratings rounded to the nearest 0.5 because:

A. 0.5 increments are required by ACA regulations

B. Displaying two decimal places (3.83 stars) would create consumer confusion and allow micro-comparisons that exceed the measurement precision of the underlying data. Rounding to 0.5 preserves the meaningful distinctions (3.5 vs. 4.0 Stars matters for QBP) while avoiding false precision.

C. The clustering algorithm only produces half-star increments

D. 0.5 rounding eliminates the effect of measure-level statistical noise

Answer: B. *The displayed Star Rating is ROUND(raw_summary_score × 2) / 2.0. A raw score of 3.73 displays as 3.5 Stars. A raw score of 3.75 displays as 4.0 Stars. This creates a critical threshold: the difference between a raw score of 3.74 and 3.75 is one Star tier and potentially $25M+ in QBP revenue. Plans within 0.10 raw score points of a half-star boundary should model exact gap closure scenarios at the individual member level.*

Q7. Describe the complete Stars pipeline from measure data collection to Summary Rating. What are the key failure points?

(Short answer)

Sample Answer:

Stars pipeline: (1) Measure data collection: HEDIS rates from claims + medical record abstraction (hybrid); CAHPS survey administration and scoring; HOS follow-up cohort matching; Administrative measures from CMS operational data (appeals, complaints, member service). (2) Data submission: submit HEDIS rates to NCQA; submit CAHPS results to CMS vendor. CMS collects administrative measure data directly. Failure point: late or incorrect HEDIS submission → measures receive 1 Star by default or are excluded. (3) Cut-point determination: CMS clusters all plan rates nationally and sets cut-points. Published in the annual Stars Technical Notes. Failure point: using last year's cut-points to project this year's scores — cut-points shift annually. (4) Measure-level star assignment: each measure rate compared to cut-points → 1–5 stars. Failure point: rates calculated on the wrong population (wrong measurement year, wrong LOB, wrong age band). (5) Domain scoring: weighted average within each domain. Failure point: incorrect stars_weight for newly added or reclassified measures. (6) Summary Rating: average of domain scores, rounded to nearest 0.5. Failure point: applying equal domain weights when CMS has specified differential domain weights for a specific plan type. (7) QBP determination: CMS applies the bonus percentage to the plan's benchmark. Failure point: not accounting for the Employer Group Waiver Plan (EGWP) exclusion from QBP. Every pipeline step should have a reconciliation check: plan's own calculation vs. CMS's posted preliminary rates (published approximately 9 months before the final Stars determination).

Q8. A plan is at 3.75 raw Stars score (displaying as 4.0 Stars). The VP of Quality wants to know which measures to protect to avoid dropping below 4.0 Stars. Write the SQL.

(Short answer)

Sample Answer:

SELECT sa.measure_id, sa.measure_description, sa.stars_domain, sa.stars_weight, sa.measure_star_score AS current_star, sa.rate_pct, cp.cut3 AS threshold_for_current_star, -- How much the rate can fall before losing a star ROUND(sa.rate_pct - cp.cut3, 2) AS buffer_above_threshold, -- Impact on Summary Rating if this measure drops 1 star ROUND((sa.stars_weight * 1.0 / ds.total_weight) * (1.0/5.0), 3) AS summary_impact_per_star_drop FROM star_assignment sa JOIN ref_star_cutpoints cp ON sa.measure_id=cp.measure_id AND cp.star_year=:meas_year JOIN domain_scores ds ON sa.stars_domain=ds.stars_domain WHERE sa.measure_star_score IN (4,5) ORDER BY buffer_above_threshold ASC, sa.stars_weight DESC. Interpretation: measures with small buffer_above_threshold (close to falling a star) AND high stars_weight are the vulnerability risk. If a 3-weighted measure at 4 Stars drops to 3 Stars, the domain score drops by 3/total_domain_weight points. Protecting these measures requires monitoring their rates monthly and maintaining the denominator quality (correct enrollment, correct age bands, correct exclusions). Present to the VP of Quality as the "hold the line" watchlist alongside the "advance" prioritization list from Section 29.4.

Q9. Describe the CMS Low-Performing Icon (LPI) and Improvement Measures policies and their analytical implications.

(Short answer)

Sample Answer:

Low-Performing Icon (LPI): CMS displays an LPI (a warning flag) on the plan finder for any plan with a measure-level star score of 1 or 2 Stars on a designated LPI measure for three consecutive years. LPI measures include high-visibility clinical measures: breast cancer screening, diabetes care, and colorectal cancer screening. Analytical implication: identify all measures where the plan has scored 1 or 2 Stars. Check the historical trend — if a measure has been at 1 or 2 Stars for two consecutive years, the plan is one year away from an LPI designation that will appear on plan finder and potentially damage enrollment. SQL: SELECT measure_id, survey_year, measure_star_score FROM fact_stars_history WHERE measure_star_score <= 2 AND measure_id IN (SELECT measure_id FROM ref_lpi_measures) ORDER BY measure_id, survey_year. Improvement Measures policy: CMS gives credit in the summary rating calculation for measures that show statistically significant improvement year-over-year, even if the measure remains at a low star level. This credit can prevent a plan from being flagged as "consistently low performing." Analytical implication: track year-over-year rate changes. A measure that improved from 55% to 63% (statistically significant at the plan's denominator size) qualifies for improvement credit even if 63% is still only 2 Stars. The analyst should calculate whether year-over-year changes are statistically significant using chi-square or z-test on the numerator/denominator counts.

Q10. Build the full gap closure ROI presentation: combine the Stars simulation with the per-gap closure cost estimate to produce a ranked investment table for the CFO.

(Short answer)

> **Sample Answer:**
>
> Combine Stars simulation (Section 29.4) with care management program cost data: WITH stars_sim AS (-- Simulation query from 29.4: measure_id, stars_weight, current_star, gaps_to_close_for_next_star, est_qbp_revenue_impact, revenue_per_gap_closed), closure_cost AS (SELECT measure_id, measure_description, avg_cost_per_gap_closed, typical_weeks_to_close FROM ref_gap_closure_costs -- plan-maintained reference: cost and timeline per measure type), combined AS (SELECT s.measure_id, s.measure_description, s.stars_domain, s.stars_weight, s.current_star, s.simulated_star, s.gaps_to_close_for_next_star, s.est_qbp_revenue_impact, c.avg_cost_per_gap_closed, ROUND(s.gaps_to_close_for_next_star * c.avg_cost_per_gap_closed,0) AS total_program_cost, ROUND(s.est_qbp_revenue_impact - s.gaps_to_close_for_next_star * c.avg_cost_per_gap_closed,0) AS net_qbp_benefit, s.revenue_per_gap_closed, c.typical_weeks_to_close FROM stars_sim s JOIN closure_cost c ON s.measure_id=c.measure_id) SELECT * FROM combined WHERE net_qbp_benefit > 0 ORDER BY net_qbp_benefit DESC. CFO presentation format: each row = one measure improvement opportunity. Columns: current_star → simulated_star; gaps to close; program cost; QBP revenue gained; net benefit; weeks to close. Top rows represent the clearest investment cases — high net benefit, low cost, short timeline. Present as "the quality investment portfolio" with a total row showing aggregate program cost vs. aggregate QBP uplift. Typical finding: 3–5 measures account for 80% of the achievable QBP revenue improvement.

Key Takeaways

What every analyst must remember from this chapter.

1 Stars pipeline: measure rates → cut-point assignment (1–5) → domain weighted average → Summary Rating (rounded to 0.5). QBP: ≥ 4.0 Stars = up to 5% bonus. Plans below 3.0 Stars for 3 consecutive years face contract termination.

2 Cut-points shift annually with the industry distribution. Always use the current year's CMS-published cut-points — never assume last year's thresholds hold. A plan that maintained 72% may drop from 4 to 3 Stars if the national distribution improved.

3 pct_pts_to_next_star × denominator / 100 = gaps_to_close_for_next_star. CEIL() rounds up — you need every fraction of a gap. The measure closest to the next threshold with the highest Stars weight = the best investment per gap.

4 Domain score = SUM(measure_star × weight) / SUM(weight). Summary Rating = average of domain scores, rounded to nearest 0.5. A raw score of 3.75+ displays as 4.0 Stars (QBP threshold). Every hundredth of a point near a boundary matters.

5 Stars simulation: recalculate domain score after improving a measure by one star. revenue_per_gap_closed = est_qbp_impact / gaps_to_close. Rank by revenue_per_gap_closed DESC for the quality investment portfolio.

6 Vulnerability analysis: measures at 4–5 Stars with small buffer above the current threshold. SQL: rate_pct - cut-point for current star level = buffer. Small buffer + high weight = risk of dropping a star and losing QBP threshold.

7 Low-Performing Icon (LPI): 1–2 Stars on a designated LPI measure for 3 consecutive years triggers a public warning flag on plan finder. Check historical star scores. Two consecutive years at 1–2 Stars = emergency remediation priority.

8 Net QBP benefit = est_qbp_revenue_impact - (gaps_to_close × avg_cost_per_gap). Rank by net_qbp_benefit DESC for the CFO investment table. Typically 3–5 measures account for 80% of achievable QBP revenue improvement.

Chapter 30: Data Quality & Governance

Six DQ dimensions · Automated DQ dashboard · NPI validation · Anomaly detection · Reference data governance

30.1 Data Quality Framework

All analytics in this book rests on data quality. A claims database with missing NPIs, duplicate members, stale reference tables, or systematically miscoded diagnoses produces incorrect HEDIS rates, wrong risk scores, and flawed financial projections. The six-dimension DQ framework provides a structured approach: Completeness (are required fields populated?), Validity (are values within defined domains?), Timeliness (is data current?), Consistency (do values agree across systems?), Uniqueness (are records free of duplicates?), and Accuracy (do values match the ground truth?).

> **DQ Gate Principle** Each dimension has a threshold below which downstream analytics cannot be trusted. When a gate fails, the pipeline halts and an alert fires. Never run HEDIS or Stars calculations on data that has not passed all DQ gates for that measurement period.

30.2 Automated DQ Dashboard

ANSI SQL — 30.2: Automated Data Quality Dashboard — All Six Dimensions (Fully Annotated)

```
-- PURPOSE: Evaluate the six data quality dimensions for the current
-- claims extract and produce a pass/fail gate for each.
-- Run at every ETL load. Fail = halt pipeline and alert Data Engineering.

-- DIMENSION 1: COMPLETENESS
-- Required fields must have non-null, non-empty values.
WITH completeness AS (
  SELECT
    'COMPLETENESS'                    AS dq_dimension,
    'Rendering NPI present'           AS dq_check,
    COUNT(*)                          AS total_records,
    SUM(CASE WHEN rendering_npi IS NULL
        OR rendering_npi = '' THEN 1 ELSE 0 END) AS fail_count,
    ROUND(100.0 * SUM(CASE WHEN rendering_npi IS NULL
        OR rendering_npi = '' THEN 1 ELSE 0 END)
      / NULLIF(COUNT(*),0), 2)          AS fail_pct,
    2.0 AS threshold_pct,  -- alert if > 2% missing
    CASE WHEN ROUND(100.0*SUM(CASE WHEN rendering_npi IS NULL
        OR rendering_npi = '' THEN 1 ELSE 0 END)
      /NULLIF(COUNT(*),0),2) <= 2.0
        THEN 'PASS' ELSE 'FAIL' END       AS gate_status
  FROM  fact_medical_claims
  WHERE EXTRACT(YEAR FROM service_date) = EXTRACT(YEAR FROM CURRENT_DATE)
   AND claim_status = 'PAID'

  UNION ALL

  -- Primary diagnosis completeness
  SELECT 'COMPLETENESS', 'Primary diagnosis code present',
    COUNT(*), SUM(CASE WHEN primary_diag IS NULL OR primary_diag='' THEN 1 ELSE 0 END),
```

```
    ROUND(100.0*SUM(CASE WHEN primary_diag IS NULL OR primary_diag='' THEN 1 ELSE 0 END)
      /NULLIF(COUNT(*),0),2),
    1.0, -- alert if > 1% missing
    CASE WHEN ROUND(100.0*SUM(CASE WHEN primary_diag IS NULL OR primary_diag='' THEN 1 ELSE 0 END)
      /NULLIF(COUNT(*),0),2) <= 1.0 THEN 'PASS' ELSE 'FAIL' END
  FROM  fact_medical_claims
  WHERE EXTRACT(YEAR FROM service_date) = EXTRACT(YEAR FROM CURRENT_DATE)
   AND claim_status = 'PAID'
),

-- DIMENSION 2: VALIDITY
-- Values must conform to defined domains and code sets.
validity AS (
  SELECT 'VALIDITY', 'ICD-10 diagnosis code in reference table',
    COUNT(*),
    -- Claims where primary_diag is NOT found in the ICD-10 reference
    SUM(CASE WHEN ref.icd10_code IS NULL THEN 1 ELSE 0 END),
    ROUND(100.0*SUM(CASE WHEN ref.icd10_code IS NULL THEN 1 ELSE 0 END)
      /NULLIF(COUNT(*),0),2),
    0.5, -- alert if > 0.5% invalid codes
    CASE WHEN ROUND(100.0*SUM(CASE WHEN ref.icd10_code IS NULL THEN 1 ELSE 0 END)
      /NULLIF(COUNT(*),0),2) <= 0.5 THEN 'PASS' ELSE 'FAIL' END
  FROM  fact_medical_claims c
  LEFT JOIN ref_icd10_codes ref ON c.primary_diag = ref.icd10_code
  WHERE EXTRACT(YEAR FROM c.service_date) = EXTRACT(YEAR FROM CURRENT_DATE)
   AND c.claim_status = 'PAID'
),

-- DIMENSION 3: TIMELINESS
-- Claims should appear within a reasonable lag of the service date.
timeliness AS (
  SELECT 'TIMELINESS', 'Claims processed within 90 days of service',
    COUNT(*),
    SUM(CASE WHEN DATEDIFF('day', service_date, paid_date) > 90
      THEN 1 ELSE 0 END),
    ROUND(100.0*SUM(CASE WHEN DATEDIFF('day', service_date, paid_date) > 90
      THEN 1 ELSE 0 END)/NULLIF(COUNT(*),0),2),
    5.0, -- alert if > 5% of claims take more than 90 days to process
    CASE WHEN ROUND(100.0*SUM(CASE WHEN DATEDIFF('day',service_date,paid_date)>90
      THEN 1 ELSE 0 END)/NULLIF(COUNT(*),0),2)<=5.0
       THEN 'PASS' ELSE 'FAIL' END
  FROM  fact_medical_claims
  WHERE EXTRACT(YEAR FROM service_date) = EXTRACT(YEAR FROM CURRENT_DATE)
   AND claim_status = 'PAID'
),

-- DIMENSION 4: CONSISTENCY
-- Values should agree across related tables.
consistency AS (
  SELECT 'CONSISTENCY', 'Member IDs in claims exist in dim_members',
    COUNT(DISTINCT c.member_id),
    COUNT(DISTINCT CASE WHEN m.member_id IS NULL THEN c.member_id END),
    ROUND(100.0*COUNT(DISTINCT CASE WHEN m.member_id IS NULL THEN c.member_id END)
      /NULLIF(COUNT(DISTINCT c.member_id),0),2),
    0.1, -- alert if > 0.1% orphan member IDs
    CASE WHEN ROUND(100.0*COUNT(DISTINCT CASE WHEN m.member_id IS NULL THEN c.member_id END)
      /NULLIF(COUNT(DISTINCT c.member_id),0),2)<=0.1
       THEN 'PASS' ELSE 'FAIL' END
  FROM  fact_medical_claims c
  LEFT JOIN dim_members m ON c.member_id = m.member_id
  WHERE EXTRACT(YEAR FROM c.service_date) = EXTRACT(YEAR FROM CURRENT_DATE)
```

```
),

-- DIMENSION 5: UNIQUENESS
-- No duplicate claim records.
uniqueness AS (
  SELECT 'UNIQUENESS', 'Duplicate claim IDs absent',
    COUNT(*),
    SUM(dup_count - 1), -- number of excess duplicate rows
    ROUND(100.0*SUM(dup_count-1)/NULLIF(COUNT(*),0),2),
    0.01, -- alert if > 0.01% duplicate claim IDs
    CASE WHEN ROUND(100.0*SUM(dup_count-1)/NULLIF(COUNT(*),0),2)<=0.01
      THEN 'PASS' ELSE 'FAIL' END
  FROM (
    SELECT claim_id, COUNT(*) AS dup_count
    FROM fact_medical_claims
    WHERE EXTRACT(YEAR FROM service_date) = EXTRACT(YEAR FROM CURRENT_DATE)
    GROUP BY claim_id
  ) dups
),

-- DIMENSION 6: ACCURACY
-- Allowed amount should not exceed billed amount (basic financial logic check).
accuracy AS (
  SELECT 'ACCURACY', 'Allowed amount <= billed amount',
    COUNT(*),
    SUM(CASE WHEN allowed_amount > billed_amount THEN 1 ELSE 0 END),
    ROUND(100.0*SUM(CASE WHEN allowed_amount > billed_amount
      THEN 1 ELSE 0 END)/NULLIF(COUNT(*),0),2),
    0.5, -- alert if > 0.5% of claims have allowed > billed
    CASE WHEN ROUND(100.0*SUM(CASE WHEN allowed_amount > billed_amount
      THEN 1 ELSE 0 END)/NULLIF(COUNT(*),0),2)<=0.5
      THEN 'PASS' ELSE 'FAIL' END
  FROM  fact_medical_claims
  WHERE EXTRACT(YEAR FROM service_date) = EXTRACT(YEAR FROM CURRENT_DATE)
   AND claim_status = 'PAID'
)
-- FINAL: Union all six dimensions into a single dashboard.
SELECT dq_dimension, dq_check, total_records, fail_count, fail_pct,
  threshold_pct, gate_status,
  -- Timestamp for audit trail
  CURRENT_TIMESTAMP AS dq_run_timestamp
FROM (
  SELECT * FROM completeness
  UNION ALL SELECT * FROM validity
  UNION ALL SELECT * FROM timeliness
  UNION ALL SELECT * FROM consistency
  UNION ALL SELECT * FROM uniqueness
  UNION ALL SELECT * FROM accuracy
) all_checks
ORDER BY gate_status DESC, fail_pct DESC; -- FAILs first, largest fail % first
```

30.3 NPI Validation and Reference Data Governance

ANSI SQL — 30.3: NPI Format Validation and NPPES Reconciliation (Fully Annotated)

```
-- PURPOSE: Validate NPIs in fact_medical_claims against two rules:
-- (1) Format: 10 digits, Luhn check digit valid.
-- (2) Active status: NPI must appear in the NPPES NPI registry download.
-- Invalid or inactive NPIs corrupt provider scorecards, network analysis,
-- HEDIS attribution, and OIG exclusion checks.
```

```
-- STEP 1: Format check -- NPI must be exactly 10 numeric characters.
WITH npi_format AS (
  SELECT rendering_npi,
      COUNT(DISTINCT claim_id) AS claim_count,
      -- Flag NPIs that are not exactly 10 digits
      CASE
        WHEN LENGTH(TRIM(rendering_npi)) <> 10 THEN 'INVALID LENGTH'
        WHEN rendering_npi ~ '[^0-9]' THEN 'NON-NUMERIC CHARACTERS'
        -- Luhn algorithm check for NPI (simplified: check digit position 10)
        WHEN CAST(RIGHT(rendering_npi,1) AS INT) <>
          MOD(10 - MOD(
            -- Sum of doubled digits (positions 1,3,5,7,9) + undoubled (2,4,6,8)
            (CAST(SUBSTRING(rendering_npi,1,1) AS INT)*2
             + CAST(SUBSTRING(rendering_npi,2,1) AS INT)
             + CAST(SUBSTRING(rendering_npi,3,1) AS INT)*2
             + CAST(SUBSTRING(rendering_npi,4,1) AS INT)
             + CAST(SUBSTRING(rendering_npi,5,1) AS INT)*2
             + CAST(SUBSTRING(rendering_npi,6,1) AS INT)
             + CAST(SUBSTRING(rendering_npi,7,1) AS INT)*2
             + CAST(SUBSTRING(rendering_npi,8,1) AS INT)
             + CAST(SUBSTRING(rendering_npi,9,1) AS INT)*2
             + 24), -- 24 = constant prefix 80840 Luhn contribution
          10), 10)    THEN 'INVALID LUHN CHECK DIGIT'
        ELSE 'VALID FORMAT'
      END AS format_status
  FROM  fact_medical_claims
  WHERE claim_status = 'PAID'
   AND EXTRACT(YEAR FROM service_date) = EXTRACT(YEAR FROM CURRENT_DATE)
  GROUP BY rendering_npi
),

-- STEP 2: Active status check -- NPI must be in the NPPES registry download.
-- ref_nppes_registry updated monthly from CMS NPPES full file download.
nppes_check AS (
  SELECT nf.rendering_npi, nf.claim_count, nf.format_status,
      CASE
        WHEN nppes.npi IS NULL THEN 'NOT IN NPPES — deactivated or invalid'
        WHEN nppes.entity_type_code = '1' THEN 'TYPE 1 — individual'
        WHEN nppes.entity_type_code = '2' THEN 'TYPE 2 — organization'
        ELSE 'ACTIVE'
      END AS nppes_status,
      nppes.provider_last_name, nppes.provider_org_name,
      nppes.taxonomy_code_1,
      nppes.deactivation_reason_code  -- null if active
  FROM  npi_format nf
  LEFT JOIN ref_nppes_registry nppes ON nf.rendering_npi = nppes.npi
)
-- STEP 3: Report all problematic NPIs.
SELECT rendering_npi, claim_count, format_status, nppes_status,
  provider_last_name, provider_org_name, taxonomy_code_1,
  CASE
    WHEN format_status <> 'VALID FORMAT'    THEN 'ACTION: fix format at source system'
    WHEN nppes_status LIKE 'NOT IN NPPES%'   THEN 'ACTION: verify with provider — may be deactivated'
    ELSE 'OK'
  END AS recommended_action
FROM  nppes_check
WHERE format_status <> 'VALID FORMAT'
  OR nppes_status LIKE 'NOT IN NPPES%'
ORDER BY claim_count DESC;  -- highest-volume bad NPIs first
```

30.4 Anomaly Detection — Claims Volume and Cost Surveillance

ANSI SQL — 30.4: Weekly Claims Volume and Cost Anomaly Detection (Fully Annotated)

```
-- PURPOSE: Detect sudden changes in weekly claims volume or allowed PMPM
-- that may indicate a data feed problem, processing error, or a real
-- clinical/financial event requiring investigation.
-- Flag weeks where volume or cost is > 2 standard deviations from 12-week mean.

WITH weekly_metrics AS (
  SELECT
    DATE_TRUNC('week', service_date)        AS week_start,
    COUNT(DISTINCT claim_id)                AS claim_count,
    SUM(allowed_amount)                     AS total_allowed,
    COUNT(DISTINCT member_id)               AS unique_members,
    ROUND(SUM(allowed_amount)
      /NULLIF(COUNT(DISTINCT member_id),0),2) AS allowed_pmpm_proxy
  FROM  fact_medical_claims
  WHERE claim_status = 'PAID'
   AND service_date >= CURRENT_DATE - INTERVAL '16' WEEK
  GROUP BY DATE_TRUNC('week', service_date)
),

-- 12-week rolling mean and standard deviation for each metric.
-- ROWS BETWEEN 11 PRECEDING AND CURRENT ROW = 12-week window.
rolling_stats AS (
  SELECT week_start, claim_count, total_allowed, allowed_pmpm_proxy,
     -- Rolling 12-week mean for claim count
     AVG(claim_count) OVER (
       ORDER BY week_start
       ROWS BETWEEN 11 PRECEDING AND CURRENT ROW) AS rolling_mean_count,
     -- Rolling 12-week standard deviation for claim count
     STDDEV(claim_count) OVER (
       ORDER BY week_start
       ROWS BETWEEN 11 PRECEDING AND CURRENT ROW) AS rolling_sd_count,
     AVG(total_allowed) OVER (
       ORDER BY week_start
       ROWS BETWEEN 11 PRECEDING AND CURRENT ROW) AS rolling_mean_allowed,
     STDDEV(total_allowed) OVER (
       ORDER BY week_start
       ROWS BETWEEN 11 PRECEDING AND CURRENT ROW) AS rolling_sd_allowed
  FROM  weekly_metrics
)
-- Flag weeks where claim count or allowed amount is > 2 SDs from rolling mean.
SELECT week_start, claim_count, total_allowed, allowed_pmpm_proxy,
  ROUND(rolling_mean_count,0) AS mean_count_12wk,
  ROUND(rolling_sd_count,0)  AS sd_count_12wk,
  ROUND((claim_count - rolling_mean_count)
    /NULLIF(rolling_sd_count,0),2)         AS count_z_score,
  ROUND(rolling_mean_allowed,0) AS mean_allowed_12wk,
  ROUND((total_allowed - rolling_mean_allowed)
    /NULLIF(rolling_sd_allowed,0),2)        AS allowed_z_score,
  -- Flag type identifies whether the anomaly is volume-based, cost-based, or both
  CASE
    WHEN ABS((claim_count-rolling_mean_count)/NULLIF(rolling_sd_count,0)) > 2
     AND ABS((total_allowed-rolling_mean_allowed)/NULLIF(rolling_sd_allowed,0)) > 2
    THEN 'FLAG BOTH — volume AND cost anomaly'
    WHEN ABS((claim_count-rolling_mean_count)/NULLIF(rolling_sd_count,0)) > 2
    THEN 'FLAG VOLUME — claims count anomaly only'
    WHEN ABS((total_allowed-rolling_mean_allowed)/NULLIF(rolling_sd_allowed,0)) > 2
    THEN 'FLAG COST — allowed amount anomaly only'
    ELSE 'Normal'
```

```
  END AS anomaly_flag
FROM rolling_stats
WHERE week_start >= CURRENT_DATE - INTERVAL '4' WEEK -- report last 4 weeks
ORDER BY week_start DESC;

-- Interpretation guide:
-- Volume anomaly + Cost anomaly: likely a data feed duplicate or double-load.
-- Volume drop only: possible data feed outage or late claims batch.
-- Cost anomaly only: possible high-cost catastrophic claim or fee schedule error.
-- Always investigate before running downstream analytics on flagged weeks.
```

Chapter 30 Review

Unit Test · Key Takeaways

Answer each question before reading the explanation.

Q1. The DQ Gate Principle means:

A. Run quality checks after each analytics report to validate results

B. Analytics pipelines halt when a DQ threshold is breached — downstream HEDIS rates, Stars simulations, and financial projections cannot be trusted when the underlying data has not passed all DQ gates. Halting is always preferable to producing and distributing incorrect results.

C. DQ gates approve data for regulatory submission once all checks pass

D. DQ gates are advisory — analysts can override them with documented rationale

Answer: B. *The cost of distributing a HEDIS rate calculated on data with 15% missing NPIs is enormous: decisions are made on incorrect information, the error propagates to regulatory submissions, and correcting it requires rerunning weeks of analytics. The DQ gate is a pre-run validation that prevents bad data from entering the analytics pipeline at all. When a gate fails, the Data Engineering team investigates and resolves the source issue before analytics proceed.*

Q2. The NPI Luhn check digit validates:

A. That the NPI is registered with NPPES

B. The mathematical integrity of the 10-digit NPI number. CMS defines a specific Luhn algorithm check digit as the 10th digit of every NPI. If the check digit does not match the calculated value from the first nine digits plus the prefix constant 24, the NPI was either entered incorrectly or fabricated.

C. That the provider's license is active in their state of practice

D. That the NPI belongs to an individual (Type 1) rather than an organization (Type 2)

Answer: B. *The Luhn algorithm is a standard checksum formula used in financial and healthcare identifiers to detect single-digit transcription errors. An NPI that fails the Luhn check was either mistyped (transposed digits, missing digit) or fabricated. Claims with Luhn-invalid NPIs cannot be attributed to a real provider — they corrupt provider scorecards, network analysis, HEDIS attribution, and OIG exclusion checks. Luhn validation catches these errors before they propagate downstream.*

Q3. A claims volume anomaly (Z-score > 2) with no corresponding cost anomaly most likely indicates:

A. A real epidemic or disease outbreak causing more members to seek care

B. A data feed or processing issue — duplicate claims being loaded, a batch being double-processed, or a missing batch from the prior week being loaded late. When volume and cost both spike proportionally, it suggests a real clinical event. Volume spike with flat cost per claim = data processing artifact.

C. A fee schedule update that changed how claims are categorized

D. A member enrollment surge that increased the denominator

Answer: B. *Anomaly diagnostic table: (1) Volume up AND cost up proportionally = real clinical event (e.g., influenza outbreak, new high-cost member joining). (2) Volume up, cost flat = likely duplicate claims loaded. (3) Volume down, cost up per claim = possible data feed outage with high-cost claims still flowing. (4) Cost up sharply with stable volume = single catastrophic claim or fee schedule error. Always route anomaly flags to Data Engineering for investigation before running downstream analytics.*

Q4. Orphan member IDs in the consistency check (claims with no matching dim_members row) cause:

A. Claims to be automatically excluded from all HEDIS denominators

B. Analytics failures across the entire system — HEDIS denominators cannot include members without dim_members records, provider scorecards lose attribution, risk stratification omits these members, and financial reporting undercounts costs. Even 0.1% orphan member IDs can affect HEDIS rates by fractions of a percentage point.

C. Member months to be double-counted in the PMPM denominator

D. The OIG exclusion check to produce false positives

Answer: B. *Orphan member IDs arise from: (1) Claims arriving before the enrollment record is loaded (timing issue). (2) Member ID format changes between the claims system and the enrollment system (mapping failure). (3) Retroactive enrollment terminations that remove the member from dim_members but leave historical claims. Each case has a different remediation. The 0.1% threshold for the consistency gate is strict because even small orphan rates corrupt HEDIS denominator construction — the CDC denominator requires a JOIN to dim_members for age and enrollment data.*

Q5. Reference table governance requires monthly updates for:

A. Only tables that change more frequently than quarterly

B. ICD-10 code sets (updated October 1 annually), CPT codes (updated January 1 annually), NPPES NPI registry (updated monthly by CMS), NDC drug codes (updated continuously), HCC crosswalk (updated with model version changes), and fee schedules (updated per contract). Stale reference tables cause diagnosis codes to appear invalid, drugs to be miscategorized, and providers to appear unregistered.

C. Only reference tables used in HEDIS calculations

D. Only federal reference tables — state-specific tables are maintained by IT

Answer: B. *Reference table staleness cascade: an ICD-10 code introduced October 1 that is not loaded into ref_icd10_codes by October 2 will cause all claims with that code to fail the Validity DQ check. If those claims represent a significant new condition cluster (e.g., a new COVID variant diagnosis code), the HCC capture gap analysis will miss those members entirely. Reference table governance is a monthly operational task that must be owned and tracked with a formal update calendar.*

Q6. The rolling 12-week window in the anomaly detection query is preferred over a fixed annual benchmark because:

A. Rolling windows require less SQL to compute

B. Annual benchmarks are inflated by holiday and seasonal patterns — a volume drop in the week of Thanksgiving appears as a massive anomaly vs. the annual mean but is perfectly normal vs. the prior four Thanksgivings. The rolling 12-week window provides a current baseline that naturally accounts for recent trends and seasonal patterns.

C. CMS requires 12-week windows for all anomaly detection

D. Rolling windows reduce the number of false positives from statistical noise

Answer: B. *Seasonal adjustment is critical in healthcare: claims volume drops every major holiday week (Thanksgiving, Christmas, Memorial Day), spikes during influenza season, and varies by benefit year reset patterns (high January deductible activity). A rolling 12-week mean adapts to these patterns dynamically. ROWS BETWEEN 11 PRECEDING AND CURRENT ROW creates a window that includes the current week plus the 11 immediately preceding weeks — exactly 12 weeks of history.*

Q7. Describe the complete reference data governance calendar for a health plan analytics team. What table, who owns the update, and what fails if it is missed?

(Short answer)

> **Sample Answer:**
> Reference data governance calendar: (1) October 1 — ICD-10-CM annual update: Owner: Clinical Informatics. Impact if missed: all claims with new diagnosis codes fail the Validity DQ check; new HCC mappings are not captured; HEDIS measures miss new exclusion codes. (2) January 1 — CPT/HCPCS annual update: Owner: Clinical Informatics. Impact: new procedure codes appear invalid; E&M upcoding detection misses new code variants; fee schedule compliance fails on new codes. (3) Monthly (first week) — NPPES NPI registry full file download: Owner: Data Engineering. Impact: deactivated providers not caught; new providers appear as invalid in NPI validation; OIG exclusion cross-reference misses NPIs that changed status. (4) Quarterly — CMS HCC crosswalk update (when CMS publishes model updates): Owner: Risk Adjustment Analytics. Impact: HCC capture gap analysis uses wrong ICD-10 to HCC mappings; RAF increment values are stale. (5) Per contract — Fee schedule updates: Owner: Network Analytics. Impact: fee schedule compliance SQL detects false overpayments/underpayments; rate achievement calculations are wrong. (6) Annually (fall) — NCQA HEDIS value sets (new measurement year specifications): Owner: Quality Analytics. Impact: HEDIS numerator logic uses wrong code sets; rates are incorrect for the new measurement year. Governance tool: maintain ref_data_update_log: table_name, expected_update_date, actual_update_date, records_before, records_after, updated_by. Alert if actual_update_date > expected_update_date + 3 days.

Q8. Write the SQL to detect duplicate member records in dim_members — different member_id values that likely represent the same physical person.

(Short answer)

> **Sample Answer:**
> SELECT a.member_id AS member_id_1, b.member_id AS member_id_2, a.member_name AS name_1, b.member_name AS name_2, a.date_of_birth, b.date_of_birth AS dob_2, a.ssn_last4, b.ssn_last4 AS ssn2, a.zip_code, b.zip_code AS zip2, ROUND(100.0 * (CASE WHEN a.date_of_birth = b.date_of_birth THEN 25 ELSE 0 END + CASE WHEN a.ssn_last4 = b.ssn_last4 THEN 40 ELSE 0 END + CASE WHEN SOUNDEX(a.member_name) = SOUNDEX(b.member_name) THEN 25 ELSE 0 END + CASE WHEN a.zip_code = b.zip_code THEN 10 ELSE 0 END) / 100.0, 0) AS match_confidence_pct FROM dim_members a JOIN dim_members b ON a.member_id < b.member_id AND a.date_of_birth = b.date_of_birth AND (a.ssn_last4 = b.ssn_last4 OR

SOUNDEX(a.member_name) = SOUNDEX(b.member_name)) WHERE a.coverage_status = 'ACTIVE' AND b.coverage_status = 'ACTIVE' ORDER BY match_confidence_pct DESC. match_confidence_pct: 85%+ = likely duplicate requiring manual review. 70–84% = possible duplicate, requires additional verification. Key fields: date_of_birth (strong identifier), SSN last 4 (strong but privacy-sensitive), SOUNDEX of name (phonetic match for name spelling variations), ZIP code (geographic proximity). Escalate high-confidence duplicates to the enrollment team. Duplicate member IDs cause double-counting in HEDIS denominators, split claims history across two IDs (breaking risk stratification), and can trigger erroneous payment for the same member twice.

Q9. Describe how to build a data lineage map for the HEDIS CDC HbA1c Control measure. Why is lineage documentation required for regulatory audits?

(Short answer)

Sample Answer:

Data lineage map for CDC HbA1c (<8%): Source system → Target table → Transformation step. (1) Enrollment system → dim_members (member_id, date_of_birth, coverage_status, line_of_business). ETL: nightly load, SCD-2 for historical changes. (2) Claims system → fact_medical_claims (member_id, service_date, procedure_code, primary_diag, allowed_amount). ETL: daily load, deduplication on claim_id. (3) Lab system / clearinghouse → fact_lab_results (member_id, loinc_code, result_date, numeric_result, result_status). ETL: bi-weekly load from reference lab feeds. (4) Enrollment → fact_member_months (member_id, membership_year, member_months). ETL: monthly aggregation from dim_members enrollment segments. (5) Attribution → dim_pcp_attribution. ETL: quarterly refresh from PCP panel assignments. CDC denominator SQL joins: dim_members (age, enrollment) + fact_medical_claims (diabetes dx, two-claim rule) + fact_member_months (continuous enrollment). CDC numerator SQL: fact_lab_results (LOINC codes, result_date, numeric_result). Lineage is required for NCQA HEDIS compliance audits because auditors need to trace every measure value back to its source record. If an auditor questions why member X is in the denominator, the analyst must show: the dim_members record showing age 52 on 12/31, the two fact_medical_claims records with E11.9 diagnosis, the fact_member_months records showing 11 months enrolled, and the absence of any exclusion criteria. Without documented lineage, this trace takes days instead of hours. NCQA auditors cite "inability to trace numerator/denominator logic to source data" as one of the most common compliance audit findings.

Q10. Explain how the six DQ dimensions interact. Give an example where a Validity failure cascades into a Consistency failure.

(Short answer)

Sample Answer:

DQ dimension interactions: Validity failure (a value violates the defined domain) almost always cascades downstream. Example: a claims system upgrade introduces a new claim type code "37" that is not yet loaded into ref_claim_type_codes. All claims with claim_type = "37" fail the Validity check. But they also produce Consistency failures: those claims appear in fact_medical_claims but their claim_type does not join to any row in ref_claim_type_codes — creating what appears to be orphaned records in the service category dimension. Those same claims may fail the Completeness check for service_category (because the service_category field is derived from the claim_type lookup and returns NULL when the lookup fails). If "37" is the code for a new inpatient claim type, those claims also fail the HEDIS TOB filter (LIKE "11%") — the Accuracy of HEDIS calculations is compromised. And because those claims cannot be attributed to a service category, they appear as a volume drop in specific service lines — triggering a false Timeliness flag when the monitoring team checks for missing data. Cascade chain: Validity → Completeness (derived NULL) → Consistency (orphaned dimension join) → Accuracy (wrong HEDIS rates) → false Timeliness flag. Resolution requires fixing the root cause (loading claim_type "37" into the reference table), then re-running the DQ dashboard to confirm all downstream gates clear before re-running analytics. This cascade is why the DQ dashboard runs in the correct dimension order: Completeness and Validity first (source data quality), then Consistency and Uniqueness (structural integrity), then Timeliness and Accuracy (derived quality). Failures in the first two dimensions will always cause apparent failures in the last four.

Key Takeaways

What every analyst must remember from this chapter.

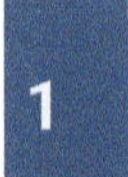
1 Six DQ dimensions: Completeness (required fields populated), Validity (values in defined domains), Timeliness (data is current), Consistency (values agree across systems), Uniqueness (no duplicates), Accuracy (values match ground truth). All six must pass before analytics pipelines run.

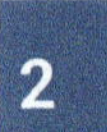
2 DQ gate principle: pipeline halts on any gate failure. Never run HEDIS, Stars, or financial analytics on data that has not passed all DQ gates for that period. Distributing incorrect results is costlier than delaying a report.

3 NPI validation two layers: (1) Format: 10 numeric digits with valid Luhn check digit. (2) Active status: NPI must appear in the monthly NPPES registry download. Invalid or deactivated NPIs corrupt provider scorecards, HEDIS attribution, and OIG exclusion checks.

4 Anomaly detection: rolling 12-week Z-score for claims volume and allowed amount. Z > 2.0 = investigate before running downstream analytics. Volume up + cost up proportionally = clinical event. Volume up + flat unit cost = duplicate data load. Volume drop = possible feed outage.

5 Reference table governance calendar: ICD-10 (October 1), CPT (January 1), NPPES (monthly), HCC crosswalk (with model updates), fee schedules (per contract), HEDIS value sets (fall). Maintain ref_data_update_log with expected vs. actual update dates.

6 Duplicate member detection: JOIN dim_members a to b WHERE a.member_id < b.member_id AND date_of_birth matches AND (SSN last 4 matches OR SOUNDEX(name) matches). match_confidence_pct ≥ 85% = likely duplicate. Duplicates split claims history and double-count HEDIS denominators.

7 Consistency gate: member IDs in claims must exist in dim_members. Threshold: 0.01% orphan member IDs. Orphan IDs cause HEDIS denominator failures, risk stratification gaps, and financial reporting errors. Root causes: timing (claims arrive before enrollment record loads), format mismatch, retroactive terminations.

8 Data lineage documentation: map every HEDIS measure input to its source table, ETL transformation, and business rule. Required for NCQA compliance audits. Any analyst must be able to trace a single member's denominator or numerator status back to the source record within minutes, not days.

Part IX -Advanced SQL & Analytics Patterns

— Chapter 31

Gap-Island · Recursive Hierarchy · Dynamic Pivot · Episode Grouper · Running IBNR · Multi-Period Trend

Chapter 31: Advanced SQL Patterns for Healthcare

Six production patterns — each solving a problem that simpler SQL cannot. Every pattern is shown in its healthcare context, not as an abstract exercise.

The six patterns in this chapter are not SQL tutorials. They are solutions to specific, recurring problems in healthcare analytics that analysts encounter when building production pipelines for HEDIS measurement, claims adjudication, risk adjustment, and financial reporting. Each pattern is presented with the exact healthcare problem it solves, a fully annotated SQL implementation, a real-world scenario showing the output, and a clear statement of what goes wrong when a simpler approach is attempted.

The patterns build on each other conceptually. Gap-island detection (Pattern 1) is the foundation for continuous enrollment logic used in every HEDIS denominator. Recursive hierarchy (Pattern 2) powers the ICD-10 code family lookups that underpin HCC capture gap analysis. Dynamic pivot (Pattern 3) produces the lag triangle used in IBNR completion factor calculation. The episode grouper (Pattern 4) implements bundled payment episode construction. Running IBNR completion (Pattern 5) ties the lag triangle to a live financial dashboard. Multi-period trend (Pattern 6) produces the annualized geometric trend that feeds actuarial rate filings. Read this chapter as a reference library: return to it whenever a pattern is needed, and adapt the annotated SQL to the specific business problem at hand.

Pattern 1

Gap-Island Detection

Continuous enrollment logic · HEDIS coverage periods · Readmission windows

31.1 The Problem: Finding Enrollment Gaps

NCQA HEDIS continuous enrollment requires that a member is enrolled for at least 11 of 12 months with no single gap exceeding 45 days. A member can have multiple enrollment segments (enrolled, termed, re-enrolled). The analyst must identify each consecutive enrollment island, measure the gap between islands, and fail members whose maximum gap exceeds 45 days. Simpler approaches — SUM(member_months) >= 11 — miss members who have two 30-day gaps (total = 60 days, not 45), which technically fails the NCQA rule.

> **Also Used For** Gap-island logic also powers: 30-day readmission window detection (find all admissions within 30 days of a prior discharge), chronic condition continuous therapy gaps (identify patients who stopped a medication for > 30 days), and care management outreach gap tracking (members who went > 90 days without contact).

ANSI SQL — 31.1: Gap-Island Enrollment Continuity — NCQA 45-Day Rule (Fully Annotated)

```
-- PROBLEM: HEDIS requires no single enrollment gap > 45 days.
-- SUM(member_months) >= 11 is insufficient — it misses members with
```

```
-- two 30-day gaps (both < 45 days individually, but total = 60 days gap).
-- This pattern finds each enrollment island and measures the inter-island gaps.

-- STEP 1: Get each member's enrollment segments.
-- Each row is one continuous enrollment period with a start and end date.
WITH enrollment_segments AS (
   SELECT member_id,
         coverage_start_date,
         coverage_end_date
   FROM  dim_member_enrollment
   WHERE membership_year = :meas_year
    AND coverage_status IN ('ACTIVE','TERMED')
   ORDER BY member_id, coverage_start_date
),

-- STEP 2: For each segment, find the previous segment's end date using LAG().
-- LAG() looks back one row within the same member_id partition.
lagged AS (
   SELECT member_id,
         coverage_start_date,
         coverage_end_date,
         LAG(coverage_end_date) OVER (
            PARTITION BY member_id         -- reset for each member
            ORDER BY coverage_start_date  -- look back to the previous segment
         ) AS prev_end_date
   FROM  enrollment_segments
),

-- STEP 3: Calculate the gap in days between consecutive enrollment islands.
-- A gap = days between the end of the prior segment and the start of the next.
-- First segment for each member has prev_end_date = NULL (no gap — it is the start).
gap_calc AS (
   SELECT member_id,
         coverage_start_date,
         coverage_end_date,
         DATEDIFF('day', prev_end_date, coverage_start_date) AS gap_days
   FROM  lagged
   WHERE prev_end_date IS NOT NULL   -- skip the first segment (no prior gap)
),

-- STEP 4: Find each member's maximum single gap and total coverage days.
member_gaps AS (
   SELECT g.member_id,
         MAX(g.gap_days)                AS max_single_gap_days,
         SUM(DATEDIFF('day',             -- total enrolled days this year
            es.coverage_start_date,
            es.coverage_end_date) + 1)    AS total_enrolled_days
   FROM  gap_calc g
   JOIN  enrollment_segments es ON g.member_id = es.member_id
   GROUP BY g.member_id
)
-- STEP 5: Apply the NCQA 45-day gap rule.
-- Fail members whose maximum single gap exceeds 45 days.
SELECT mg.member_id, m.member_name,
   mg.max_single_gap_days,
   mg.total_enrolled_days,
   CASE
      WHEN mg.max_single_gap_days <= 45 THEN 'ENROLLED — gap ≤ 45 days (NCQA pass)'
      WHEN mg.max_single_gap_days > 45  THEN 'EXCLUDED — gap > 45 days (NCQA fail)'
   END AS enrollment_status
FROM  member_gaps mg
```

```
JOIN dim_members m ON mg.member_id = m.member_id
ORDER BY mg.max_single_gap_days DESC;

-- WHY THIS MATTERS: A member with two 25-day gaps passes SUM(member_months)>=11
-- but fails MAX(gap_days) <= 45 -- they are correctly excluded from the denominator.
-- Using the simplified rule overstates the HEDIS denominator and deflates the rate.
```

Healthcare Application — 30-Day Readmission Window: The same gap-island pattern identifies readmissions. Each inpatient discharge is an "island anchor." The gap between discharge_date and the next admission_date is measured. If gap_days <= 30 AND the readmission is not a planned procedure, the second admission is a readmission event. The NCQA All-Cause Readmission (PCR) measure uses exactly this logic.

Pattern 2

Recursive Hierarchy Traversal

ICD-10 code families · Provider group roll-ups · Organizational attribution

31.2 The Problem: Navigating ICD-10 Code Families

ICD-10-CM codes are organized as a hierarchy: chapter → block → category → subcategory → subclassification. The HCC crosswalk maps code families using prefixes — E11 (type 2 diabetes) encompasses E11.0, E11.1, E11.21, E11.22 ... E11.9 and all their subcode variants. Analysts also use recursive hierarchy for provider organizational roll-ups: individual provider → practice group → health system → IPA network. A flat LIKE 'E11%' join works for two levels but fails for multi-level hierarchies maintained as parent-child reference tables.

ANSI SQL — 31.2: Recursive CTE — ICD-10 Chapter Hierarchy Traversal (Fully Annotated)

```
-- PROBLEM: ref_icd10_hierarchy is a parent-child table.
-- Each row: child_code, parent_code, level (Chapter / Block / Category / Subcategory).
-- To find ALL codes belonging to "Diabetes mellitus" (E08-E13 block),
-- we must traverse the hierarchy downward recursively from the block level.
-- A flat LIKE join cannot handle variable-depth hierarchies.

-- STEP 1: Recursive CTE — start at the anchor node, then recurse downward.
WITH RECURSIVE icd_tree AS (

  -- ANCHOR: Start at the target parent node (e.g., Diabetes block E08-E13).
  SELECT
    code_id,
    icd_code,
    code_description,
    parent_code_id,
    hierarchy_level,
    0 AS depth              -- depth 0 = the starting (anchor) node
  FROM ref_icd10_hierarchy
  WHERE icd_code = 'E08-E13'    -- the block we want to expand

  UNION ALL

  -- RECURSIVE MEMBER: Join children to the current level of the tree.
  -- The CTE references itself — this is what makes it recursive.
  SELECT
    child.code_id,
    child.icd_code,
    child.code_description,
    child.parent_code_id,
    child.hierarchy_level,
```

```
    parent.depth + 1          -- each recursion increments depth by 1
  FROM  ref_icd10_hierarchy child
  -- Join: child's parent = current level's code_id
  JOIN  icd_tree parent ON child.parent_code_id = parent.code_id
  WHERE parent.depth < 5          -- safety guard: prevent infinite loops
)
-- STEP 2: Use the expanded tree to find all member claims with any
-- diabetes code in the entire family — regardless of specificity depth.
SELECT DISTINCT c.member_id, m.member_name,
  c.primary_diag,
  t.icd_code AS matched_family_code,
  t.code_description,
  t.depth AS family_depth,
  c.service_date
FROM  fact_medical_claims c
-- Join on code prefix: claim code starts with the family code
JOIN  icd_tree t ON c.primary_diag LIKE t.icd_code || '%'
JOIN  dim_members m ON c.member_id = m.member_id
WHERE c.claim_status = 'PAID'
 AND t.hierarchy_level IN ('Subcategory','Subclassification') -- leaf nodes only
 AND EXTRACT(YEAR FROM c.service_date) = :meas_year
ORDER BY c.member_id, t.depth;

-- HEALTHCARE APPLICATIONS:
-- (1) HCC code family capture: expand any ICD-10 block to all leaf codes,
--     then join to claims — more accurate than hardcoded LIKE patterns.
-- (2) Provider organizational roll-up: provider → practice → system.
--     Replace ref_icd10_hierarchy with ref_provider_hierarchy.
-- (3) Benefit plan hierarchy: plan → product → benefit → sub-benefit.
```

Provider Hierarchy Application: the same recursive CTE traverses the provider organizational hierarchy from individual NPI → practice group TIN → health system parent → IPA network. A query asking "total allowed cost for all providers in Northwell Health" recursively expands from the health system node to every practice group and individual NPI within it — producing an accurate system-level financial summary without manually maintaining a flat list of NPIs.

Pattern 3

Dynamic Pivot — IBNR Lag Triangle

Claims lag triangle · Completion factors · Actuarial data preparation

31.3 The Problem: Pivoting Variable-Width Lag Columns

The IBNR lag triangle (Chapter 14) cross-tabulates service months against elapsed months since service. The number of lag columns varies — a 36-month triangle has 36 columns. Hardcoding MAX(CASE WHEN lag = 1 THEN pmpm END) ... MAX(CASE WHEN lag = 36 THEN pmpm END) is fragile: when the analysis window changes, all 36 CASE statements must be rewritten. The dynamic pivot pattern generates the column list programmatically, then executes it as a single prepared statement — making the triangle width a runtime parameter, not a code constant.

ANSI SQL — 31.3: Dynamic Pivot — IBNR Lag Triangle (Fully Annotated)

```
-- PROBLEM: The lag triangle has a variable number of columns (one per lag month).
-- Hardcoded CASE WHEN lag = 1 ... lag = 36 breaks when the window changes.
-- Solution: generate the column definitions dynamically, then EXECUTE them.

-- STEP 1: Build the base data — cumulative PMPM at each lag month per service month.
-- This is the same CTE used in Chapter 14, Section 14.3.
WITH monthly_paid AS (
```

```
  SELECT
    DATE_TRUNC('month', service_date)         AS svc_month,
    DATE_TRUNC('month', paid_date)            AS paid_month,
    SUM(allowed_amount)                       AS paid_in_month
  FROM fact_medical_claims
  WHERE claim_status = 'PAID'
   AND service_date >= CURRENT_DATE - INTERVAL '36' MONTH
  GROUP BY 1, 2
),
cumulative_pmpm AS (
  SELECT
    mp.svc_month,
    DATEDIFF('month', mp.svc_month, mp.paid_month)  AS lag_months,
    -- Running cumulative sum within each service month
    SUM(mp.paid_in_month) OVER (
      PARTITION BY mp.svc_month
      ORDER BY mp.paid_month
      ROWS BETWEEN UNBOUNDED PRECEDING AND CURRENT ROW
    ) / NULLIF(mm.total_mm, 0)                AS cumulative_pmpm
  FROM monthly_paid mp
  JOIN (
    SELECT DATE_TRUNC('month',month_start) AS svc_month,
        SUM(member_months) AS total_mm
    FROM fact_member_months
    WHERE line_of_business = 'COMMERCIAL'
    GROUP BY 1
  ) mm ON mp.svc_month = mm.svc_month
)
-- STEP 2 (Static version — shown for clarity):
-- Each lag month becomes a column using MAX(CASE WHEN lag = N THEN pmpm END).
-- This is replaced by the dynamic version in production (Step 3).
SELECT svc_month,
  MAX(CASE WHEN lag_months =  1 THEN ROUND(cumulative_pmpm,2) END) AS lag_1m,
  MAX(CASE WHEN lag_months =  3 THEN ROUND(cumulative_pmpm,2) END) AS lag_3m,
  MAX(CASE WHEN lag_months =  6 THEN ROUND(cumulative_pmpm,2) END) AS lag_6m,
  MAX(CASE WHEN lag_months =  9 THEN ROUND(cumulative_pmpm,2) END) AS lag_9m,
  MAX(CASE WHEN lag_months = 12 THEN ROUND(cumulative_pmpm,2) END) AS lag_12m,
  MAX(CASE WHEN lag_months = 18 THEN ROUND(cumulative_pmpm,2) END) AS lag_18m,
  MAX(CASE WHEN lag_months = 24 THEN ROUND(cumulative_pmpm,2) END) AS lag_24m
FROM cumulative_pmpm
GROUP BY svc_month
ORDER BY svc_month;

-- STEP 3 (Dynamic version — Snowflake / PostgreSQL pattern):
-- Generate the CASE WHEN list dynamically from the data, then EXECUTE it.
/*
DO $$
DECLARE
  col_list TEXT;
  sql_stmt TEXT;
BEGIN
  -- Build column list: "MAX(CASE WHEN lag_months=1 THEN ROUND(cumulative_pmpm,2) END) AS lag_1m"
  -- for every distinct lag month found in the data (up to 36)
  SELECT STRING_AGG(
    'MAX(CASE WHEN lag_months=' || lag_months ||
    ' THEN ROUND(cumulative_pmpm,2) END) AS lag_' || lag_months || 'm',
    ', ' ORDER BY lag_months
  ) INTO col_list
  FROM (SELECT DISTINCT lag_months FROM cumulative_pmpm
      WHERE lag_months BETWEEN 1 AND 36) lags;

  -- Assemble and execute the full pivot query
```

```
    sql_stmt := 'SELECT svc_month, ' || col_list ||
            ' FROM cumulative_pmpm GROUP BY svc_month ORDER BY svc_month';
    EXECUTE sql_stmt;
END $$;
*/

-- COMPLETION FACTOR DERIVATION (from the static version):
-- completion_factor_at_Nm = AVG(lag_Nm / lag_24m) across all matured months.
-- Matured = months where lag_24m IS NOT NULL (24+ months of development).
-- IBNR_multiplier = 1 / completion_factor.
-- Apply to current-month lag_1m to estimate the true final PMPM.
```

Pattern 4

Clinical Episode Grouper

Bundled payment episodes · DRG-based acute care episodes · Episode cost benchmarking

31.4 The Problem: Attributing All Care to an Anchor Event

Clinical episode grouping (Chapter 19) links every claim that belongs to a clinical episode — defined by an anchor event plus a window — to a single episode record. The challenge: a member can have multiple overlapping episode types simultaneously (e.g., a hip replacement during the same window as a readmission for CHF). The correct logic anchors on the qualifying procedure, then collects all claims within the episode window regardless of whether they relate to a different concurrent condition, because all costs within the episode window are the surgeon's financial responsibility under the bundle.

ANSI SQL — 31.4: Clinical Episode Grouper with Overlap Handling (Fully Annotated)

```
-- PROBLEM: A member may have multiple anchor events in the same year.
-- Each anchor starts its own episode window (e.g., 90 days post-procedure).
-- Claims within overlapping windows must be attributed to the correct anchor.
-- Rule: each claim belongs to the EARLIEST anchor whose window contains it.

-- STEP 1: Identify all anchor events (qualifying procedures) for the year.
WITH anchor_events AS (
    SELECT
        c.claim_id                  AS anchor_claim_id,
        c.member_id,
        c.rendering_npi             AS performing_npi,
        c.service_date              AS anchor_date,
        c.procedure_code            AS anchor_procedure,
        bp.bundle_type,
        bp.target_price,
        bp.episode_window_days,
        -- Episode end date = anchor date + window length
        c.service_date + bp.episode_window_days AS episode_end_date
    FROM fact_medical_claims c
    JOIN ref_bundle_procedures bp ON c.procedure_code = bp.procedure_code
    WHERE c.claim_status = 'PAID'
     AND EXTRACT(YEAR FROM c.service_date) = :perf_year
),

-- STEP 2: For each non-anchor claim, find all anchors whose window contains it.
-- A claim can fall within multiple episode windows if the member had
-- two qualifying procedures close together (e.g., bilateral knee replacements).
candidate_attribution AS (
    SELECT
        all_claims.claim_id,
        all_claims.member_id,
```

```sql
        all_claims.service_date,
        all_claims.allowed_amount,
        ae.anchor_claim_id,
        ae.anchor_date,
        ae.bundle_type,
        ae.target_price,
        ae.performing_npi,
        -- Rank anchors by anchor_date: earliest anchor gets priority
        ROW_NUMBER() OVER (
            PARTITION BY all_claims.claim_id  -- one ranking per claim
            ORDER BY ae.anchor_date ASC       -- earliest anchor = rank 1
        ) AS anchor_priority
    FROM  fact_medical_claims all_claims
    JOIN  anchor_events ae
      ON all_claims.member_id = ae.member_id
     -- Claim falls within this episode window
     AND all_claims.service_date BETWEEN ae.anchor_date
                             AND ae.episode_end_date
     AND all_claims.claim_status = 'PAID'
),

-- STEP 3: Keep only the highest-priority (earliest anchor) attribution per claim.
-- This resolves overlapping episodes: each claim belongs to exactly one episode.
attributed_claims AS (
    SELECT *
    FROM  candidate_attribution
    WHERE anchor_priority = 1    -- earliest anchor wins for overlapping windows
),

-- STEP 4: Aggregate total episode cost and compare to target price.
-- Readmission flag: inpatient claim after the anchor date = complication signal.
episode_summary AS (
    SELECT
        ac.anchor_claim_id,
        ac.bundle_type,
        ac.performing_npi,
        ac.target_price,
        SUM(ac.allowed_amount)              AS total_episode_cost,
        ac.target_price - SUM(ac.allowed_amount) AS episode_savings,
        -- Readmission: any inpatient claim after the anchor date (not the anchor itself)
        COUNT(DISTINCT CASE
            WHEN fc.type_of_bill LIKE '11%'
             AND fc.claim_id <> ac.anchor_claim_id
            THEN fc.claim_id END)           AS readmission_count
    FROM  attributed_claims ac
    JOIN  fact_medical_claims fc ON ac.claim_id = fc.claim_id
    GROUP BY ac.anchor_claim_id, ac.bundle_type,
             ac.performing_nni, ac.target_price
)
SELECT es.anchor_claim_id, es.bundle_type,
    p.provider_full_name AS surgeon,
    es.target_price, es.total_episode_cost,
    ROUND(es.episode_savings,0) AS episode_savings,
    es.readmission_count,
    CASE WHEN es.episode_savings < 0
         THEN 'OVERRUN — review for outlier protection'
         ELSE 'Within target' END AS financial_status
FROM  episode_summary es
JOIN  dim_providers p ON es.performing_npi = p.npi
ORDER BY es.episode_savings ASC;  -- largest overruns first
```

```
-- KEY DESIGN DECISION: ROW_NUMBER() with anchor_priority = 1 ensures
-- each claim belongs to exactly one episode even when windows overlap.
-- Alternative approaches (e.g., splitting cost proportionally across
-- overlapping anchors) are less defensible in provider contract disputes.
```

Pattern 5

Running IBNR Completion — Window Functions

Live PMPM estimation · Completion factor application · Financial dashboard accuracy

31.5 The Problem: Adjusting Incomplete Recent Months in a Live Dashboard

Every financial dashboard that shows PMPM by service month must address IBNR: recent months have only received a fraction of their eventual claims. A dashboard showing October PMPM at $285 when the true estimated final is $678 will trigger false "favorable" alerts and incorrect decisions. The window function pattern applies completion factors dynamically — each month's observed PMPM is divided by the appropriate completion factor based on how many months have elapsed since service, producing an IBNR-adjusted PMPM that is clearly labeled as an estimate.

ANSI SQL — 31.5: Running IBNR Completion — Window Function Application (Fully Annotated)

```
-- PROBLEM: Recent service months are incomplete. Displaying raw PMPM
-- for months < 6 months old misleads financial decision-makers.
-- Solution: apply pre-computed completion factors using CASE WHEN on lag_months.
-- Completion factors are from the lag triangle (Pattern 3).

-- STEP 1: Calculate observed PMPM for each service month.
-- Observed = what has been paid so far, regardless of data maturity.
WITH observed_pmpm AS (
  SELECT
    DATE_TRUNC('month', c.service_date)      AS svc_month,
    ROUND(SUM(c.allowed_amount)
      / NULLIF(SUM(mm.member_months), 0), 2) AS observed_pmpm,
    -- Months elapsed since this service month
    DATEDIFF('month',
      DATE_TRUNC('month', c.service_date),
      DATE_TRUNC('month', CURRENT_DATE))    AS months_elapsed
  FROM  fact_medical_claims c
  JOIN  fact_member_months mm
    ON mm.member_id = c.member_id
   AND mm.membership_year = EXTRACT(YEAR FROM c.service_date)
  WHERE c.claim_status = 'PAID'
   AND c.line_of_business = 'COMMERCIAL'
   AND c.service_date >= CURRENT_DATE - INTERVAL '24' MONTH
  GROUP BY DATE_TRUNC('month', c.service_date)
),

-- STEP 2: Pre-computed completion factors from the lag triangle.
-- These are calculated monthly and stored in ref_ibnr_completion_factors.
-- Each row: lag_months, service_category, completion_factor (0-1 scale).
-- completion_factor = 0.42 means: at this lag, 42% of final PMPM is received.
completion_factors AS (
  SELECT lag_months, service_category,
     completion_factor,
     -- IBNR multiplier = 1 / completion_factor
     1.0 / NULLIF(completion_factor, 0) AS ibnr_multiplier
  FROM  ref_ibnr_completion_factors
  WHERE line_of_business = 'COMMERCIAL'
),
```

```sql
-- STEP 3: Apply the completion factor for the appropriate lag.
-- Match each service month to its completion factor based on months_elapsed.
-- Use a running window to see PMPM trending across the past 24 months.
ibnr_adjusted AS (
  SELECT
    op.svc_month,
    op.months_elapsed,
    op.observed_pmpm,
    cf.completion_factor,
    cf.ibnr_multiplier,
    -- IBNR-adjusted PMPM = observed / completion_factor
    ROUND(op.observed_pmpm * cf.ibnr_multiplier, 2) AS ibnr_adjusted_pmpm,
    -- Label each month by data maturity for transparency in dashboards
    CASE
      WHEN op.months_elapsed >= 12 THEN 'FINAL — fully developed'
      WHEN op.months_elapsed >= 6  THEN 'NEAR-FINAL — 90%+ developed'
      WHEN op.months_elapsed >= 3  THEN 'DEVELOPING — apply IBNR adjustment'
      ELSE                              'IMMATURE — estimate only'
    END AS data_maturity_label
  FROM  observed_pmpm op
  -- Join on months_elapsed: use the completion factor for this exact lag
  LEFT JOIN completion_factors cf
    ON cf.lag_months = op.months_elapsed
   AND cf.service_category = 'TOTAL'  -- aggregate completion factor
),

-- STEP 4: Add a rolling 3-month average of the IBNR-adjusted PMPM
-- to smooth out month-to-month volatility in the dashboard.
final_dashboard AS (
  SELECT
    svc_month, months_elapsed,
    observed_pmpm, completion_factor, ibnr_adjusted_pmpm,
    data_maturity_label,
    -- 3-month rolling average using window function over the time series
    ROUND(AVG(ibnr_adjusted_pmpm) OVER (
      ORDER BY svc_month
      ROWS BETWEEN 2 PRECEDING AND CURRENT ROW
    ), 2) AS rolling_3m_avg_adjusted_pmpm,
    -- Year-over-year comparison: same month last year
    LAG(ibnr_adjusted_pmpm, 12) OVER (
      ORDER BY svc_month
    ) AS prior_year_same_month_pmpm
  FROM  ibnr_adjusted
)
SELECT
  TO_CHAR(svc_month, 'YYYY-MM')        AS month,
  observed_pmpm,
  ROUND(completion_factor * 100, 1) || '%' AS pct_developed,
  ibnr_adjusted_pmpm,
  rolling_3m_avg_adjusted_pmpm,
  prior_year_same_month_pmpm,
  ROUND(ibnr_adjusted_pmpm
    - prior_year_same_month_pmpm, 2)   AS yoy_pmpm_change,
  data_maturity_label
FROM  final_dashboard
ORDER BY svc_month DESC;

-- DASHBOARD CONTRACT:
-- Always show data_maturity_label alongside ibnr_adjusted_pmpm.
-- Never display ibnr_adjusted_pmpm for IMMATURE months as a final number.
```

```
-- The rolling_3m_avg smooths high-volatility recent months.
-- Year-over-year comparison uses adjusted PMPM for both years -- apples to apples.
```

Pattern 6

Multi-Period Geometric Trend

Actuarial trend calculation · Rate filing inputs · Service category decomposition

31.6 The Problem: Annualizing Trend Across Unequal Periods

Medical cost trend (Chapter 15) must be expressed as an annualized geometric rate: POWER(end/start, 1.0/years) - 1. Arithmetic averaging — (end - start) / start / years — understates trend when growth compounds. The multi-period pattern calculates trend simultaneously across multiple service categories and multiple look-back periods (1-year, 2-year, 3-year), then stacks them for actuarial review. The SQL uses self-joins across measurement years and CROSS JOIN LATERAL (or equivalent) to generate multiple trend intervals in a single query.

ANSI SQL — 31.6: Multi-Period Geometric Trend — Actuarial Rate Filing Output (Fully Annotated)

```
-- PROBLEM: Rate filing requires trend at multiple look-back periods
-- (1yr, 2yr, 3yr) for each service category, all in one table.
-- Arithmetic averaging understates compounding trend.
-- Solution: self-join annual metrics across years, compute POWER() formula.

-- STEP 1: Annual PMPM, utilization rate, and unit cost per service category.
-- This is the foundational metric table used across all trend periods.
WITH annual_metrics AS (
  SELECT
    EXTRACT(YEAR FROM c.service_date)                AS yr,
    p.service_category,
    -- PMPM: total allowed / total enrolled member months
    ROUND(SUM(c.allowed_amount)
      / NULLIF(SUM(mm.member_months), 0), 2)          AS pmpm,
    -- Utilization: claims per 1,000 member months
    ROUND(1000.0 * COUNT(DISTINCT c.claim_id)
      / NULLIF(SUM(mm.member_months), 0), 1)          AS util_per_1k,
    -- Unit cost: average allowed per claim
    ROUND(SUM(c.allowed_amount)
      / NULLIF(COUNT(DISTINCT c.claim_id), 0), 0)     AS unit_cost
  FROM  fact_medical_claims c
  JOIN  ref_procedure_codes p  ON c.procedure_code = p.procedure_code
  JOIN  fact_member_months  mm
    ON c.member_id = mm.member_id
   AND mm.membership_year = EXTRACT(YEAR FROM c.service_date)
  WHERE c.claim_status = 'PAID'
   AND c.line_of_business = 'COMMERCIAL'
   -- Include all years needed for the 3-year look-back
   AND EXTRACT(YEAR FROM c.service_date)
     BETWEEN EXTRACT(YEAR FROM CURRENT_DATE) - 3
       AND EXTRACT(YEAR FROM CURRENT_DATE)
  GROUP BY 1, 2
),

-- STEP 2: Current year metrics (the "end" of each trend period).
current_yr AS (
  SELECT * FROM annual_metrics
  WHERE yr = EXTRACT(YEAR FROM CURRENT_DATE)
),
```

```sql
-- STEP 3: Self-join to each base year (1, 2, and 3 years prior).
-- Each join produces the "start" for that trend interval.
-- POWER(end/start, 1.0/n) - 1 = geometric compound annual trend.
trend_1yr AS (
  SELECT cy.service_category,
       cy.pmpm AS pmpm_current, py.pmpm AS pmpm_prior,
       cy.util_per_1k AS util_current, py.util_per_1k AS util_prior,
       cy.unit_cost AS uc_current, py.unit_cost AS uc_prior,
       -- 1-year trend: no POWER needed (n=1), just (end/start) - 1
       ROUND(cy.pmpm / NULLIF(py.pmpm, 0) - 1, 4)       AS pmpm_trend_1yr,
       ROUND(cy.util_per_1k / NULLIF(py.util_per_1k,0) - 1, 4) AS util_trend_1yr,
       ROUND(cy.unit_cost / NULLIF(py.unit_cost,0) - 1, 4)     AS cost_trend_1yr
  FROM  current_yr cy
  JOIN  annual_metrics py
    ON cy.service_category = py.service_category
   AND py.yr = EXTRACT(YEAR FROM CURRENT_DATE) - 1
),

trend_2yr AS (
  SELECT cy.service_category,
       -- 2-year geometric: POWER(end/start, 0.5) - 1
       ROUND(POWER(cy.pmpm / NULLIF(py.pmpm,0), 0.5) - 1, 4) AS pmpm_trend_2yr,
       ROUND(POWER(cy.util_per_1k / NULLIF(py.util_per_1k,0), 0.5) - 1, 4) AS util_trend_2yr,
       ROUND(POWER(cy.unit_cost / NULLIF(py.unit_cost,0), 0.5) - 1, 4) AS cost_trend_2yr
  FROM  current_yr cy
  JOIN  annual_metrics py
    ON cy.service_category = py.service_category
   AND py.yr = EXTRACT(YEAR FROM CURRENT_DATE) - 2
),

trend_3yr AS (
  SELECT cy.service_category,
       -- 3-year geometric: POWER(end/start, 1/3) - 1
       ROUND(POWER(cy.pmpm / NULLIF(py.pmpm,0), 1.0/3.0) - 1, 4) AS pmpm_trend_3yr,
       ROUND(POWER(cy.util_per_1k / NULLIF(py.util_per_1k,0), 1.0/3.0) - 1, 4) AS util_trend_3yr,
       ROUND(POWER(cy.unit_cost / NULLIF(py.unit_cost,0), 1.0/3.0) - 1, 4) AS cost_trend_3yr
  FROM  current_yr cy
  JOIN  annual_metrics py
    ON cy.service_category = py.service_category
   AND py.yr = EXTRACT(YEAR FROM CURRENT_DATE) - 3
)
-- STEP 4: Assemble the full rate filing trend table.
-- All three look-back periods side by side per service category.
-- Actuary selects the most appropriate trend point for filing.
SELECT
  cy.service_category,
  cy.pmpm              AS pmpm_current_yr,
  -- 1-year trends
  ROUND(t1.pmpm_trend_1yr * 100, 2) AS pmpm_trend_1yr_pct,
  ROUND(t1.util_trend_1yr * 100, 2) AS util_trend_1yr_pct,
  ROUND(t1.cost_trend_1yr * 100, 2) AS cost_trend_1yr_pct,
  -- 2-year geometric trends (preferred for rate filing)
  ROUND(t2.pmpm_trend_2yr * 100, 2) AS pmpm_trend_2yr_pct,
  ROUND(t2.util_trend_2yr * 100, 2) AS util_trend_2yr_pct,
  ROUND(t2.cost_trend_2yr * 100, 2) AS cost_trend_2yr_pct,
  -- 3-year geometric trends (smooths COVID-era distortions)
  ROUND(t3.pmpm_trend_3yr * 100, 2) AS pmpm_trend_3yr_pct,
  ROUND(t3.util_trend_3yr * 100, 2) AS util_trend_3yr_pct,
  ROUND(t3.cost_trend_2yr * 100, 2) AS cost_trend_3yr_pct,
  -- Blended trend: average of 2yr and 3yr (common actuarial practice)
  ROUND(((t2.pmpm_trend_2yr + t3.pmpm_trend_3yr) / 2.0) * 100, 2)
                  AS blended_pmpm_trend_pct
```

```
FROM current_yr cy
LEFT JOIN trend_1yr t1 ON cy.service_category = t1.service_category
LEFT JOIN trend_2yr t2 ON cy.service_category = t2.service_category
LEFT JOIN trend_3yr t3 ON cy.service_category = t3.service_category
ORDER BY cy.pmpm DESC; -- highest-cost categories first

-- VALIDATION CHECK:
-- blended_pmpm_trend should approximately equal:
-- (1 + blended_util_trend) × (1 + blended_cost_trend) - 1
-- If this multiplicative relationship does not hold within ±0.5pp,
-- investigate for member mix changes, DRG grouper upgrades,
-- or benefit design changes that distort the decomposition.
```

Chapter 31 Review

Unit Test · Key Takeaways

Answer each question before reading the explanation.

Q1. Gap-island detection using LAG() is required (rather than SUM(member_months) >= 11) because:

A. LAG() is faster than aggregate functions on large tables

B. SUM(member_months) >= 11 permits members with two 30-day gaps (each < 45 days but combined = 60 days) to pass when they should fail the NCQA rule. LAG() computes each inter-island gap individually so the maximum single gap can be compared to the 45-day threshold.

C. SUM(member_months) does not account for plan type differences

D. The NCQA rule requires LAG() to be explicitly used in denominator SQL

Answer: B. *Concrete example: a member enrolled Jan–Feb (2 months), gap March 1–April 29 (59 days), enrolled May–December (8 months). SUM = 10 months — this member fails the 11-month test but would pass it if they had one fewer gap day. MAX(gap_days) = 59 > 45 → correctly excluded. A member with Jan–Apr (4 months), gap May 1–May 30 (29 days), Jun–Dec (7 months) has SUM = 11 months and MAX(gap_days) = 29 ≤ 45 → correctly included. Both cases require the gap-island pattern.*

Q2. The RECURSIVE CTE anchor member must be separated from the recursive member by:

A. A WHERE clause filtering on depth = 0

B. UNION ALL — the anchor defines the starting rows; the recursive member joins the CTE to itself using UNION ALL to add each successive level. UNION (without ALL) would deduplicate rows and break the recursion.

C. A PARTITION BY clause on the hierarchy level

D. A separate CTE defined before the recursive one

Answer: B. *Recursive CTE structure: WITH RECURSIVE tree AS (anchor UNION ALL recursive_member). The anchor executes once and produces the seed rows. The recursive member executes repeatedly, joining back to tree, until no new rows are produced. The depth guard (WHERE depth < N) prevents infinite loops in circular hierarchies. UNION instead of UNION ALL would deduplicate at each level, potentially terminating the recursion prematurely when the same code appears in multiple branches.*

Q3. The dynamic pivot pattern (Pattern 3) generates the column list at runtime because:

A. Dynamic SQL runs faster than hardcoded CASE WHEN statements

B. The number of lag months in the IBNR triangle is a runtime parameter — it changes when the analysis window changes from 24 to 36 months, or when a new service category is added. Hardcoded CASE WHEN requires manual rewriting for every window change. Dynamic SQL reads the distinct lag values from the data and generates the correct column list automatically.

C. CASE WHEN cannot handle NULL values in lag month columns

D. Regulatory submissions require dynamically generated pivot queries

Answer: B. *The static version (shown for clarity in Pattern 3) is perfectly valid for a fixed 24-month triangle. The dynamic version is production-appropriate because: (1) the lag window changes when historical data accumulates, (2) different lines of business may have different credible lag windows, (3) adding a new service category to the analysis does not require code changes. The STRING_AGG pattern builds the CASE WHEN list by aggregating a template string over all distinct lag values, then executes it with EXECUTE.*

Q4. In the episode grouper (Pattern 4), ROW_NUMBER() with anchor_priority = 1 solves:

A. The problem of claims appearing in multiple fact tables

B. The overlapping episode window problem — when a member has two qualifying procedures close together, any claims in the overlap period could belong to either episode. ROW_NUMBER() ranks anchors by anchor_date ASC;

taking only rank = 1 assigns each claim to the earliest qualifying anchor, making the attribution deterministic and defensible in provider contract disputes.

C. The problem of the same claim being counted twice in the total episode cost

D. The challenge of identifying readmissions within 90 days of the anchor

Answer: B. *The "earliest anchor wins" rule is one of several valid attribution conventions. Others include: "most expensive anchor wins" (assigns the claim to the episode where it has the highest financial impact), "most clinically related anchor wins" (requires clinical coding rules), and "proportional split" (divides the claim cost across all qualifying anchors by window overlap). The earliest anchor rule is most common because it is deterministic, auditable, and mirrors the way clinical pathways are structured: the first qualifying procedure initiates the episode of care.*

Q5. The IBNR completion factor application (Pattern 5) multiplies observed_pmpm by ibnr_multiplier rather than adding a fixed adjustment because:

A. Additive adjustments are not permitted in GAAP financial reporting

B. IBNR is proportional to the volume of underlying services — a month with twice the enrollment needs roughly twice the IBNR reserve. Multiplicative adjustment (observed × 1/completion_factor) scales the reserve correctly. An additive constant would over-reserve low-enrollment months and under-reserve high-enrollment months.

C. Multiplicative adjustments are required by CMS for all financial dashboards

D. The completion factor is always greater than 1.0 so addition would create negative values

Answer: B. *The proportionality insight: if inpatient has 42% completion at 1 month, that means 58% of inpatient PMPM is still in transit regardless of whether the plan has 10,000 or 100,000 members. The absolute IBNR reserve scales with enrollment. A 10,000-member plan has a smaller absolute IBNR reserve than a 100,000-member plan for the same service, but the same completion percentage. Multiplicative adjustment handles this correctly: observed_pmpm × (1/0.42) produces the right estimated final PMPM for any enrollment level.*

Q6. The multi-period geometric trend query uses POWER(end/start, 1.0/n) - 1 rather than arithmetic averaging (end - start)/start/n because:

A. POWER() is a built-in function so it executes faster

B. Geometric compounding is the economically correct model for trend. If PMPM grows by 10% in year 1 and 10% in year 2, the 2-year geometric trend = POWER(end/start, 0.5) - 1. The arithmetic average (10% + 10%)/2 = 10% is the same — but if year 1 is +15% and year 2 is +5%, arithmetic = 10.0% while geometric = POWER(1.15 × 1.05, 0.5) - 1 = 9.89%. The arithmetic method ignores compounding and consistently overstates trend when growth is uneven.

C. POWER() avoids divide-by-zero errors that arithmetic formulas produce

D. Geometric trend is required by NCQA for all rate filing submissions

Answer: B. *The compounding difference matters in rate filings. A plan that uses arithmetic trend and overstates by 0.2% annually, applied to a $400M book of business, overprices premiums by $800,000 per year — creating adverse selection as competitors price more accurately. Conversely, understatement through arithmetic averaging (when trend is accelerating) leads to chronic underpricing. Actuaries universally use geometric trend; the analyst must match this convention precisely.*

Q7. Describe how the gap-island pattern extends beyond enrollment logic to power the NCQA All-Cause Readmission (PCR) measure SQL. What additional exclusions must be applied?

(Short answer)

> **Sample Answer:**
> PCR readmission SQL using gap-island: (1) Anchor: identify all inpatient acute discharges (TOB 11x, discharge_status in (01,02,03,06,81,86,87,88,90,91,92,93,94)) = the index admissions. (2) LAG() pattern: for each member, use LAG(discharge_date) OVER (PARTITION BY member_id ORDER BY admission_date) to find the prior discharge. (3) Gap calculation: DATEDIFF('day', prior_discharge_date, current_admission_date) = readmission_gap. (4) Readmission flag: gap <= 30 days AND the current admission is not an excluded planned procedure. (5) Exclusions per NCQA PCR spec: planned procedures (CABG, knee/hip replacement, other elective surgeries from NCQA planned procedure value sets), admissions following a discharge from an acute psychiatric facility, admissions for COVID-19 (NCQA pandemic exclusion), and obstetric admissions. SQL: LEFT JOIN ref_planned_procedures pp ON current_claim.procedure_code = pp.procedure_code WHERE pp.procedure_code IS NULL (exclude planned). Also: WHERE current_diag NOT LIKE 'O%' (exclude obstetric). The gap-island LAG() pattern naturally handles members with multiple admissions — each admission looks back exactly one row to its predecessor within the same member partition, computing the gap correctly regardless of how many admissions the member had during the year.

Q8. Explain how the recursive hierarchy pattern would be adapted for provider organizational roll-up analytics. Write the SQL structure for a health system → hospital → practice group → individual NPI hierarchy.

(Short answer)

> **Sample Answer:**
> Provider hierarchy recursive CTE: WITH RECURSIVE provider_tree AS (-- ANCHOR: start at the health system level SELECT org_id, org_name, parent_org_id, org_level, 0 AS depth, org_id AS root_system_id FROM ref_provider_hierarchy WHERE org_level

= 'HEALTH_SYSTEM' AND org_name = :target_system UNION ALL -- RECURSIVE: expand to child organizations SELECT child.org_id, child.org_name, child.parent_org_id, child.org_level, parent.depth + 1, parent.root_system_id FROM ref_provider_hierarchy child JOIN provider_tree parent ON child.parent_org_id = parent.org_id WHERE parent.depth < 4) -- max 4 levels deep -- Use the expanded tree: join to NPIs at the leaf level (individual providers) SELECT pt.root_system_id, hs.org_name AS health_system, pt.org_name AS org_unit, pt.org_level, np.npi, np.provider_full_name, SUM(c.allowed_amount) AS total_allowed, COUNT(DISTINCT c.claim_id) AS claim_count FROM provider_tree pt JOIN ref_provider_npi_mapping npm ON pt.org_id = npm.org_id -- maps org units to their NPIs JOIN dim_providers np ON npm.npi = np.npi LEFT JOIN fact_medical_claims c ON np.npi = c.rendering_npi AND EXTRACT(YEAR FROM c.service_date) = :yr AND c.claim_status = 'PAID' JOIN ref_provider_hierarchy hs ON pt.root_system_id = hs.org_id GROUP BY pt.root_system_id, hs.org_name, pt.org_name, pt.org_level, np.npi, np.provider_full_name ORDER BY total_allowed DESC. Use case: "What is the total allowed cost for all providers affiliated with Northwell Health?" — the recursive expansion replaces the need to maintain a flat NPI list that would need manual updating every time a practice joins or leaves the system.

Q9. Describe the production deployment considerations for the running IBNR completion dashboard (Pattern 5). How should incomplete months be labeled and what governance process is required?

(Short answer)

Sample Answer:

Production deployment requirements for Pattern 5: (1) Completion factor table governance: ref_ibnr_completion_factors must be recalibrated quarterly using the most recent 24 months of lag triangle data. The calibration runs the Pattern 3 lag triangle, averages completion factors across matured months (lag >= 12), and loads the updated factors. Never use completion factors calibrated more than 3 months ago — the underlying claim mix and processing speed may have shifted. (2) Dashboard labeling contract: every IBNR-adjusted PMPM cell must display the data_maturity_label alongside the number. Labels: FINAL (lag >= 12): no adjustment applied, show observed PMPM as-is. NEAR-FINAL (lag 6–11): adjustment < 15%, label as "estimated." DEVELOPING (lag 3–5): adjustment 15–40%, label prominently as "IBNR-adjusted estimate." IMMATURE (lag 0–2): adjustment > 40%, label as "preliminary estimate — do not use for decisions." (3) Governance process: the dashboard must have a data currency indicator showing the extract date and the most recent service month where claims were received. If the indicator is > 5 business days stale, auto-display a "DATA STALE — do not use for decisions" banner. (4) Reconciliation: monthly, the prior month's IBNR-adjusted estimate is compared to the actual PMPM once it is fully developed. If the estimate was off by > 10%, the completion factor for that lag period is recalibrated. This feedback loop improves accuracy over time. (5) User education: a dashboard footnote must explain what IBNR means and why the adjusted PMPM differs from the raw number. Without this, executives will assume the adjustment is an error and override it — producing the exact misinformation problem the adjustment was designed to prevent.

Q10. A rate filing actuary needs the multi-period trend table (Pattern 6) but asks why the 1-year trend for inpatient shows +18% while the 2-year geometric shows +6%. Explain the most likely cause and how the analyst investigates it.

(Short answer)

Sample Answer:

A 1-year trend of +18% combined with a 2-year geometric of +6% means the current year jumped sharply but the year before current had a large decline. 2-year geometric: POWER(current/two_years_ago, 0.5) - 1 = 6%. This implies: current/two_years_ago = 1.06^2 = 1.124 → 12.4% total growth over 2 years. But 1-year: current/prior_year = 1.18. Therefore: prior_year/two_years_ago = 1.124/1.18 = 0.953 → prior year was DOWN 4.7% vs. the year before it. The most likely healthcare cause: COVID-19 utilization distortion. Many plans saw inpatient utilization collapse in 2020–2021 (avoided care, elective procedure cancellations) followed by a sharp rebound in 2022–2023. A 1-year trend measured off the depressed COVID-era base is artificially inflated. Investigation SQL: SELECT yr, pmpm, util_per_1k, unit_cost FROM annual_metrics WHERE service_category = 'INPATIENT' ORDER BY yr. If the pattern shows: 2019=$320, 2020=$240 (COVID collapse), 2021=$260, 2022=$308 — a 1-year trend from 2021 to 2022 = +18.5%, but the 3-year trend from 2019 to 2022 = POWER(308/320, 1/3) - 1 = -1.2% — the plan is still below pre-COVID inpatient PMPM. Recommendation to actuary: use 3-year or blended trend (average of 2yr and 3yr) for the rate filing to smooth the COVID distortion. Document the COVID adjustment rationale explicitly in the filing narrative. State insurance regulators expect an explanation for trend outliers.

Key Takeaways

What every analyst must remember from this chapter.

1 Gap-island (Pattern 1): LAG(coverage_end_date) OVER (PARTITION BY member_id ORDER BY coverage_start_date). MAX(gap_days) > 45 = NCQA exclusion. SUM(member_months) >= 11 is insufficient — it misses members with multiple sub-45-day gaps whose total exceeds the threshold.

2 Recursive CTE (Pattern 2): ANCHOR UNION ALL RECURSIVE_MEMBER. Depth guard (WHERE depth < N) prevents infinite loops. Use for ICD-10 code family expansion, provider organizational hierarchy roll-up, and benefit plan hierarchy traversal.

3 Dynamic pivot (Pattern 3): generate the CASE WHEN column list via STRING_AGG over distinct lag values, then EXECUTE the assembled SQL. Makes the lag triangle window a runtime parameter rather than a code constant — essential for production pipelines.

4 Episode grouper (Pattern 4): ROW_NUMBER() OVER (PARTITION BY claim_id ORDER BY anchor_date ASC) resolves overlapping episode windows. anchor_priority = 1 assigns each claim to the earliest qualifying anchor — deterministic, auditable, defensible in contract disputes.

5 Running IBNR (Pattern 5): ibnr_adjusted_pmpm = observed_pmpm × (1 / completion_factor). Use multiplicative (not additive) adjustment — IBNR scales proportionally with enrollment volume. Always label data_maturity alongside adjusted PMPM. Never present IMMATURE months as final numbers.

6 Multi-period geometric trend (Pattern 6): POWER(end/start, 1.0/n) - 1. n=1 is just (end/start)−1; n=2 uses POWER(end/start, 0.5)−1; n=3 uses POWER(end/start, 1.0/3.0)−1. Arithmetic averaging overstates trend when growth is uneven. Actuary selects from 1yr, 2yr, 3yr, and blended.

7 COVID-era trend distortion: 1-year trend measured off a depressed COVID base overstates the sustainable trend. Always present 3-year and blended trend alongside 1-year in rate filing tables. Document the COVID adjustment rationale explicitly in the filing narrative.

8 Pattern selection guide: enrollment continuity → Gap-Island. Code family expansion / org hierarchy → Recursive CTE. Variable-width cross-tab → Dynamic Pivot. Multi-claim episode attribution → Episode Grouper with ROW_NUMBER(). Incomplete recent period → IBNR Completion. Actuarial trend → Multi-Period Geometric POWER().

Appendices A–G: Reference Compendium

DDL · HEDIS Quick Ref · Drug Codes · Official Sources · Validation · Glossary · Cheat Sheet

The appendices serve as a standing reference that analysts return to throughout their work. They are not required reading before any chapter — they are looked up when a specific need arises: when a schema question surfaces, when a formula needs confirmation, when a term requires a precise definition, or when a validation check needs to be verified against a canonical list.

Appendix A: DDL Scripts & Data Model

Core tables used throughout this book — schema definitions and column-level descriptions

The schemas below define the canonical tables referenced in every SQL example in this book. Actual production environments will differ in naming conventions, data types, and partitioning strategies. Use these as a structural template. All tables assume ANSI SQL-compatible data types. Timestamp/Date types should be adjusted for your platform (DATE, TIMESTAMP, DATETIME).

A.1 Core Fact Tables

DDL — fact_medical_claims (Core Claims Fact Table)

```
CREATE TABLE fact_medical_claims (
  claim_id              VARCHAR(30)  NOT NULL,  -- unique claim identifier
  member_id             VARCHAR(20)  NOT NULL,  -- FK to dim_members
  rendering_npi         CHAR(10),               -- performing provider NPI (Type 1)
  billing_npi           CHAR(10),               -- billing entity NPI (Type 1 or 2)
  billing_tin           VARCHAR(10),            -- tax ID for fee schedule joins
  service_date          DATE         NOT NULL,  -- date of service (DOS)
  paid_date             DATE,                   -- date claim was adjudicated
  procedure_code        VARCHAR(10),            -- CPT or HCPCS code
  primary_diag          VARCHAR(10),            -- ICD-10-CM primary diagnosis
  diag_2                VARCHAR(10),            -- secondary diagnosis
  diag_3                VARCHAR(10),            -- tertiary diagnosis
  primary_drg           VARCHAR(5),             -- DRG for inpatient claims
  type_of_bill          VARCHAR(4),             -- UB-04 TOB (e.g., 111x, 131x)
  revenue_code          VARCHAR(4),             -- UB-04 revenue code
  claim_status          VARCHAR(20),            -- PAID, DENIED, REVERSED, VOID
  claim_frequency_code  CHAR(1),                -- 8 = void/cancel transaction
  discharge_status_code VARCHAR(2),             -- UB-04 patient discharge status
  billed_amount         NUMERIC(12,2),          -- provider charge (billed)
  allowed_amount        NUMERIC(12,2),          -- contractual allowed amount
  paid_amount           NUMERIC(12,2),          -- plan payment (allowed minus member cost-sharing)
  units_of_service      NUMERIC(8,2),           -- units billed on claim line
  line_of_business      VARCHAR(30),            -- COMMERCIAL, MEDICARE_ADVANTAGE, MEDICAID
  service_locality      VARCHAR(10),            -- geographic locality for Medicare rate lookups
  denial_reason_code    VARCHAR(10),            -- CARC code for denied claims
  appeal_status         VARCHAR(20),            -- NONE, PENDING, OVERTURNED, UPHELD
  payer_id              VARCHAR(20),            -- payer identifier for RCM analytics
  CONSTRAINT pk_medical_claims PRIMARY KEY (claim_id)
```

```
);
```

DDL — fact_pharmacy_claims · fact_member_months · fact_lab_results

```
CREATE TABLE fact_pharmacy_claims (
  claim_id              VARCHAR(30) NOT NULL,
  member_id             VARCHAR(20) NOT NULL,
  prescribing_npi       CHAR(10),          -- prescribing provider NPI
  dispensing_pharmacy_npi CHAR(10),        -- dispensing pharmacy NPI
  dispensing_date       DATE      NOT NULL, -- date prescription dispensed
  ndc_code              VARCHAR(11),       -- 11-digit National Drug Code
  days_supply           INT,               -- days of medication supplied
  quantity_dispensed    NUMERIC(10,3),
  plan_paid_amount      NUMERIC(10,2),     -- plan portion of drug cost
  member_cost_share     NUMERIC(10,2),     -- copay/coinsurance member paid
  claim_status          VARCHAR(20),
  CONSTRAINT pk_rx_claims PRIMARY KEY (claim_id)
);

CREATE TABLE fact_member_months (
  member_id       VARCHAR(20)  NOT NULL,
  membership_year INT          NOT NULL,     -- calendar year
  month_start     DATE,                      -- first day of enrollment month
  member_months   NUMERIC(4,2) DEFAULT 1,    -- 1.0 = full month enrolled
  line_of_business VARCHAR(30),
  plan_id         VARCHAR(20),
  CONSTRAINT pk_member_months PRIMARY KEY (member_id, membership_year, month_start)
);

CREATE TABLE fact_lab_results (
  result_id      VARCHAR(30) NOT NULL,
  member_id      VARCHAR(20) NOT NULL,
  rendering_npi  CHAR(10),
  loinc_code     VARCHAR(10),              -- LOINC code identifying the test
  result_date    DATE,
  numeric_result NUMERIC(10,3),            -- numeric result value
  result_unit    VARCHAR(20),              -- unit of measure (%, mg/dL, etc.)
  result_status  VARCHAR(10),              -- FINAL, PRELIMINARY, CORRECTED
  CONSTRAINT pk_lab_results PRIMARY KEY (result_id)
);
```

A.2 Core Dimension Tables

DDL — dim_members · dim_providers · dim_pcp_attribution

```
CREATE TABLE dim_members (
  member_id            VARCHAR(20)  NOT NULL,
  member_name          VARCHAR(100),
  date_of_birth        DATE,
  gender               CHAR(1),        -- M, F, U
  zip_code             VARCHAR(10),
  county_fips          VARCHAR(5),
  phone                VARCHAR(20),
  preferred_language   VARCHAR(50),
  coverage_status      VARCHAR(10),    -- ACTIVE, TERMED
  line_of_business     VARCHAR(30),
  plan_id              VARCHAR(20),
  dual_eligible_flag   CHAR(1),        -- Y/N
  lis_flag             CHAR(1),        -- Y/N Low Income Subsidy
  disability_flag      CHAR(1),        -- Y/N
  race_ethnicity_self_reported VARCHAR(50),
```

```
  race_ethnicity_bisg       VARCHAR(50),       -- BISG probabilistic estimate
  ssn_last4             CHAR(4),           -- last 4 of SSN (masked)
  death_date             DATE,
  attributed_pcp_npi         CHAR(10),
  CONSTRAINT pk_members PRIMARY KEY (member_id)
);

CREATE TABLE dim_providers (
  npi             CHAR(10)   NOT NULL,     -- 10-digit NPI
  billing_tin         VARCHAR(10),
  provider_full_name   VARCHAR(150),
  provider_last_name   VARCHAR(100),
  provider_org_name    VARCHAR(150),
  specialty_group      VARCHAR(80),
  specialty_code       VARCHAR(10),          -- NUCC taxonomy code
  provider_type        VARCHAR(30),          -- PHYSICIAN, FACILITY, TELEHEALTH
  network_status       VARCHAR(20),          -- IN_NETWORK, OUT_OF_NETWORK
  accepting_new_patients CHAR(1),
  county_fips         VARCHAR(5),
  county             VARCHAR(80),
  hospital_name        VARCHAR(150),
  CONSTRAINT pk_providers PRIMARY KEY (npi)
);

CREATE TABLE dim_pcp_attribution (
  member_id          VARCHAR(20) NOT NULL,
  attributed_pcp_npi CHAR(10)    NOT NULL,
  attribution_year   INT         NOT NULL,
  attribution_method VARCHAR(30),               -- CLAIMS_BASED, VOLUNTARY
  CONSTRAINT pk_pcp_attr PRIMARY KEY (member_id, attribution_year)
);
```

Appendix B: HEDIS Administrative Measure Quick Reference

Denominator criteria · Numerator events · Key exclusions · Measurement year look-back

Each row summarizes the denominator population, numerator qualifying event, key exclusions, and look-back window for the most commonly implemented HEDIS administrative measures. NCQA publishes complete technical specifications annually — always verify against the current-year specification before HEDIS submission.

Measure	Denominator Population	Numerator Event	Key Exclusions	Look-Back
CDC — HbA1c Tested	18–75, diabetes dx, ≥11 mo enrolled	Any HbA1c lab (LOINC 4548-4 etc.) during the year	Gestational diabetes only, ESRD/dialysis, death	Current year
CDC — HbA1c Control (<8%)	Same as HbA1c Tested	HbA1c result < 8.0%	Same as above	Current year
CDC — Eye Exam	Same as HbA1c Tested	Retinal/dilated eye exam CPT or bilateral retinal photo	Same as above	Current year OR prior year
CDC — Kidney Health Eval	Same as HbA1c Tested	eGFR test OR urine albumin/creatinine ratio (LOINC codes)	Same as above	Current year

BCS – Breast Cancer Screening	Women 52–74, ≥11 mo enrolled (current OR prior year)	Mammogram (CPT 77065–77067) in the 27-month look-back period	Bilateral mastectomy (any time prior)	27 months (current + prior year)
CCS – Cervical Cancer Screening	Women 24–64, ≥11 mo enrolled	Cervical cytology or high-risk HPV test within 3 or 5 years (depending on test type)	Hysterectomy with no residual cervix	3 or 5 years
COL – Colorectal Cancer Screening	50–75, ≥11 mo enrolled	FOBT (1 yr), FIT-DNA (1–3 yr), flexible sigmoidoscopy (5 yr), CT colonography (5 yr), colonoscopy (10 yr)	Colorectal cancer diagnosis, total colectomy	Variable (1–10 yr per test type)
CBP – Controlling Blood Pressure	18–85, hypertension dx, ≥11 mo enrolled	Outpatient BP reading < 140/90 (from medical record)	ESRD, pregnancy, death – hybrid measure	Current year
MDD – Diabetes Medication Adherence	≥18, diabetes dx on oral antidiabetics, ≥11 mo enrolled	PDC ≥ 80% across the year	None specified	Current year
FUH – Follow-Up After Hospitalization	6+, BH inpatient discharge, ≥30 days enrolled post-discharge	Outpatient BH visit within 7 days (FUH-7) or 30 days (FUH-30)	Death within 30 days post-discharge	30-day post-discharge window
AMB – Ambulatory Care Visits	All enrolled, no age restriction	ED visits or outpatient visits per 1,000 member months (utilization measure, not a rate)	None	Current year
PCR – All-Cause Readmission	18+, inpatient discharge, ≥31 days enrolled	Acute inpatient readmission within 30 days of discharge	Planned procedures (value set), obstetric admissions, death < 30 days post-discharge	30-day post-discharge window

Appendix C: Oncology Drug Code Reference

Key HCPCS J-codes · Oral oncolytic NDC families · Biosimilar reference codes

Oncology claims analytics requires mapping HCPCS J-codes (administered drugs billed on medical claims) and NDC codes (oral oncolytics billed on pharmacy claims) to their drug families and mechanism of action. This reference covers the most commonly encountered oncology drug codes. Full HCPCS and NDC code sets are published annually by CMS and the FDA respectively.

HCPCS / NDC	Drug Name (Brand)	Class & Primary Indication
J9035	Bevacizumab (Avastin)	Angiogenesis inhibitor – colorectal, NSCLC, glioblastoma
J9045	Carboplatin	Platinum-based chemotherapy – ovarian, lung, head/neck
J9060	Cisplatin	Platinum-based chemotherapy – bladder, testicular, cervical
J9171	Docetaxel (Taxotere)	Taxane – breast, NSCLC, prostate, gastric
J9178	Epirubicin	Anthracycline – breast cancer (EC/FEC regimens)
J9190	Fluorouracil (5-FU)	Antimetabolite – colorectal, head/neck, breast
J9217	Leuprolide acetate (Lupron)	LHRH agonist – prostate cancer hormone therapy
J9228	Ipilimumab (Yervoy)	CTLA-4 checkpoint inhibitor – melanoma, RCC
J9299	Nivolumab (Opdivo)	PD-1 inhibitor – melanoma, NSCLC, RCC, urothelial

J9306	Pertuzumab (Perjeta)	HER2-targeted — breast cancer (with trastuzumab)
J9310	Rituximab (Rituxan)	CD20-targeted — NHL, CLL, RA
J9355	Trastuzumab (Herceptin)	HER2-targeted — breast cancer, gastric cancer
J9358	Pembrolizumab (Keytruda)	PD-1 inhibitor — multiple solid tumors, MSI-H
J9999	Chemotherapy, NOS	Unclassified — requires medical record for drug identification
NDC 59148-0022-xx	Imatinib (Gleevec) oral	BCR-ABL inhibitor — CML, GIST (oral oncolytic)
NDC 00003-0150-xx	Lenalidomide (Revlimid) oral	Immunomodulatory — multiple myeloma, MDS, MCL
NDC 00781-3199-xx	Ibrutinib (Imbruvica) oral	BTK inhibitor — CLL, MCL, WM (oral oncolytic)

Oral Oncolytic Parity Many states have enacted oral chemotherapy parity laws requiring health plans to cover oral oncolytics (NDC-billed pharmacy claims) at the same cost-sharing level as IV chemotherapy (J-code medical claims). Analytics must monitor both claim streams for the same member episode to ensure parity compliance and accurate episode cost attribution.

Appendix D: Official Sources of Truth

Where to obtain authoritative reference data — URLs and update frequencies

Every reference table in this book must be sourced from an authoritative publisher. The table below identifies the canonical source, update frequency, and data format for each critical reference dataset. Substituting unofficial or outdated reference data is the most common source of HEDIS compliance audit findings and HCC submission errors.

Reference Dataset	Authoritative Source	Update Frequency & Notes
ICD-10-CM Diagnosis Codes	CMS — cms.gov/medicare/coding-billing/icd-10-codes	Annual (Oct 1). FY update adds, revises, invalidates codes. Load within 2 business days of release.
CPT Procedure Codes	AMA — ama-assn.org/practice-management/cpt	Annual (Jan 1). AMA license required. Load by December 15 for January 1 readiness.
HCPCS Level II Codes	CMS — cms.gov/medicare/coding-billing/healthcare-common-procedure-system	Quarterly updates. J-codes for drugs change frequently as new biologics receive codes.
NPI Registry (NPPES)	CMS — download.cms.gov/nppes/NPI_Files.html	Monthly full file + weekly deactivation file. Load within 5 business days of monthly release.
OIG Exclusion List	OIG — exclusions.oig.hhs.gov	Monthly updates. Weekly monitoring required for claims pre-payment edits.
CMS HCC Crosswalk (v28)	CMS — cms.gov/medicare/health-plans/medicareadvtgspecratestats	Annual. Model coefficients update with each payment year. v28 blend ratios in transition years.
NCQA HEDIS Value Sets	NCQA — ncqa.org/hedis/measures	Annual (fall). Requires NCQA license. Load before January 1 of measurement year.
CMS Star Rating Cut-Points	CMS — cms.gov/medicare/health-plans/plan-performance-data	Annual (October preview, January final). Use for Stars simulation and gap prioritization.
NDC Drug Codes	FDA — fda.gov/drugs/drug-approvals-databases/national-drug-code-directory	Continuous. Weekly update recommended. Critical for pharmacy analytics and opioid monitoring.
Medicare Fee Schedule	CMS — cms.gov/medicare/payment/physician-fee-schedule	Annual (Jan 1) with quarterly updates. Locality codes required for geographic adjustment.
Area Deprivation Index (ADI)	University of Wisconsin — neighborhoodatlas.medicine.wisc.edu	Annual. ZIP-level and census block group-level. Free for research use.

AHRQ PQI Specifications	AHRQ — qualityindicators.ahrq.gov	Annual updates. ICD-10 code sets for each PQI measure. Exclusion DRG lists change annually.
CAHPS Survey Instruments	AHRQ — cahps.ahrq.gov	Annual updates. Administration is via CMS-approved survey vendor for MA plans.
NCCI Edits	CMS — cms.gov/medicare/coding-billing/national-correct-coding-initiative-edits	Quarterly. Column 1 / Column 2 edit pairs and modifier indicators. Essential for unbundling detection.

Appendix E: Four Pillars of Healthcare SQL Validation

Structural · Referential · Business Rule · Temporal — a checklist for every production query

Every SQL query that feeds a production dashboard, a regulatory submission, or a financial report must pass four validation pillars before its results are distributed. These checks should be embedded as assertions or automated unit tests in the analytics pipeline — not performed manually after the fact.

Pillar 1 Structural Validation — Does the query produce a well-formed result set?

Check	Validation SQL & Expected Result
Row count sanity	HEDIS denominator should contain between 80% and 120% of last year's count. Alert if COUNT(*) < 0.80 × prior_year_count OR > 1.20 × prior_year_count.
No NULL in critical fields	SELECT COUNT(*) FROM result WHERE member_id IS NULL OR measure_id IS NULL. Result must = 0.
No duplicate grain keys	SELECT member_id, measure_id, COUNT(*) FROM result GROUP BY 1,2 HAVING COUNT(*) > 1. Result must return 0 rows.
Rate within valid range	All rates must be between 0% and 100%. SELECT * FROM result WHERE rate_pct < 0 OR rate_pct > 100. Result must = 0 rows.
Denominator >= numerator	SELECT * FROM result WHERE numerator > denominator. Result must = 0 rows — numerator is always a subset of denominator.

Pillar 2 Referential Validation — Do all keys resolve?

Check	Validation SQL & Expected Result
Member IDs resolve	SELECT COUNT(*) FROM result r LEFT JOIN dim_members m ON r.member_id=m.member_id WHERE m.member_id IS NULL. Must = 0.
NPIs in NPPES	SELECT COUNT(DISTINCT rendering_npi) FROM fact_medical_claims WHERE rendering_npi NOT IN (SELECT npi FROM ref_nppes_registry). Alert if > 2%.
ICD-10 codes valid	SELECT COUNT(*) FROM fact_medical_claims c LEFT JOIN ref_icd10_codes r ON c.primary_diag=r.icd10_code WHERE r.icd10_code IS NULL AND c.primary_diag IS NOT NULL. Alert if > 0.5%.
LOINC codes in reference	SELECT COUNT(*) FROM fact_lab_results l LEFT JOIN ref_loinc r ON l.loinc_code=r.loinc_code WHERE r.loinc_code IS NULL. Alert if > 1%.
Fee schedule coverage	SELECT COUNT(*) FROM fact_medical_claims c LEFT JOIN ref_fee_schedule fs ON c.billing_tin=fs.billing_tin AND c.procedure_code=fs.procedure_code AND c.service_date BETWEEN fs.effective_date AND COALESCE(fs.expiration_date,'2099-12-31') WHERE fs.allowed_amount IS NULL AND c.claim_status='PAID'. Report weekly.

Pillar 3 Business Rule Validation — Do values conform to domain logic?

Check	Validation SQL & Expected Result
Allowed ≤ Billed	SELECT COUNT(*) FROM fact_medical_claims WHERE allowed_amount > billed_amount AND claim_status='PAID'. Alert if > 0.5%.
Service date ≤ Paid date	SELECT COUNT(*) FROM fact_medical_claims WHERE paid_date < service_date. Must = 0 — claims cannot be paid before service rendered.
No service after death	SELECT COUNT(*) FROM fact_medical_claims c JOIN dim_members m ON c.member_id=m.member_id WHERE c.service_date > m.death_date AND m.death_date IS NOT NULL. Must = 0.
Age-consistent diagnoses	SELECT COUNT(*) FROM result WHERE gender='M' AND primary_diag LIKE 'O%'. Must = 0 — obstetric codes cannot appear on male members.
Inpatient TOB consistency	SELECT COUNT(*) FROM fact_medical_claims WHERE type_of_bill LIKE '11%' AND primary_drg IS NULL AND claim_status='PAID'. Alert if > 1% — inpatient claims should have a DRG.

Pillar 4 Temporal Validation — Is data current and correctly bounded?

Check	Validation SQL & Expected Result
IBNR completeness flag	Flag any service month where months_elapsed < 3 as IMMATURE in all dashboards. Never present raw PMPM for months < 3 months old without an IBNR adjustment.
Measurement year boundary	SELECT COUNT(*) FROM fact_hedis_gaps WHERE measurement_year <> :meas_year. Must = 0 — confirm the query is scoped to the correct year.
Reference tables current	SELECT table_name, MAX(last_updated_date), :run_date - MAX(last_updated_date) AS days_stale FROM ref_data_update_log GROUP BY table_name HAVING days_stale > :threshold. Alert on any reference table exceeding its staleness threshold.
Claims extract currency	SELECT MAX(service_date), DATEDIFF('day', MAX(service_date), CURRENT_DATE) AS lag_days FROM fact_medical_claims WHERE claim_status='PAID'. Alert if lag_days > 7 — extract may be stale.
HEDIS snapshot date	Confirm measurement_snapshot_date in ref_hedis_run_log matches the date the HEDIS algorithms were last executed. Any re-run must log a new snapshot date for audit trail.

Appendix F: Comprehensive Healthcare Glossary

150+ terms — clinical, financial, regulatory, and technical

Terms are listed alphabetically. Acronyms are cross-referenced to their full form. Each definition is written from the perspective of the healthcare data analyst — emphasizing how the term is used in SQL, financial models, or regulatory filings rather than providing a clinical or legal definition.

Term	Definition
ADI	Area Deprivation Index. A composite socioeconomic deprivation score by ZIP or census block derived from census variables including income, education, employment, and housing quality. Higher rank = more disadvantaged. Used as an SDOH proxy in risk stratification and health equity analytics.
Allowed Amount	The contractual amount a health plan is obligated to pay for a covered service — the fee schedule rate for in-network providers, or the plan's non-par rate for out-of-network. Always use allowed_amount (not billed or paid) as the rate filing and PMPM base. Paid_amount = allowed minus member cost-sharing.
BISG	Bayesian Improved Surname Geocoding. A probabilistic method that assigns race/ethnicity from a member's surname and ZIP code using Census Bureau data. Improves

	race/ethnicity data completeness from ~30% (self-reported) to ~65–75%. Used for health equity stratification when self-reported data is unavailable.
Bundled Payment	An alternative payment model in which a single target price covers all services within a clinically defined episode of care (e.g., total hip replacement + 90-day post-acute care). The plan and provider share savings below the target price; the provider shares financial risk for overruns.
CARC	Claim Adjustment Reason Code. A standardized code on an Explanation of Benefits (EOB) or remittance advice that explains why a claim was denied, adjusted, or paid differently than billed. CARC 97 = bundled service; CARC 29 = timely filing exceeded. Used in RCM denial root-cause analysis.
CAHPS	Consumer Assessment of Healthcare Providers and Systems. A standardized survey instrument measuring patient experience of care across composites: Getting Care Quickly, How Well Doctors Communicate, Customer Service, Rating of Health Plan, and Rating of Personal Doctor. Administered annually by CMS-approved vendors. CAHPS scores contribute to CMS Star Ratings.
Capitation	A fixed monthly payment per enrolled member to a provider or provider group, regardless of how many services the member uses. The provider bears full financial risk for the enrolled population's healthcare costs. Contrast with fee-for-service (payment per claim).
CCI	Charlson Comorbidity Index. A weighted score summing 17 chronic conditions (weights 1–6) to quantify comorbidity burden and predict 1-year mortality. Used in risk stratification composite scores. CCI 0 = no major comorbidities; CCI ≥ 5 = severe burden. SQL: GROUP BY member_id, condition_name + MAX(weight) before summing to prevent double-counting.
CMS	Centers for Medicare & Medicaid Services. The federal agency within HHS that administers Medicare, Medicaid, CHIP, and the ACA Marketplace. CMS sets payment rates, quality reporting requirements, Star Ratings methodology, and risk adjustment rules for Medicare Advantage plans.
Completion Factor	The proportion of a service month's eventual final PMPM that has been received at a given lag period. From the IBNR lag triangle: completion_factor_at_1m = AVG(cumulative_pmpm_at_1m / final_pmpm). IBNR multiplier = 1 / completion_factor. Applied to incomplete recent months in financial dashboards.
CPT	Current Procedural Terminology. The AMA-maintained code set for medical procedures and services billed on CMS 1500 professional claims. Updated annually January 1. E&M codes (99201–99215) are the most analytically significant for upcoding detection.
Credibility (Z)	Z = MIN(1, SQRT(n / 1082)). The actuarial weight given to a plan's own experience versus an external benchmark. Full credibility at 1,082 member months (90% confidence, ±5% precision). Used in rate filing PMPM blending: credibility_weighted_pmpm = Z × plan_pmpm + (1-Z) × benchmark_pmpm.
Days in A/R	Accounts Receivable metric: total_AR_balance / (annual_gross_charges / 365). Measures how many days of revenue are outstanding. Benchmarks: < 30 days for physician groups, < 45 for community hospitals, < 60 for teaching hospitals. Rising days-in-A/R indicates denial rate increase or billing backlog.
DRG	Diagnosis-Related Group. A CMS payment classification for inpatient acute hospitalizations. Each admission is assigned one DRG based on primary diagnosis, secondary diagnoses, procedures, and patient demographics. The DRG determines the fixed payment rate the plan pays the hospital under a DRG-based contract.
EDPS	Encounter Data Processing System. The current CMS system for receiving Medicare Advantage encounter data (complete 837 transactions) for risk adjustment. Replaced RAPS in 2016. All HCC credit for MA plans flows through EDPS-accepted submissions. Errors in EDPS submissions directly reduce capitation payments in the following year.
Episode Grouper	A clinical algorithm that groups all claims related to a clinical episode — defined by an anchor event plus a time window — into a single episode record with a total cost. Used for bundled payment settlement, episode benchmarking, and provider cost profiling. SQL: anchor → ROW_NUMBER() for overlap resolution → SUM(allowed_amount) per anchor.
HEDIS	Healthcare Effectiveness Data and Information Set. NCQA's standardized quality measurement set of 90+ measures spanning preventive care, chronic disease management, behavioral health, and patient safety. Used for health plan accreditation,

	employer plan selection, and CMS Star Ratings. Published annually with updated technical specifications.
HCC	Hierarchical Condition Category. A CMS risk adjustment diagnostic classification. ICD-10-CM codes map to HCC codes; HCC codes have RAF increments that add to a member's total risk score. Higher RAF = higher capitation payment to the MA plan. HCC capture gap = HCC in claims but not submitted via EDPS.
HEI	Health Equity Index. A CMS additive measure incorporated into MA Star Ratings that rewards plans for improving HEDIS performance specifically for historically underserved members (dual-eligible, LIS, disability, BISG-designated race/ethnicity groups). Calculated separately from the main Stars score but can contribute to the overall rating.
HOS	Health Outcomes Survey. A CMS-administered two-year longitudinal survey for Medicare Advantage members measuring physical (PCS) and mental (MCS) health component scores at baseline and 24-month follow-up. Plans are scored on the percentage of members who maintained or improved relative to their expected trajectory based on CMS regression equations.
IBNR	Incurred But Not Reported. Claims for services already provided but not yet received or processed by the plan. Recent service months have incomplete claims data because of processing lag. IBNR completion factors (from the lag triangle) convert incomplete observed PMPM to an estimated final PMPM. Inpatient claims have the longest IBNR lag (35–45% complete at 1 month); pharmacy the shortest (85–90%).
ICD-10-CM	International Classification of Diseases, 10th Revision, Clinical Modification. The US standard for diagnosis coding on all medical claims. Updated annually October 1 by CMS/NCHS. Code structure: letter prefix (A–Z) + 2 numeric digits + period + up to 4 additional characters. E11.9 = type 2 diabetes without complications.
LOINC	Logical Observation Identifiers Names and Codes. A universal code system for laboratory tests, clinical measurements, and observations. Maintained by Regenstrief Institute. Used in HEDIS lab-based measures (HbA1c: LOINC 4548-4; LDL: 13457-7). Required for all FHIR-based clinical data exchange.
Luhn Algorithm	A modular arithmetic checksum formula used to validate 10-digit NPIs. The 10th digit of every NPI is a check digit calculated from the first 9 digits plus a constant (24). Luhn validation in SQL detects mistyped, transposed, or fabricated NPIs before they corrupt provider scorecards and OIG exclusion checks.
MHPAEA	Mental Health Parity and Addiction Equity Act. Federal law requiring that prior authorization, treatment limitations, and nonquantitative treatment limits (NQTLs) for behavioral health and SUD benefits are no more restrictive than those for comparable medical/surgical benefits. Analytics: compare BH vs. medical PA denial rates and processing times.
MLR	Medical Loss Ratio. Claims paid / premium revenue. ACA floors: 85% for large group (50+ employees), 80% for small group/individual. Plans below the floor must rebate the difference to members. MLR above 100% = underwriting loss. Monitor weekly; flag when MLR trended above floor for 3+ consecutive months.
NCCI	National Correct Coding Initiative. CMS-defined edits specifying pairs of CPT codes that cannot be billed together because one code is included in the comprehensive code. Unbundling = billing both codes separately to collect higher combined payment. NCCI edits are organized as Column 1 (comprehensive) and Column 2 (component) code pairs.
NCQA	National Committee for Quality Assurance. Independent non-profit that accredits health plans and manages HEDIS. NCQA accreditation levels: Excellent, Commendable, Accredited, Provisional, Denied. MA plans with NCQA accreditation receive CMS deemed status, reducing regulatory burden. Commercial employers widely require NCQA accreditation for plan inclusion.
NPI	National Provider Identifier. A unique 10-digit identifier for every healthcare provider in the US, assigned by CMS through the NPPES system. Type 1 = individual clinician (rendering_npi in claims). Type 2 = organization/facility (billing_npi). Required on all Medicare, Medicaid, and most commercial claims.
NPPES	National Plan and Provider Enumeration System. The CMS-administered registry of all active NPIs. Monthly full file download available free at download.cms.gov. Use for NPI validation (active status check), provider specialty lookup, and OIG exclusion cross-reference. Load monthly into ref_nppes_registry.

PDC	Proportion of Days Covered. A pharmacy adherence metric: days covered by a medication fill / days in the measurement period. PDC ≥ 80% = adherent (HEDIS numerator met for adherence measures). Uses calendar-join SQL to avoid double-counting overlapping fills. Distinct from MPR (Medication Possession Ratio), which allows double-counting.
PMPM	Per Member Per Month. The foundational unit of healthcare cost analysis. PMPM = total allowed amount / total member months. Always use member months from fact_member_months as the denominator — never derive it from claims alone. PMPM enables cost comparison across populations of different sizes and time periods.
PQI	Prevention Quality Indicator. AHRQ-developed measures of ambulatory care quality: inpatient admissions for conditions (diabetes, CHF, COPD, asthma, hypertension) that, with appropriate outpatient care, rarely require hospitalization. High PQI rates indicate primary care access gaps. Rate per 100,000 member months. Exclude obstetric DRGs per AHRQ methodology.
Prior Authorization (PA)	A utilization management process requiring clinical review and plan approval before certain services are covered. CMS 2026 rule: urgent PA ≤ 72 hours, standard ≤ 7 calendar days. Analytics: turnaround compliance, denial rates, MHPAEA parity (BH vs. medical), gold carding eligibility (≥ 90% approval rate).
QBP	Quality Bonus Payment. CMS bonus paid to MA plans with Star Ratings ≥ 4.0 Stars. Worth up to 5% of the plan's CMS benchmark revenue. A plan with $500M in MA revenue at 4.5 Stars earns ~$25M in QBP annually. The primary financial incentive driving the Stars analytics pipeline.
RADV	Risk Adjustment Data Validation. CMS audit process that selects ~200 MA members per contract and requires the plan to produce medical records supporting every submitted HCC. Unsupported HCCs result in payment clawbacks extrapolated to the entire contract. Plans must maintain RADV readiness: digital documentation index for all submitted HCCs.
RAF	Risk Adjustment Factor. A numeric score representing a member's expected healthcare cost relative to the average Medicare beneficiary (RAF = 1.0). Calculated from submitted HCC codes. Higher RAF = higher CMS capitation payment. RAF = sum of all applicable HCC increments + demographic factor. The plan's average RAF drives its total MA revenue.
RAPS	Risk Adjustment Processing System. Legacy CMS system for MA encounter data submission, accepting simplified encounter summary records. Replaced by EDPS (complete 837 data) from 2016 onward. RAPS is still referenced in historical context but no longer accepts new submissions for risk adjustment credit.
Stars Rating	CMS annual quality rating for Medicare Advantage plans on a 1–5 star scale. Based on HEDIS, CAHPS, HOS, and administrative measures across five domains. Summary Rating rounded to nearest 0.5. Plans ≥ 4.0 Stars qualify for QBP. Plans < 3.0 Stars for 3 consecutive years face contract termination. Cut-points set annually by CMS clustering algorithm.
Stop-Loss	Reinsurance protecting health plans from catastrophic claims. Specific stop-loss: per-member annual threshold (e.g., $250K). Aggregate stop-loss: plan-wide total claims threshold (e.g., 120% of expected). Monitor specific stop-loss weekly (members approaching threshold); aggregate monthly. Submit specific stop-loss claims immediately when threshold is met.
TOB	Type of Bill. A 3–4 digit code on UB-04 institutional claims identifying the facility type and claim classification. First two digits: 11x = inpatient acute, 13x = outpatient hospital, 23x = ambulatory surgery, 32x = home health, 81x = hospice. Critical for HEDIS TOB filters (LIKE '11%' for inpatient) and PQI avoidable admission identification.
Total Cost of Care	The complete cost of healthcare services for an attributed population including medical claims (allowed_amount) AND pharmacy claims (plan_paid_amount). Critical in VBC analytics: excluding pharmacy allows providers to game shared savings by shifting costs to the pharmacy channel. Always UNION ALL both claim streams for the denominator population.
VBC	Value-Based Care. Payment models that link provider reimbursement to quality outcomes and cost efficiency rather than volume of services. Spectrum: pay-for-reporting → pay-for-performance → shared savings → bundled payment → full capitation. Analytics: shared savings = benchmark_pmpm vs. actual_pmpm; quality gate; risk corridor. Requires total cost of care (medical + pharmacy).
Wilson CI	Wilson Confidence Interval. Preferred over normal approximation for proportions near 0% or 100% and small denominators. Formula: $(n \times p + z^2/2 \pm z \times \sqrt{n \times p \times (1-p) + z^2/4}) / (n+z^2)$.

	SQL approximation: 1.92 ≈ $z^2/2$, 3.84 ≈ z^2. Used for stratified HEDIS reporting and health equity disparity flagging with small racial/ethnic subgroup denominators (n < 100).
Z-Code	ICD-10-CM codes Z00–Z99 documenting factors influencing health status that are not diseases. Z55–Z65 specifically capture social determinants: Z59.0 = homelessness, Z59.4 = food insecurity, Z60.2 = living alone, Z63.4 = death of family member. Severely under-captured in claims (<5% of visits). When present, they are highly actionable for social work referral and care management routing.

Appendix G: Formula, SQL & Quick Reference Cheat Sheet ★ NEW

The most-used formulas and SQL patterns — one page per domain

This cheat sheet collects the formulas and SQL patterns most frequently needed in day-to-day healthcare analytics work. Organized by domain. Formulas are written as they appear in SQL.

G.1 Financial Metrics

Metric	Formula / SQL
PMPM	SUM(allowed_amount) / SUM(member_months)
MLR	SUM(claims) / SUM(premium_revenue)
Days in A/R	SUM(ar_balance) / (SUM(annual_charges) / 365.0)
Annualized N-year trend	POWER(pmpm_end / NULLIF(pmpm_start,0), 1.0/N) - 1
Blended trend (util × cost)	(1 + util_trend) × (1 + cost_trend) - 1
Credibility weight Z	MIN(1.0, SQRT(member_months / 1082.0))
Credibility-weighted PMPM	Z × plan_pmpm + (1-Z) × benchmark_pmpm
IBNR multiplier	1.0 / NULLIF(completion_factor, 0)
IBNR-adjusted PMPM	observed_pmpm × ibnr_multiplier
Pooling charge PMPM	SUM(MAX(0, ytd_allowed - threshold)) / total_mm
Large claim excess SQL	GREATEST(0, ytd_allowed - :threshold) AS pooled_excess
Stop-loss 80% alert SQL	CASE WHEN ytd_allowed >= threshold*0.80 THEN 'ALERT' END

G.2 Risk Adjustment & HCC

Metric	Formula / SQL
RAF = member total risk	SUM of all HCC raf_increments + demographic factor
HCC revenue gap (annual)	raf_increment × monthly_capitation_rate × 12
Risk index (VBC benchmark)	current_avg_raf / base_avg_raf
Risk-adjusted PMPM	actual_pmpm / avg_panel_raf
CCI score SQL	SUM(MAX(cci_weight) per condition_name) — GROUP BY member, condition before summing
HCC gap detection SQL	LEFT JOIN submitted_hccs WHERE sh.member_id IS NULL

G.3 Quality — HEDIS & Stars

Metric	Formula / SQL
HEDIS rate	numerator / denominator × 100
PDC (adherence)	SUM(distinct covered days) / measurement_period_days
Stars domain score	SUM(measure_star × weight) / SUM(weight)
Stars summary rating	AVG(domain_scores) — rounded to nearest 0.5
Gaps to close for next star	CEIL((target_rate/100 × denominator) - numerator)
Revenue per gap closed	est_qbp_revenue_impact / gaps_to_close
CAHPS question score	Always=100, Usually=67, Sometimes=33, Never=0
Wilson CI lower	100×((N+1.92) - 1.96×SQRT(N×(1-N/D)+0.96)) / (D+3.84)
Disparity flag	rate_pct < overall_rate - 5 percentage points
HEI focus population	dual_eligible OR LIS OR disability OR BISG race (Black/Hispanic/AIAN/NHOPI)

G.4 Provider & Network Analytics

Metric	Formula / SQL
Rate achievement vs Medicare	SUM(plan_allowed) / SUM(medicare_rate)
Excess above 1.50× Medicare	SUM(CASE WHEN rate_achievement>1.50 THEN plan_allowed - medicare_rate*1.50 ELSE 0 END)
Fee schedule JOIN (SCD-2)	service_date >= effective_date AND service_date < COALESCE(expiration_date, '2099-12-31')
Referral leakage flag	network_status = 'OUT_OF_NETWORK' for specialist claims of attributed panel members
OIG exclusion JOIN	JOIN ref_oig_exclusions ON (rendering_npi = npi OR billing_tin = tin) AND exclusion_date <= service_date AND (reinstatement_date IS NULL OR reinstatement_date > service_date)
Gold card eligibility	approval_rate >= 90% AND total_requests >= 20 over last 12 months
PA urgent compliance	DATEDIFF('hour', request_date, decision_date) <= 72
PA standard compliance	DATEDIFF('day', request_date, decision_date) <= 7

G.5 Advanced SQL Pattern Quick Reference

Pattern	Implementation Note
Gap-island enrollment gap	LAG(end_date) OVER (PARTITION BY member_id ORDER BY start_date) → DATEDIFF(start, prev_end) = gap_days → MAX(gap_days) > 45 = NCQA exclusion
Recursive ICD-10 expansion	WITH RECURSIVE tree AS (anchor UNION ALL child JOIN tree ON child.parent = tree.code_id WHERE depth < 5) → join claims on LIKE tree.code || '%'
Dynamic pivot column list	STRING_AGG('MAX(CASE WHEN lag=' || lag || ' THEN pmpm END) AS lag_' || lag || 'm', ', ' ORDER BY lag) → EXECUTE assembled SQL
Episode overlap resolution	ROW_NUMBER() OVER (PARTITION BY claim_id ORDER BY anchor_date ASC) → WHERE anchor_priority = 1
Rolling 12-week anomaly	STDDEV(x) OVER (ORDER BY week ROWS BETWEEN 11 PRECEDING AND CURRENT ROW) → Z = (x - mean) / sd → flag |Z| > 2
Year-over-year same period	LAG(pmpm, 12) OVER (ORDER BY svc_month) AS prior_year_same_month
Running 3-month average	AVG(pmpm) OVER (ORDER BY svc_month ROWS BETWEEN 2 PRECEDING AND CURRENT ROW)

Point-in-time member age	DATEDIFF('year', date_of_birth, DATE(:year || '-12-31')) AS age_at_year_end
Null-safe equality check	COALESCE(a, '__NULL__') = COALESCE(b, '__NULL__') – compares NULLs as equal
Prevent divide-by-zero	/ NULLIF(denominator, 0) — returns NULL instead of error when denominator = 0

G.6 Benchmark Quick Reference

Metric	Benchmark Value	Analyst Note
IBNR completion at 1 month	Inpatient: 35–42% · Outpatient: 48–55% · Professional: 58–65% · Pharmacy: 85–92%	Multiply observed PMPM by reciprocal to estimate final PMPM
E&M upcoding flag	Z-score > 2.0 SD above specialty peer high-complexity rate	Minimum 100 E&M visits for statistical validity
Opioid diversion flag	3+ prescribers OR 3+ pharmacies in 90-day rolling window	HIGH = both; MODERATE = either; clinical review required
Days in A/R benchmarks	Physician group: < 30 · Community hospital: < 45 · Teaching hospital: < 60	Rising trend = denial rate or billing issue
30-day readmission benchmarks	CHF: 23–25% · COPD: 19–22% · Pneumonia: 17–19% · All-cause: 14–16%	CMS penalizes excess readmissions vs. expected rate
Stars QBP threshold	≥ 4.0 Stars = QBP eligible (up to 5% of benchmark)	Plans < 3.0 Stars × 3 consecutive years face contract termination
HEDIS denominators	Continuous enrollment: ≥ 11 of 12 months enrolled · Max single gap: ≤ 45 days	Two-claim rule for chronic conditions (2 outpatient OR 1 inpatient/ED)
ADI disadvantage threshold	ADI national rank ≥ 80 = highest disadvantage quintile (Q5)	Use for SDOH risk scoring and health equity outreach targeting
Full credibility threshold	1,082 member months (Z = 1.0) at 90% CI, ±5% precision	Z = MIN(1, SQRT(n / 1082)) for partial credibility
NCQA min stratum size	30 members for internal reporting · 11 members per NCQA HEDIS submission	Label sub-threshold strata as "insufficient data"

www.ingramcontent.com/pod-product-compliance
Lightning Source LLC
LaVergne TN
LVHW061202120826
845149LV00011B/1880
* 9 7 8 1 9 7 1 4 4 7 1 9 3 *